Epilepsy: Diagnosis and Treatment

Epilepsy: Diagnosis and Treatment

Edited by Maisy Kirk

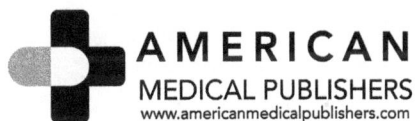

AMERICAN
MEDICAL PUBLISHERS
www.americanmedicalpublishers.com

American Medical Publishers,
41 Flatbush Avenue,
1st Floor, New York,
NY 11217, USA

Visit us on the World Wide Web at:
www.americanmedicalpublishers.com

ISBN: 978-1-63927-294-5

Cataloging-in-Publication Data

Epilepsy : diagnosis and treatment / edited by Maisy Kirk.
p. cm.
Includes bibliographical references and index.
ISBN 978-1-63927-294-5
1. Epilepsy. 2. Epilepsy--Diagnosis. 3. Epilepsy--Treatment. 4. Brain--Diseases.
5. Developmental disabilities. I. Kirk, Maisy.

RC372 .E65 2022

616.853--dc23

Table of Contents

Preface

Epilepsy is a disorder of nervous system that is characterized by recurring epileptic seizure. A seizure is a period of symptoms that happens because of abnormal excessive neuronal activity in the cortex of the brain. It may vary from short to long periods of forceful and uncontrolled shaking movements. Most of the time these movements last for less than two minutes but it takes some time for the person to return to the normal state. Epileptic seizures can cause physical injuries and the patient may sometimes face loss of bladder control. Low blood sugar, alcohol intake, brain infection, or low blood sodium may cause provoked seizures. Unprovoked seizures may happen due to stress or lack of sleep. The cause of epilepsy can be genetic or acquired. An electroencephalogram test helps in finding the source and cause of epilepsy. This book presents researches and studies performed by experts across the globe. It provides comprehensive insights into epilepsy disease, and its diagnosis and treatment. The readers would gain knowledge that would broaden their perspective about this disorder.

The information contained in this book is the result of intensive hard work done by researchers in this field. All due efforts have been made to make this book serve as a complete guiding source for students and researchers. The topics in this book have been comprehensively explained to help readers understand the growing trends in the field.

I would like to thank the entire group of writers who made sincere efforts in this book and my family who supported me in my efforts of working on this book. I take this opportunity to thank all those who have been a guiding force throughout my life.

Editor

1

Temporal profiles of age-dependent changes in cytokine mRNA expression and glial cell activation after status epilepticus in postnatal rat hippocampus

Juha T Järvelä[1], Francisco R Lopez-Picon[1,2†], Anna Plysjuk[1†], Saku Ruohonen[1] and Irma E Holopainen[1,3*]

Abstract

Background: Status epilepticus (SE) is proposed to lead to an age-dependent acute activation of a repertoire of inflammatory processes, which may contribute to neuronal damage in the hippocampus. The extent and temporal profiles of activation of these processes are well known in the adult brain, but less so in the developing brain. We have now further elucidated to what extent inflammation is activated by SE by investigating the acute expression of several cytokines and subacute glial reactivity in the postnatal rat hippocampus.

Methods: SE was induced by an intraperitoneal (i.p.) injection of kainic acid (KA) in 9- and 21-day-old (P9 and P21) rats. The mRNA expression of interleukin-1 beta (IL-1β), tumor necrosis factor-alpha (TNF-α), interleukin-10 (IL-10), matrix metalloproteinase-9 (MMP-9), glial-derived neurotrophic factor (GDNF), interferon gamma (IFN-γ), and transforming growth factor-beta 1 (TGF-β1) were measured from 4 h up to 3 days after KA injection with real-time quantitative PCR (qPCR). IL-1β protein expression was studied with ELISA, GFAP expression with western blotting, and microglial and astrocyte morphology with immunohistochemistry 3 days after SE.

Results: SE increased mRNA expression of IL-1β, TNF-α and IL-10 mRNA in hippocampus of both P9 and P21 rats, their induction being more rapid and pronounced in P21 than in P9 rats. MMP-9 expression was augmented similarly in both age groups and GDNF expression augmented only in P21 rats, whereas neither IFN-γ nor TGF-β1 expression was induced in either age group. Microglia and astrocytes exhibited activated morphology in the hippocampus of P21 rats, but not in P9 rats 3 d after SE. Microglial activation was most pronounced in the CA1 region and also detected in the basomedial amygdala.

Conclusion: Our results suggest that SE provokes an age-specific cytokine expression in the acute phase, and age-specific glial cell activation in the subacute phase as verified now in the postnatal rat hippocampus. In the juvenile hippocampus, transient increases in cytokine mRNA expression after SE, in contrast to prolonged glial reactivity and region-specific microglial activity after SE, suggest that the inflammatory response is changed from a fulminant and general initial phase to a more moderate and specific subacute response.

* Correspondence: irma.holopainen@utu.fi
† Contributed equally
[1]Department of Pharmacology, Drug Development, and Therapeutics, Institute of Biomedicine, University of Turku, Itäinen Pitkäkatu 4B, FIN-20014 Turku, Finland
Full list of author information is available at the end of the article

Background

Status epilepticus (SE) has been shown to cause induction of the innate immunity system in brain, including hippocampus. In adult rats, several inflammatory mediators are activated in response to SE. These include upregulation of cyclooxygenase-2 (COX-2) and cytokines, e. g. interleukin-1β (IL-1β), tumor necrosis factor-α (TNF-α), and interleukin-6 (IL-6), together with morphological and functional changes in glial cells, i.e. microglia and astrocytes, from resting to active states after either pilocarpine- or kainic acid- (KA) induced seizures [1-3]. Furthermore, upon activation by seizures, cytokine (e.g. IL-1β, TNF-α, and IL-6) expression is increased in both glial cell types [4]. It has been suggested that these responses could contribute to excitotoxic neuronal damage in the hippocampus, a brain region especially susceptible to injury caused by SE [5-7].

In contrast to adult brain, SE-induced acute activation of inflammatory processes seems to be age-specifically regulated in the developing postnatal rat brain, e.g. postnatal-day 21 (P21) rats exhibit pronounced inflammatory responses (increases in COX-2 and pro-inflammatory cytokine expression, and glial cell reactivity) within 24 h after SE in hippocampus whereas this is not seen in P9 rats [6,8]. Additionally, SE-induced neuronal damage has been shown to differ according to age; younger brain being more resistant to seizure-induced damage than older brain [9,10]. In the hippocampus of juvenile rats, neuronal damage caused by a single episode of SE is localized in the CA1 or CA3 pyramidal cell regions [6,8]. Although more thoroughly studied in the adult rat brain, classical pro-inflammatory cytokines (IL-1β, TNF-α, and IL-6) have been found to be upregulated within a few hours after SE in juvenile hippocampus as well [6]. However, whether SE leads to augmented expression of other cytokines involved in inflammation has remained unaddressed in the developing hippocampus. Such factors include anti-inflammatory cytokines, matrix metalloproteinases, growth factors and interferons. The anti-inflammatory cytokine, interleukin-10 (IL-10), can suppress pro-inflammatory cytokine signalling in macrophages and microglia by inhibiting STAT-1α activation [11], and IL-10 expression is upregulated after excitotoxic lesions in P9 rat brain [12]. Matrix metalloproteinases (MMP) are known to regulate the metabolism of the pericellular environment and, in particular, MMP-9 activity is increased after KA-induced SE in the hippocampus of adult rats [13]. Furthermore, transforming growth factor-β1 (TGF-β1) has been proposed to protect neurons from rapid KA-induced excitotoxicity, possibly by inhibiting the rise in intracellular Ca^{2+} [14], and on the other hand, to contribute to remodelling of brain after injury by regulating expression of MMP-9 in astrocytes and inducing

their migration [15]. Glial cell-derived neurotrophic factor (GDNF) is a potent survival factor for several types of neurons, and its mRNA expression is increased in adult rat hippocampus 6-24 h after intraperitoneal (i.p.) KA injection [16]. In addition, interferon-γ (IFN-γ) has been suggested to have a neuroprotective function as well, since it may induce neurotrophic growth factor (NGF) production in activated astrocytes obtained from rat brain that has been lesioned by intracerebral 6-hydroxydopamine injection [17]. Also, the temporal behaviour of glial cells after SE is incompletely known in P9 and P21 rat hippocampus, since there are no *in vivo* studies at these ages in which the reactivity of glial cells has been investigated beyond 24 h after KA-induced SE.

The current study was designed to obtain more detailed information of the temporal and developmental profiles of inflammatory processes activated by SE. For this purpose, we investigated mRNA expression of the cytokines IL-1β, TNF-α, IL-10, MMP-9, GDNF, IFN-γ, and TGF-β1 with real-time quantitative PCR (qPCR) in P9 and P21 rats 4-24 h, and also in P21 rats 3 d after KA-induced SE. Additionally, IL-1β protein expression was measured 8 h after SE in P21 rats. Immunohistochemistry was used to investigate microglial and astrocyte morphology subacutely (3 days) after SE, and the observed changes were quantified by counting microglial cells with active morphology and by GFAP western blotting, respectively.

Methods

Experimental animals in kainic acid-induced status epilepticus

All animal experiments were conducted in accordance with the guidelines of the European Community Council Directives 86/609/EEC, and had the approval of the Office of the Regional Government of Western Finland. All efforts were made to minimize the pain, discomfort, and number of experimental animals.

The procedure of KA-induced SE was carried out as recently described in detail [18]. Since two age groups (P9 and P21) of Sprague-Dawley rats were used, the procedure applied for each group is described separately. Group 1: P9 rat pups were weighted, and a single dose of KA (1.2 mg/kg) (Tocris Cookson Ltd., Avomouth, UK) was given i.p. Within 20-30 min after the injection, the pups first manifested stiffening, scratching, head nodding, and forelimb clonus with further progression to generalized tonic-clonic seizures within 45-60 min, which continued intermittently for 3-4 h after the KA injection. The mortality of the rat pups was negligible. After the cessation of seizures, the pups were taken back to the cages with their mother, and used for the qPCR and immunocytochemical studies 4 h, 8 h, 24 h and 3 days after the KA injection. Instead of KA injection, P9 control rats received the comparable volume of 0.9% NaCl as given to the KA-treated rats. The KA-treated and their age-matched control rats were separated from their mothers for an equivalent amount of time. Group 2: P21 rats were weighted, and a single dose of KA (7 mg/kg) was given (i.p.). Within 20-30 min, rats first showed scratching, chewing, and myoclonic jerks followed by wet dog shakes, head nodding, forelimb clonus, and rearing and falling. Behavioural signs of generalized tonic-clonic seizures occurred within 45-60 min, which continued intermittently for 3-4 h after the KA injection. The mortality within this age group was negligible as well. Rats were used for the qPCR, immunocytochemical and ELISA studies 4 h, 8 h, 24 h, and 3 days after the KA injection. Instead of KA injection, P21 control rats received the comparable volume of 0.9% NaCl as given to the KA-injected rats, but were otherwise treated as their age-matched treated rats. Rats were visually followed-up for about 2 h after the cessation of behavioural seizure signs, and taken back to their cages. All KA-injected rats of both age groups included in this study manifested the behavioural seizure signs as described above.

Immunocytochemistry

Immunocytochemistry was performed as previously described in detail for neurofilament proteins with some modifications [18]. Briefly, rats (n = 3 in both age groups of treated and control rats) were deeply anesthetized with 50 mg/kg of pentobarbital, and fixed by transcardiac perfusion with 4% paraformaldehyde in phosphate-buffered saline (PBS, pH 7.4). Brains were rapidly removed, postfixed at +4°C, processed with the antigen retrieval protocol [19], cryoprotected in 30% sucrose in PBS at +4°C, frozen, and kept at -80°C until used. For immunostaining, brains were cryosectioned in 40 µm slices, collected in Tris buffered-saline (TBS, pH 7.4) containing 0.1% Triton X-100, and immediately processed in a free-floating system. First, slices were incubated in a blocking solution (BS) containing 3% bovine serum albumin (BSA), 0.1% Triton X-100 in TBS (pH 7.4), and thereafter with the primary antibodies against Iba1 (1:1000, Wako, Japan) or GFAP (1:1000, Sigma, St Louis, MO, USA) overnight at +4°C in BS. After washings, slices were incubated with a biotin SP-conjugated secondary antibody (1:1000), followed by incubation with the avidin-peroxidase conjugate (Vectastain ABC Kit, Vector Laboratories, Burlingame, CA). Staining was detected using 3,3'-diaminobenzidinetetrahydrochloride (DAB) (Sigma) as a chromogen. In each experiment, KA-treated and control brains were processed simultaneously to minimize the possible interexperimental differences in the staining. Three to four

slices, in which the primary antibody was omitted but which were otherwise treated as indicated above, served as negative controls. The immunoreactivity was examined with a Leica DMR microscope (Heerbrugg, Germany) under bright field; pictures were captured using an Olympus U-TV1 X digital camera (Olympus Optical, Tokyo, Japan), and further processed with Adobe Photoshop Elements (version 3.0) and Corel Draw (version 11.0).

In a subset of experiments with the primary antibody against GFAP (1:1000, Sigma), slices were further incubated with a fluorescent secondary antibody Alexa 488 (Invitrogen, Carlsbad, CA, USA), which was diluted (1:1000) in TBS containing 3% BSA and 0.1% Triton X-100. After the staining, slides were dehydrated, coverslipped, and examined with the Leica DMR microscope using the appropriate fluorescence filter. The images were further processed with Corel Draw (version 11.0).

Real-time quantitative PCR

For qPCR, hippocampi (n = 5-6 in each time-point) were taken from P9 and P21 rats 4 h, 8 h or 24 h after KA injection, and those from saline-injected control groups of the two ages. Additionally, a group of P21 rats, in which hippocampi were prepared 3 days after SE, was used for qPCR, together with their own age-matched control group. Rats were decapitated, hippocampi quickly isolated, immediately frozen in -196°C liquid nitrogen, and stored at -70°C until used. For the experiments, frozen hippocampi were thawed, homogenized with Ultra-Turrax, and the total RNA extraction was carried out with Qiagen RNeasy mini kit (Qiagen, Hilden, Germany) using the protocol supplied by the manufacturer. Total RNA was reverse transcribed to cDNA by M-MuLV Reverse Transcriptase RNase H+ (including RNase inhibitor) (Finnzymes, Espoo, Finland).

PCR was performed using TaqMan One-Step qPCR Master Mix Reagents Kit (Applied Biosystems, Foster City, CA, USA). Amplification was carried out with the ABI 7300 Real-Time PCR System (Applied Biosystems) with a two-step PCR protocol (preincubation of 10 min at +95°C followed by 40 cycles at +95°C for 15 sec, and for 1 min at +60°C). All cytokine primers and probes were designed using the Primer Express software (Applied Biosystems) avoiding contaminating genomic DNA amplification by positioning one of the primers or a probe over the exon/intron boundary. The cytokine cDNA was amplified using the primers and probes as given in Table 1.

mRNA quantification results were normalized using rat ribosomal 18s RNA (rRNA) (Applied Biosystems) as an endogenous control. Before the study, the stability of rRNA expression in the samples was validated with an experiment in which different concentrations of a

Table 1 The sequences of primers and probes used to amplify cytokine cDNA

Cytokine	5′ primer	3′ primer	Probe
GDNF	GCCACCATCAAAAGACTGAAAAG	CGGTTCCTCTCTCTTCGAGGA	TCACCAGATAAACAAGCGGCGGCA
IFN-γ	TCGAATCGCACCTGATCACTA	GGGTTGTTCACCTCGAACTTG	CATCCTTTTTTGCTTTACTGTTGCTGAGAAG
IL-1β	GAAAGACGGCACACCCACC	AAACCGCTTTTCCATCTTCTTCT	TGCAGCTGGAGAGTGTGGATCCCAAAC
IL-10	CCCTCTGGATACAGCTGCG	GCTCCACTGCCTTGCTTTTATT	CGCTGTCATCGATTTCTCCCCTGTGA
MMP-9	GTATGGTCGTGGCTCTAAACCTG	TCGGCTGTGGTTCAGCTG	CCCAAGGCCTCCAGCCACCAC
TGF-β1	TGAGTGGCTGTCTTTTGACGTC	CCTGTATTCCGTCTCCTTGGTT	CTGGAGTTGTCCGGCAGTGGCTGA
TNF-α	GACCCTCACACTCAGATCATCTTCT	ACGCTGGCTCAGCCACTC	TAGCCCACGTCGTAGCAAACCACCAA

The probes were labeled with FAM at the 5′ end and with TAMRA at the 3′ end.

sample mRNA were used and rRNA expression was measured. The stability of rRNA also in stress conditions has been previously tested [20]. In all studies, each sample was run in triplicate, and the comparative threshold (CT) method (= ΔΔCT method) was used to examine the relative quantification of the samples (Relative Quantitation computer software, Applied Biosystems). Fold-expression changes were calculated using the equation $2^{-\Delta\Delta CT}$.

ELISA
For IL-1β ELISA, three control rats and four KA-injected P21 rats (8 h after injection) were used. Rats were decapitated and hippocampi quickly isolated, placed in ice-cold homogenization buffer containing 50 mM Tris-HCl (pH 7.4), 1% sodium dodecyl sulphate (SDS), 2 mM EDTA, 1 mM phenylmethylsulphonyl-fluoride (PMSF), and 0.7 mM dithiothreitol, homogenized (Ultra-Turrax T25, Janke and Kunkel, Staufen, Germany), boiled, and centrifuged at +4°C. The supernatants were frozen and stored at -80°C until used. Total protein concentration of the samples was measured using a Lowry-based assay (Bio-Rad, CA, USA). A commercial ELISA kit (Raybiotech, Norcross, GA, USA) was used, and the protocol supplied by the manufacturer was followed. Results are calculated as pg of IL-1β/mg of total protein.

Western blotting
Western blotting studies were performed as previously described in detail with slight modifications [18]. Briefly, two separate sets of P21 rats, three to four rats at each time point in each set, were used for western blotting studies at 1 and 3 days after KA injection. Different age-matched controls were used for both time-points. Rats were decapitated and hippocampi were rapidly removed and placed in ice-cold homogenization buffer containing 50 mM Tris-HCl, 1% SDS, 2 mM EDTA, 1 mM PMSF, and 0.7 mM DTT (pH 7.4). Thereafter, hippocampi were homogenized, boiled, and centrifuged at +4°C. The supernatants were collected and stored at -70°C until used. Total protein concentration of the samples was

measured using the Lowry based Biorad DC Protein assay (Bio-Rad, CA, USA). For SDS-PAGE, equal amounts of protein were applied to each lane of 7.5% acrylamide mini gels, separated by electrophoresis, and transferred to a polyvinylidene fluoride membranes, which were then incubated overnight at +4°C with the monoclonal GFAP primary antibody (Sigma) diluted 1:4500. After that, the membranes were washed and incubated with HRP-conjugated secondary antibody (1:4000) for 1 h at room temperature. The signal was obtained using a chemiluminiscence ECL system (Amersham, Buckinghamshire, UK), and exposed to a film (Hyperfilm ECL, Amersham) that was then developed, and the optical signals were quantified with Image J 1.20s (NIH, USA). The control level was set at 100%, and changes in expression are given as percentage of controls. Western blotting studies were repeated four times with the two sets of rats. Actin (1:4500) (Sigma-Aldrich Inc) was used as a loading control for western blotting.

Statistical analysis
Statistical significance of differences between groups was analyzed with one-way ANOVA with Tukey's test as a post test for experiments in which there were three or more groups. Differences between the two age groups at the studied time-points were analyzed with two-way ANOVA. Statistical significance of differences in experiments having two groups was analyzed with Student's unpaired t-test. All statistical analyses were performed using the GraphPad Prism software program (version 4.0, GraphPad Software, San Diego, CA, USA). The level of significance was set at p < 0.05.

Results
Age-dependent changes in cytokine mRNA expression
mRNA expression of IL-1β, TNF-α, IL-10, MMP-9, GDNF, IFN-γ, and TGF-β1 was investigated 4, 8 and 24 h following KA injection in P9 and P21 rat hippocampi. Additionally, mRNA expression of these cytokines was also studied 3 d after KA injection in P21 rats.

IL-1β mRNA expression in P21 rat hippocampi already showed a pronounced increase 4 h after KA

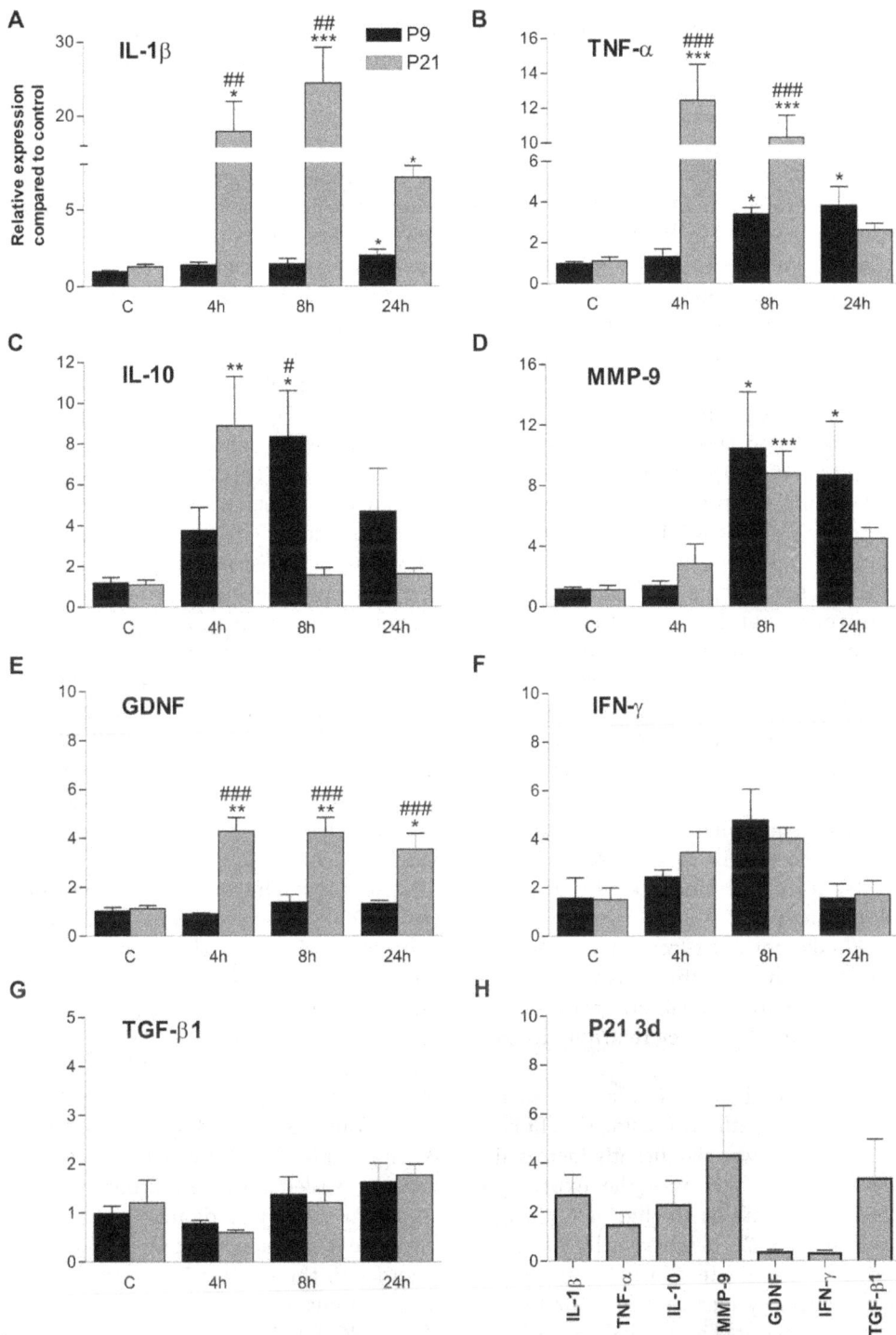

Figure 1 Cytokine mRNA expression patterns in immature and juvenile hippocampus after KA-induced SE. Relative quantification of IL-1β (A), TNF-α (B), IL-10 (C), MMP-9 (D), GDNF (E), IFN-γ (F), and TGF-β1 (G) mRNA expression 4, 8 and 24 h after KA-injection in P9 and P21 rat hippocampi, and 3 d after KA-injection in P21 rat hippocampi (H) measured with real-time PCR. Note the significant increases from control levels in both age groups, more pronounced and faster induction of IL-1β, TNF-α and IL-10 mRNA expression in P21 compared to P9 rats, and the increase in GDNF expression only in P21 rats. Note also the return of cytokine mRNA expression in P21 rats to control levels 3 d after KA injection. Data are given as mean ± S.E.M. *p < 0.05, compared to age-matched control (one-way ANOVA); **p < 0.01, compared to age-matched control (one-way ANOVA). ***p < 0.001, compared to age-matched control (one-way ANOVA); ##p < 0.01, compared to the other age at the same time-point (two-way ANOVA); ###p < 0.001, compared to the other age at the same time-point (two-way ANOVA). Abbreviations: C, control; P, postnatal.

injection, peaked at 8 h, when it was almost 25-fold higher compared to that of controls, and still remained significantly higher than in the control group at 24 h (Figure 1A). In contrast, in P9 rats, IL-1β mRNA expression did not significantly change from the control group 4 h or 8 h after KA injection, while at 24 h its expression was slightly but significantly augmented. To confirm the increased expression after SE at the protein level, IL-1β protein expression in the hippocampus of P21 rats was studied with ELISA 8 h after KA injection. The concentration of IL-1β protein was 95.3 ± 7.8 pg/mg (mean ± SEM, n = 3) in the control group, and was significantly (p < 0.05, unpaired t-test) increased to 124.3 ± 10.1 pg/mg (mean ± SEM, n = 4) in the KA-treated group (8 h after injection).

TNF-α mRNA expression closely followed the temporal expression profile of IL-1β (Figure 1B). In P21 rat hippocampi, TNF-α mRNA expression already showed a pronounced increase 4 h after KA injection, at which time it peaked, and thereafter decreased to control levels, its expression not being significantly different from that of control rats at 24 h. In P9 rats, TNF-α mRNA expression was significantly increased over the first 8 h after KA injection, and remained elevated up to 24 h. It is of importance to note that the augmented expression of this cytokine 8 h after KA injection was significantly more pronounced in P21 rats (10-fold) than in P9 rats (3 to 4-fold).

IL-10 mRNA had a somewhat different expression pattern compared to those of IL-1β and TNF-α (Figure 1C). In P21 rats, its expression was significantly increased at 4 h but thereafter it sharply decreased, and at 8 h its expression did not differ from that of the control level. In P9 rats, however, the increase in IL-10 mRNA expression was more gradual, first reaching significance 8 h after SE, and thereafter returning to control levels by 24 h.

The two age groups had more similarities in the MMP-9 mRNA expression patterns (Figure 1D). In both age groups, this expression was significantly increased 8 h after KA. However, in P21 rats the expression decreased to levels comparable to that of their age-matched control group at 24 h, whereas in P9 rats it remained significantly augmented. In P21 rats, GDNF expression was significantly increased at 4 h after KA injection, and remained elevated at 8 h and 24 h (Figure 1E), whereas in P9 rat hippocampi its expression remained unaltered after SE at all time-points studied. In both age groups, the expression of neither IFN-γ (Figure 1F) nor TGF-β1 (Figure 1G) was significantly augmented compared to their respective age-matched controls at any time-point studied.

To study whether the SE-induced increase in expressions of the studied cytokines was prolonged beyond the acute phase, their mRNA expression was also measured 3 d after SE in P21 rats and in their age-matched control group. However, the expression levels of all cytokines studied did not significantly differ from those of controls 3 d after SE (Figure 1H).

Age-dependent glial cell reactivity after SE

In order to investigate subacute glial cell reactivity after SE in hippocampus, the morphology of microglia and astrocytes was studied with immunohistochemistry 3 d after SE in both age groups. There were no discernible differences in Iba immunostaining in hippocampus between control and KA-treated P9 rats, as microglia retained their resting appearance after KA treatment in both groups (Figurs 2A-D). In contrast, in KA-treated P21 rats, the morphology of microglial cells changed from the resting appereance of the control hippocampi to an active appearance. Activated microglial cells were characterized by enlarged cell bodies and thicker processes in increased numbers (Figurs 2E-H). Microglial activation was detected to some extent throughout the hippocampus, but it is of importance to note that Iba1 immunoreactivity and morphological changes were most prominent in the microglia within the CA1 region. To quantify this, microglia with active appearance in the CA1 region were counted, in a blinded manner, in P21 rats from areas as indicated by the boxes in Figurs 2E and 2G. The number of microglia with an active appearance was 4.5 ± 0.6 (mean ± SEM, n = 4) in the control group and 14.8 ± 0.9 (mean ± SEM, n = 4) in the KA-treated group. This increase was statistically significant (p < 0.0001, Student's unpaired t-test). Also in the amygdala of P21 rats, similar microglial activation was observed 3 d after SE (Figurs 2I-J). In P9 rats, no morphological changes indicating microglial activation were observed in the amygdala (data not shown).

GFAP immunostaining of P9 rat hippocampi did not reveal any changes between controls and KA-treated rats 3 d after SE, including the CA1 region (Figurs 3A-B). In contrast, in KA-treated P21 rats, GFAP immunostaining revealed enlarged cell bodies and thickened processes in astrocytes denoting activated morphology throughout the hippocampus, including the CA1 region, whereas in the control P21 rats astroglial cells in the hippocampus had thin processes and a small cell bodies (Figurs 3C-D). The apparent increase in GFAP expression in P21 rats was confirmed with western blotting, and GFAP protein expression was found to be significantly increased 3 d after SE, but not yet 1 d after SE (Figurs 3E-F).

Discussion

The main findings of our study, in which immature and juvenile rats had KA-induced SE, were the following:

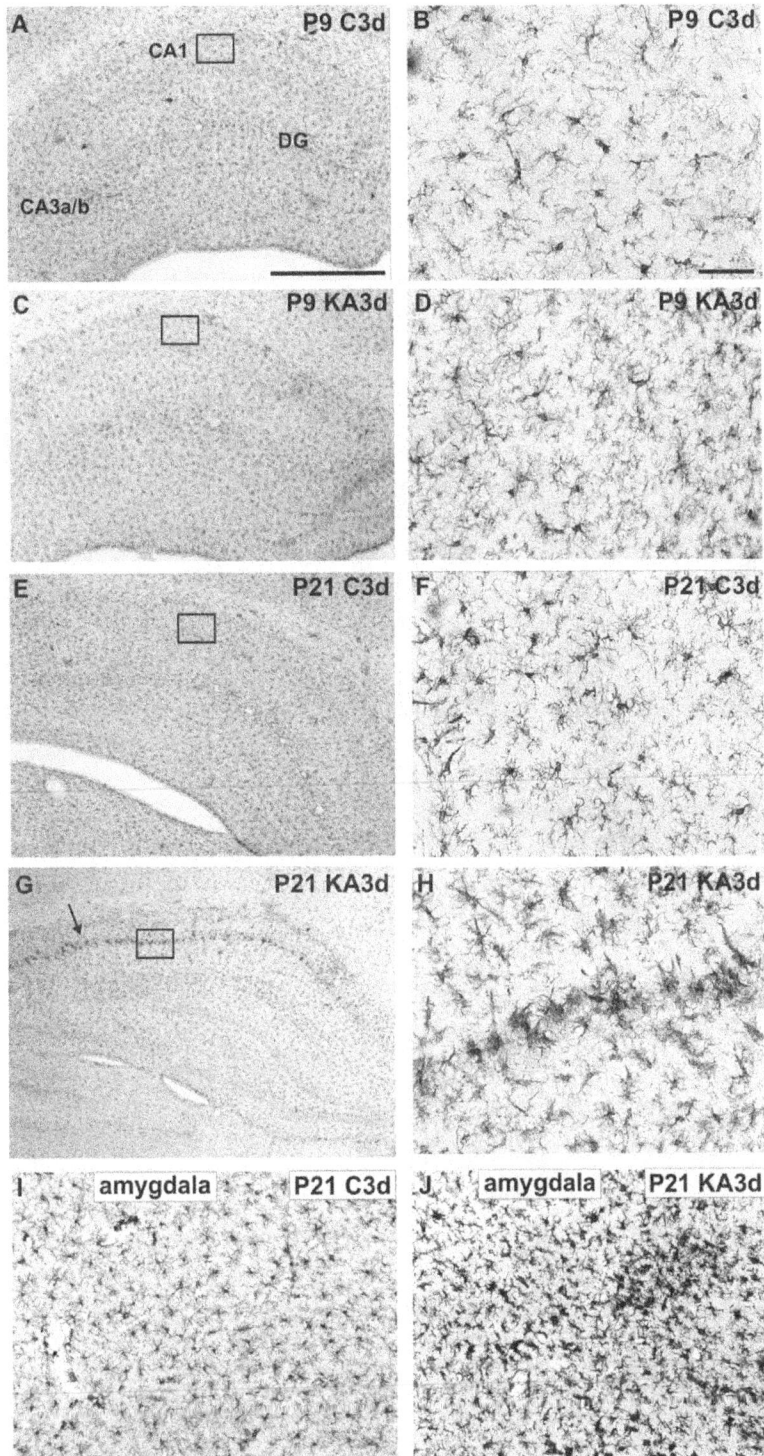

Figure 2 Microglial morphology in immature and juvenile hippocampus 3 d after SE. Representative Iba1 immunostaining images of hippocampus for a P9 (A-B) and a P21 (E-F) control rat, and a KA-treated P9 (C-D) and P21 (G-H) rat 3 d after SE, and those of the basomedial amygdala of a control (I) and a KA-treated (J) P21 rat 3 d after SE. The box in the CA1 region in A, C, E, and G is shown with a higher magnification in B, D, F and H, respectively. Note the morphological changes in microglia in the CA1 region (arrow, G) with more pronounced Iba1 immunoreactivity and thickened processes in the KA-treated P21 rat, and the lack of change in P9 rats. Note also the morphological changes of the microglia in amygdala of the P21 rat. Abbreviations: C, control; KA, KA-treated; P, postnatal. Scale bars: 1 mm in A, applicable also for C, E and G; 50 μm in B, applicable also for D, F, H, I and J.

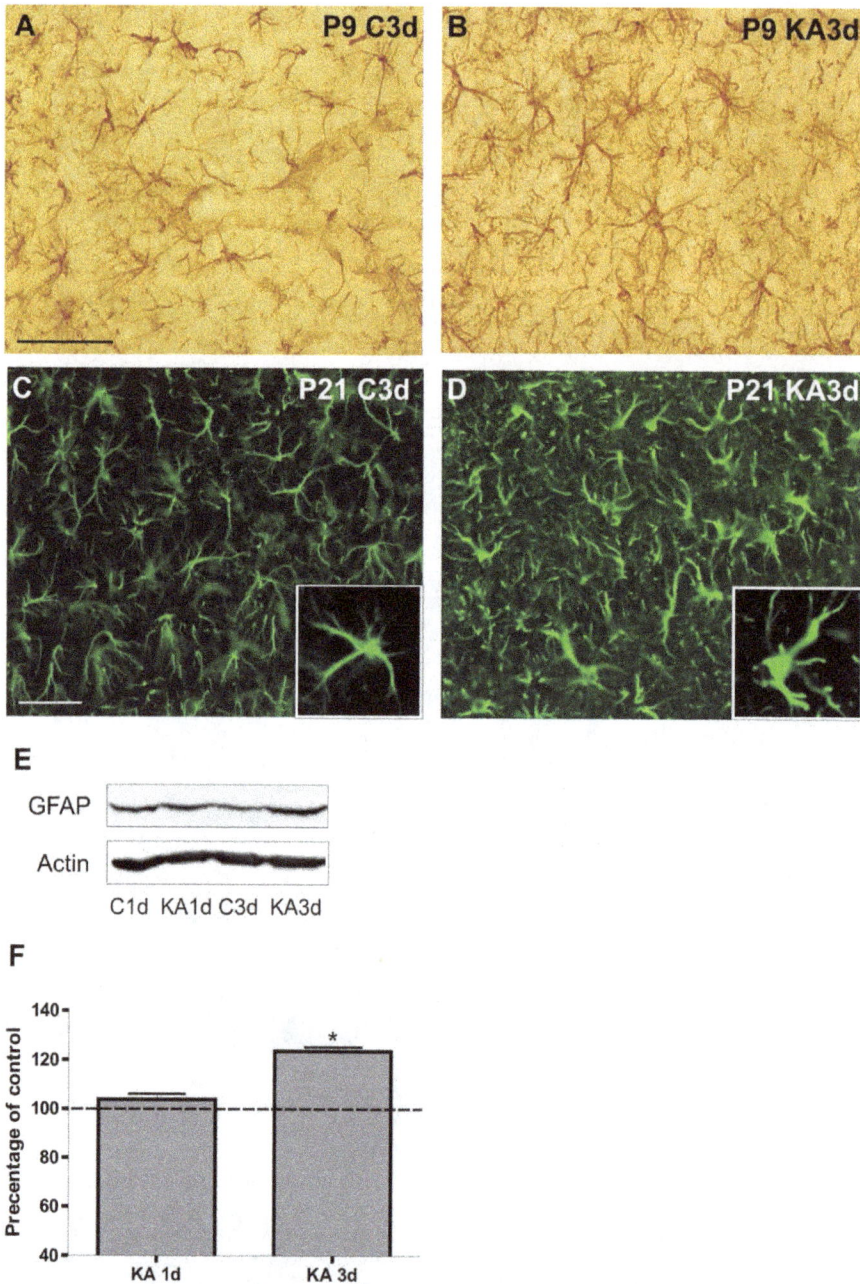

Figure 3 Astrocyte morphology in immature and juvenile hippocampus 3 d after SE. Representative images of GFAP immunostainings in the CA1 region of hippocampus for a P9 (A) and a P21 (C) control rat, and a KA-treated P9 (B) and P21 (D) rat 3 d after SE. The box in C and D shows a GFAP-positive cell at higher magnification. Note the prominent morphological changes in astrocytes with thickened, heavily GFAP-positive processes in the KA-treated P21 rat, and the lack of any changes in the P9 rats. A representative western blot (E) and its semi-quantitative analysis (F) of GFAP expression in P21 rat hippocampus in age-matched controls and 1 and 3 d after KA-induced SE. *$p < 0.05$, compared to the age-matched control group (one-way ANOVA). Abbreviations: C, control; KA, KA-treated; P, postnatal. Scale bars: 50 μm in A, applicable also for B; 50 μm in C, applicable also for D.

First, the expression of a number of cytokine mRNAs was induced in both juvenile (P21) and immature (P9) rats after SE; second, the time course and levels of increase in cytokine mRNA expression after SE varied according to the age of rats; third, glial cells exhibited an active appearance in P21 juvenile rats subacutely (3 d) after SE, especially microglia within the CA1 region, while in P9 immature rats glial cells retained their resting appearance. These topics are discussed more thoroughly below.

Expression of cytokines after SE

It has previously been shown in developing hippocampus that IL-1β mRNA expression is augmented in P15 and P21 rats but not in P9 rats 4 h after KA-induced SE, while TNF-α and IL-6 mRNA expression are increased only in P21 rats [6]. Our recent results are in accordance with these findings and further show that the induction of IL-1β and TNF-α mRNA expression is more prolonged (8 and/or 24 h after SE) in P21 rats and, although to a lesser extent, also occurs in P9 rats. Furthermore, in a previous study in which excitotoxic lesions were induced via NMDA injection in the right sensorimotor cortex of P9 rats, IL-1β and TNF-α protein expression was induced in sensorimotor cortex, corpus callosum, and internal capsule 4 h - 24 h after injection [21]. However, to our knowledge, until now there has been no evidence of any SE-induced cytokine gene expression in P9 rats. Our current results suggest that IL-1β and TNF-α mRNA expression is increased more rapidly and is more pronounced after SE in the more mature juvenile hippocampus compared to a delayed and weak induction in the immature hippocampus. Thus, the time-course and intensity of augmented IL-1β and TNF-α mRNA expression after SE in P21 rat hippocampus resembles that of adult rats [2], which implies that this response is already mature in juvenile rats. It is noteworthy that, compared to controls, the increases in IL-1β protein expression 8 h after KA injection in P21 rats are much lower than the increases in IL-1β mRNA expression at the same time-point. However, the selected time-point probably does not represent the peak in IL-1β protein expression after KA, which is likely to occur later. Furthermore, the result does confirm the tendency of increased mRNA expression to be translated into an increase at the protein level, albeit not on a one-to-one basis. As the mRNA expression levels of many other cytokines were also highly upregulated, it is reasonable to suggest that these are followed by increases in their corresponding protein expressions, although these increases might be significantly lower and occur at later time-points than the mRNA changes.

In addition to neurodegeneration, the classical pro-inflammatory cytokines have been suggested to contribute to epileptogenesis [4]. For example, transgenic mice overexpressing IL-6 showed increased sensitivity to seizures [22], and chronic IL-1β expression has recently been associated with the development of spontaneous limbic seizures after prolonged febrile seizures in P11 rats [23]. Conversely, the IL-1 receptor antagonist (IL-1Ra) mediates anticonvulsant effects in adult rodents in a number of limbic seizure models (i.e. intrahippocampal KA and bicuculline injection, and electrical kindling) [24]. The initial pronounced upregulation of pro-inflammatory cytokine mRNAs seen in juvenile rats in our current study might therefore be an early factor promoting epileptogenesis. While these cytokines can be produced by both glial cell types after seizures, there could be some subtle differences between the glial cell types as to which cytokines they produce, at least in certain seizure models. For example, 12 h after soman-induced seizures in adult rats, IL-1β was observed to be expressed by activated microglia, whereas IL-6 was expressed by astrocytes in the hippocampus, piriform cortex and thalamus [25].

mRNA expression of the anti-inflammatory cytokine IL-10, which has so far been less studied in both immature and mature brain after SE, was augmented in both age groups. In an earlier study in P9 rats, in which excitotoxic brain injury was caused by an intracerebral NMDA injection, IL-10 and its receptor were upregulated in glial cells, suggesting a protective role for IL-10 in excitotoxicity [12]. In our current study, IL-10 expression was increased in concert with the pro-inflammatory cytokines IL-1β and TNF-α, which is in line with the earlier observation that IL-10 expression may be induced simultaneously with pro-inflammatory cytokines in the brain following an insult [26]. Although the pathways of cytokine expression regulation are intricate, the finding that induction of IL-10 mRNA expression was quite moderate and short-lived compared to the more pronounced and prolonged induction of IL-1β and TNF-α mRNA in P21 rats favours the idea that pro-inflammatory cytokine expression might overcome IL-10 expression after SE at this age. In contrast, in P9 rats, IL-10 mRNA expression showed a more pronounced induction than that of IL-1β or TNF-α, which suggests that, at this age, IL-10 might inhibit activated microglial cells and thus suppress expression of pro-inflammatory cytokines after SE more effectively than in P21 animals. Furthermore, microglial cells expressing IL-10 have been shown to attenuate neurodegeneration in hippocampal cultures when apoptosis is promoted with NMDA [27]. This enables the hypothesis that microglia might self-limit their response via negative feedback by producing IL-10 and thus can have either pro-inflammatory or anti-inflammatory functions, depending on circumstances.

Also MMP-9 mRNA expression increased in both age groups after SE. In *in vitro* conditions, MMP-9 has been shown to be produced by activated microglia [28], and cytokines are proposed to regulate MMP-9 activity in astrocytes [29]. In an earlier study, increased MMP-9 activity was observed 8 h after KA-induced seizures in adult rats, and this was linked with neuronal death as confirmed in KA-treated organotypic hippocampal slice cultures (prepared from P11 rats and cultured for 14 days) [30]. In our current study, MMP-9 mRNA expression increased in both P21 and P9 rats and, as previous studies have shown that P9 rats do not exhibit any detectable neuronal damage from KA-induced SE [6,8], this suggests that MMP-9 mRNA upregulation after SE alone is not sufficient to induce neuronal damage in the P21 rat hippocampus. MMP-9 might have a more central role in epileptogenesis, as MMP-9 knockout mice show lower sensitivity to epileptogenesis after pentylene-tetrazole kindling-induced seizures, while the sensitivity of transgenic rats overexpressing MMP-9 is higher [31].

GDNF mRNA expression is augmented in the adult rat hippocampus 6-24 h after KA-induced SE [16]. In our study in developing rats, GDNF was the only studied cytokine whose mRNA was increased exclusively in P21 rats after SE. In another earlier study, in which SE was induced with KA in adult rats, adenoviral-vector-delivered GDNF, introduced before KA injection, increased Bcl-2 expression and reduced the number of apoptotic cells in the CA3 and dentate gyrus (DG) regions of the hippocampus compared to the rats, which did not receive GDNF [32]. This suggests that GDNF has a neuroprotective role in KA-induced SE. Furthermore, GDNF is proposed to suppress seizures in temporal lope epilepsy models (e.g. kindling) in adult rats [33]. Our results indicate that GDNF upregulation after SE is a mechanism that has reached an adult level of maturity in P21 rats.

The expression of IFN-γ and TGF-β1 mRNA did not significantly change after SE in either age group. In a recent study in adult rats, IFN-γ mRNA expression was increased in astrocytes of the hippocampus 24 h after lithium-pilocarpine-induced SE while the expression of its receptor was upregulated in neurons and, furthermore, neutralization of the IFN-γ receptor aggravated injury suggesting a protective role for IFN-γ [34]. Also, the expression of TGF-β1 mRNA has been shown to be increased in response to KA-induced SE in microglial cells in the hippocampus of adult rats [35]. However, TGF-β1 has recently been suggested to contribute to epileptogenesis induced by albumin after blood-brain barrier breakdown in adult rats [36]. Our current findings suggest that these mechanisms, which are activated by SE in the adult hippocampus, are still underdeveloped in the juvenile P21 rat hippocampus.

Our present results together with earlier findings of other groups suggest that the more mature innate immunity system elicits a fulminant inflammatory response after SE, in which the pro-inflammatory reaction is marked. In contrast, the immature system evokes only a mild pro-inflammatory response, but a marked anti-inflammatory reaction. We propose that in the immature brain either the ability to induce acute inflammatory reaction is underdeveloped or its emphasis is on anti-inflammatory properties. Moreover, the inflammatory reaction in developing hippocampus is likely to at

least partly contribute to age-dependent susceptibility to SE-induced neuronal injury and recurrence of seizures. However, other factors, such as molecular and functional differences in receptors and ion channels between the immature and adult rodent brain, may be of equal or even greater importance in determining changes in the seizure threshold [37].

Glial cell activation after SE at the acute and the subacute phase

Glial cells, i.e. microglia and astrocytes, are age-dependently activated (in P21 and P15, but not in P9) in the postnatal rat hippocampus up to 24 h after KA-induced SE [6]. Additionally, short-term microglial (a few days) and long-term (beyond 40 days) astrocytic activation have been observed after KA-induced seizures in P15 rats, and this has been proposed to contribute to neuronal injury, neurobehavioral impairment, and increased susceptibility to seizures [38]. Our results further address this and show that also subacutely, 3 days after seizures, both types of glial cells remain activated in P21 rats and that glial cells remain inactivated in P9 rats also at this subacute phase. Furthermore, astrocyte activity seems to increase over time after SE in P21 rats, since GFAP expression was now significantly increased 3 d after SE, but not yet 1 d after SE. This further supports the notion that the more mature brain elicits a more prominent inflammatory response after SE, which may be in part due to a diminished ability of glial cells to self-limit their response. Additionally, it is of importance to note that the most pronounced subacute microglial activation was localized to the CA1 pyramidal cell layer in P21 rats after KA treatment, which is the region damaged by KA-induced SE in rats of this age [8]. In contrast, an earlier study has shown that microglia are equally activated in all hippocampal regions 4 h and 24 h after onset of SE in P21 rats [6]. Our results therefore suggest that the generalized microglial response in hippocampus seems to be gradually and specifically concentrated on the damaged CA1 region at the subacute phase in P21 rats, whereas the astrocytic response remains ubiquitous in the hippocampus. Furthermore, our recent transcriptomic study indicated pronounced upregulation of the GFAP gene in the CA1 region together with neuronal damage in P21 rats 7 days after SE [39], which denotes long-term astrocyte activation specifically in the damaged area.

In contrast to prolonged glial cell reaction, increased expression of cytokine mRNAs is transient and, as our results show, at three days after SE in P21 rat hippocampi, cytokine mRNA expression has returned to control levels. This suggests that activated glial cells in juvenile hippocampus may have functions other than cytokine production during the subacute phase. Indeed,

Temporal profiles of age-dependent changes in cytokine mRNA expression and glial cell activation after...

11

microglial response has been shown to be diverse after their activation, and can include both neurodegenerative and neuroprotective functions [40]. The induction of COX-2 expression in adult and P21 rat brain has been shown to be transient as well, since its expression returns to the control level within three days after SE [6,41]. This further suggests that after the initial acute phase (which seems to last up to 24 h - 3 d), there is a change in the inflammatory response provoked by KA-induced SE in juvenile hippocampus, with attenuation of the pronounced, and perhaps exaggerated, expression of inflammatory mediators and modulation of microglial reactivity from widespread activation to a targeted response in the damaged area.

In our study, microglial activation was now detected in P21 rats 3 d after SE also in the basomedial amygdala, which together with the hippocampus is a part of the limbic system and suffers neuronal damage after KA-induced SE [6]. Furthermore, the expression of COX-2 and c-Fos has been shown to be markedly increased in P21 rats after SE in amygdala, this again in tandem with hippocampus [8,42]. Thus, after the acute phase post-SE, the inflammatory response at the subacute phase seems to be more accurately targeted to damaged areas of limbic structures in juvenile rat brain.

Conclusions
In conclusion, SE transiently induced mRNA expression of a number of cytokines in both immature and more mature juvenile rat hippocampus. In general, the increases in cytokine mRNA expressions were more pronounced and rapid in juvenile brain than in immature brain. Glial cells still exhibited an active appearance subacutely after SE in juvenile hippocampus while retaining their resting appearance in immature hippocampus. In juvenile hippocampus, the transient augmentation of cytokine mRNA expression after SE, in contrast to the persistence of glial cell reaction including region-specific microglial activity at the subacute phase, suggests a regulated shift from a fulminant and general initial reaction towards a more moderate and precisely targeted response.

Acknowledgements
Financial support from the Academy of Finland (Project number 8117438) and the Arvo and Lea Ylppö Foundation to IEH, and the Turku Graduate School of Biomedical Sciences (TuBS), the Turku University Foundation, and the Finnish Cultural Foundation to JTJ are gratefully acknowledged.

Author details
[1]Department of Pharmacology, Drug Development, and Therapeutics, Institute of Biomedicine, University of Turku, Itäinen Pitkäkatu 4B, FIN-20014 Turku, Finland. [2]Turku PET Center, Preclinical imaging, Tykistökatu 6A, 4th Floor, FIN-20520 Turku, Finland. [3]Medicity Research Laboratory, Tykistökatu 6A, 4th Floor, Institute of Biomedicine, University of Turku, FIN-20014 Turku, Finland.

Authors' contributions
JTJ conceived and designed the study, carried out qPCR, ELISA and immunohistochemical experiments, performed statistical analyzes, and drafted and revised the manuscript. AP carried out most of the qPCR and some of the immunochemical experiments, and FRL carried out the animal treatments. SR designed and supplied the primers and probes used in PCR experiments. IEH supervised the study, and participated in designing the study, and in drafting and revising the manuscript. All authors read and approved the final manuscript.

Competing interests
The authors declare that they have no competing interests.

References
1. Tocco G, Freire-Moar J, Schreiber SS, Sakhi SH, Aisen PS, Pasinetti GM: Maturational regulation and regional induction of cyclooxygenase-2 in rat brain: implications for Alzheimer's disease. *Exp Neurol* 1997, 144:339-349.
2. De Simoni MG, Perego C, Ravizza T, Moneta D, Conti M, Marchesi F, De Luigi A, Garattini S, Vezzani A: Inflammatory cytokines and related genes are induced in the rat hippocampus by limbic status epilepticus. *Eur J Neurosci* 2000, 12:2623-2633.
3. Shapiro LA, Wang L, Ribak CE: Rapid astrocyte and microglial activation following pilocarpine-induced seizures in rats. *Epilepsia* 2008, 49(Suppl 2):33-41.
4. Vezzani A, Balosso S, Ravizza T: The role of cytokines in the pathophysiology of epilepsy. *Brain Behav Immun* 2008, 22:797-803.
5. Kunz T, Oliw EH: The selective cyclooxygenase-2 inhibitor rofecoxib reduces kainate-induced cell death in the rat hippocampus. *Eur J Neurosci* 2001, 13:569-575.
6. Rizzi M, Perego C, Aliprandi M, Richichi C, Ravizza T, Colella D, Veliskova J, Moshe SL, De Simoni MG, Vezzani A: Glia activation and cytokine increase in rat hippocampus by kainic acid-induced status epilepticus during postnatal development. *Neurobiol Dis* 2003, 14:494-503.
7. Kawaguchi K, Hickey RW, Rose ME, Zhu L, Chen J, Graham SH: Cyclooxygenase-2 expression is induced in rat brain after kainate-induced seizures and promotes neuronal death in CA3 hippocampus. *Brain Res* 2005, 1050:130-137.
8. Järvelä JT, Lopez-Picon FR, Holopainen IE: Age-dependent cyclooxygenase-2 induction and neuronal damage after status epilepticus in the postnatal rat hippocampus. *Epilepsia* 2008, 49:832-841.
9. Scantlebury MH, Heida JG, Hasson HJ, Veliskova J, Velisek L, Galanopoulou AS, Moshe SL: Age-dependent consequences of status epilepticus: animal models. *Epilepsia* 2007, 48(Suppl 2):75-82.
10. Holopainen IE: Seizures in the developing brain: cellular and molecular mechanisms of neuronal damage, neurogenesis and cellular reorganization. *Neurochem Int* 2008, 52:935-947.
11. Qin H, Wilson CA, Roberts KL, Baker BJ, Zhao X, Benveniste EN: IL-10 inhibits lipopolysaccharide-induced CD40 gene expression through induction of suppressor of cytokine signaling-3. *J Immunol* 2006, 177:7761-7771.
12. Gonzalez P, Burgaya F, Acarin L, Peluffo H, Castellano B, Gonzalez B: Interleukin-10 and interleukin-10 receptor-I are upregulated in glial cells after an excitotoxic injury to the postnatal rat brain. *J Neuropathol Exp Neurol* 2009, 68:391-403.
13. Zhang JW, Deb S, Gottschall PE: Regional and differential expression of gelatinases in rat brain after systemic kainic acid or bicuculline administration. *Eur J Neurosci* 1998, 10:3358-3368.
14. Prehn JH, Miller RJ: Opposite effects of TGF-beta 1 on rapidly- and slowly-triggered excitotoxic injury. *Neuropharmacology* 1996, 35:249-256.
15. Hsieh HL, Wang HH, Wu WB, Chu PJ, Yang CM: Transforming growth factor-beta1 induces matrix metalloproteinase-9 and cell migration in astrocytes: roles of ROS-dependent ERK- and JNK-NF-kappaB pathways. *J Neuroinflammation* 2010, 7:88.
16. Humpel C, Hoffer B, Stromberg I, Bektesh S, Collins F, Olson L: Neurons of the hippocampal formation express glial cell line-derived neurotrophic factor messenger RNA in response to kainate-induced excitation. *Neuroscience* 1994, 59:791-795.

17. Wu VW, Nishiyama N, Schwartz JP: A culture model of reactive astrocytes: increased nerve growth factor synthesis and reexpression of cytokine responsiveness. *J Neurochem* 1998, **71**:749-756.

18. Lopez-Picon F, Puustinen N, Kukko-Lukjanov TK, Holopainen IE: Resistance of neurofilaments to degradation, and lack of neuronal death and mossy fiber sprouting after kainic acid-induced status epilepticus in the developing rat hippocampus. *Neurobiol Dis* 2004, **17**:415-426.

19. Fritschy JM, Weinmann O, Wenzel A, Benke D: Synapse-specific localization of NMDA and GABA(A) receptor subunits revealed by antigen-retrieval immunohistochemistry. *J Comp Neurol* 1998, **390**:194-210.

20. Derks NM, Muller M, Gaszner B, Tilburg-Ouwens DT, Roubos EW, Kozicz LT: Housekeeping genes revisited: different expressions depending on gender, brain area and stressor. *Neuroscience* 2008, **156**:305-309.

21. Acarin L, Gonzalez B, Castellano B: Neuronal, astroglial and microglial cytokine expression after an excitotoxic lesion in the immature rat brain. *Eur J Neurosci* 2000, **12**:3505-3520.

22. Samland H, Huitron-Resendiz S, Masliah E, Criado J, Henriksen SJ, Campbell IL: Profound increase in sensitivity to glutamatergic- but not cholinergic agonist-induced seizures in transgenic mice with astrocyte production of IL-6. *J Neurosci Res* 2003, **73**:176-187.

23. Dube CM, Ravizza T, Hamamura M, Zha Q, Keebaugh A, Fok K, Andres AL, Nalcioglu O, Obenaus A, Vezzani A, Baram TZ: Epileptogenesis provoked by prolonged experimental febrile seizures: mechanisms and biomarkers. *J Neurosci* 2010, **30**:7484-7494.

24. Vezzani A, Moneta D, Richichi C, Aliprandi M, Burrows SJ, Ravizza T, Perego C, De Simoni MG: Functional role of inflammatory cytokines and antiinflammatory molecules in seizures and epileptogenesis. *Epilepsia* 2002, **43(Suppl 5)**:30-35.

25. Johnson EA, Kan RK: The acute phase response and soman-induced status epilepticus: temporal, regional and cellular changes in rat brain cytokine concentrations. *J Neuroinflammation* 2010, **7**:40.

26. Zhai QH, Futrell N, Chen FJ: Gene expression of IL-10 in relationship to TNF-alpha, IL-1beta and IL-2 in the rat brain following middle cerebral artery occlusion. *J Neurol Sci* 1997, **152**:119-124.

27. Laing JM, Aurelian L: DeltaRR vaccination protects from KA-induced seizures and neuronal loss through ICP10PK-mediated modulation of the neuronal-microglial axis. *Genet Vaccines Ther* 2008, **6**:1.

28. Gottschall PE, Yu X, Bing B: Increased production of gelatinase B (matrix metalloproteinase-9) and interleukin-6 by activated rat microglia in culture. *J Neurosci Res* 1995, **42**:335-342.

29. Gottschall PE, Yu X: Cytokines regulate gelatinase A and B (matrix metalloproteinase 2 and 9) activity in cultured rat astrocytes. *J Neurochem* 1995, **64**:1513-1520.

30. Jourquin J, Tremblay E, Decanis N, Charton G, Hanessian S, Chollet AM, Le Diguardher T, Khrestchatisky M, Rivera S: Neuronal activity-dependent increase of net matrix metalloproteinase activity is associated with MMP-9 neurotoxicity after kainate. *Eur J Neurosci* 2003, **18**:1507-1517.

31. Wilczynski GM, Konopacki FA, Wilczek E, Lasiecka Z, Gorlewicz A, Michaluk P, Wawrzyniak M, Malinowska M, Okulski P, Kolodziej LR, Konopka W, Duniec K, Mioduszewska B, Nikolaev E, Walczak A, Owczarek D, Gorecki DC, Zuschratter W, Ottersen OP, Kaczmarek L: Important role of matrix metalloproteinase 9 in epileptogenesis. *J Cell Biol* 2008, **180**:1021-1035.

32. Yoo YM, Lee CJ, Lee U, Kim YJ: Neuroprotection of adenoviral-vector-mediated GDNF expression against kainic-acid-induced excitotoxicity in the rat hippocampus. *Exp Neurol* 2006, **200**:407-417.

33. Kanter-Schlifke I, Georgievska B, Kirik D, Kokaia M: Seizure suppression by GDNF gene therapy in animal models of epilepsy. *Mol Ther* 2007, **15**:1106-1113.

34. Ryu HJ, Kim JE, Kim MJ, Kwon HJ, Suh SW, Song HK, Kang TC: The protective effects of interleukin-18 and interferon-gamma on neuronal damages in the rat hippocampus following status epilepticus. *Neuroscience* 2010, **170**:711-721.

35. Morgan TE, Nichols NR, Pasinetti GM, Finch CE: TGF-beta 1 mRNA increases in macrophage/microglial cells of the hippocampus in response to deafferentation and kainic acid-induced neurodegeneration. *Exp Neurol* 1993, **120**:291-301.

36. Cacheaux LP, Ivens S, David Y, Lakhter AJ, Bar-Klein G, Shapira M, Heinemann U, Friedman A, Kaufer D: Transcriptome profiling reveals TGF-beta signaling involvement in epileptogenesis. *J Neurosci* 2009, **29**:8927-8935.

37. Rakhade SN, Jensen FE: Epileptogenesis in the immature brain: emerging mechanisms. *Nat Rev Neurol* 2009, **5**:380-391.

38. Somera-Molina KC, Robin B, Somera CA, Anderson C, Stine C, Koh S, Behanna HA, Van Eldik LJ, Watterson DM, Wainwright MS: Glial activation links early-life seizures and long-term neurologic dysfunction: evidence using a small molecule inhibitor of proinflammatory cytokine upregulation. *Epilepsia* 2007, **48**:1785-1800.

39. Lauren HB, Lopez-Picon FR, Brandt AM, Rios-Rojas CJ, Holopainen IE: Transcriptome analysis of the hippocampal CA1 pyramidal cell region after kainic acid-induced status epilepticus in juvenile rats. *PLoS One* 2010, **5**:e10733.

40. Hanisch UK, Kettenmann H: Microglia: active sensor and versatile effector cells in the normal and pathologic brain. *Nat Neurosci* 2007, **10**:1387-1394.

41. Jung KH, Chu K, Lee ST, Kim J, Sinn DI, Kim JM, Park DK, Lee JJ, Kim SU, Kim M, Lee SK, Roh JK: Cyclooxygenase-2 inhibitor, celecoxib, inhibits the altered hippocampal neurogenesis with attenuation of spontaneous recurrent seizures following pilocarpine-induced status epilepticus. *Neurobiol Dis* 2006, **23**:237-246.

42. Joseph SA, Lynd-Balta E, O'Banion MK, Rappold PM, Daschner J, Allen A, Padowski J: Augmented cyclooxygenase-2 expression in olfactory-limbic forebrain following kainate-induced seizures. *Neuroscience* 2006, **140**:1051-1065.

2

NADPH oxidases as potential pharmacological targets against increased seizure susceptibility after systemic inflammation

Wan-Yu Huang[1,2], Shankung Lin[3], Hsuan-Ying Chen[3], Ya-Ping Chen[3], Ting-Yu Chen[3], Kuei-Sen Hsu[1*] and Hung-Ming Wu[3,4,5*] (iD)

Abstract

Background: Systemic inflammation associated with sepsis can induce neuronal hyperexcitability, leading to enhanced seizure predisposition and occurrence. Brain microglia are rapidly activated in response to systemic inflammation and, in this activated state, release multiple cytokines and signaling factors that amplify the inflammatory response and increase neuronal excitability. NADPH oxidase (NOX) enzymes promote microglial activation through the generation of reactive oxygen species (ROS), such as superoxide anion. We hypothesized that NOX isoforms, particularly NOX2, are potential targets for prevention of sepsis-associated seizures.

Methods: To reduce NADPH oxidase 2-derived ROS production, mice with deficits of NOX regulatory subunit/NOX2 organizer $p47^{phox}$ ($p47^{phox-/-}$) or NOX2 major subunit $gp91^{phox}$ ($gp91^{phox-/-}$) were used or the NOX2-selective inhibitor diphenyleneiodonium (DPI) was used to treat wild-type (WT) mice. Systemic inflammation was induced by intraperitoneal injection of lipopolysaccharide (LPS). Seizure susceptibility was compared among mouse groups in response to intraperitoneal injection of pentylenetetrazole (PTZ). Brain tissues were assayed for proinflammatory gene and protein expression, and immunofluorescence staining was used to estimate the proportion of activated microglia.

Results: Increased susceptibility to PTZ-induced seizures following sepsis was significantly attenuated in $gp91^{phox-/-}$ and $p47^{phox-/-}$ mice compared with WT mice. Both $gp91^{phox-/-}$ and $p47^{phox-/-}$ mice exhibited reduced microglia activation and lower brain induction of multiple proconvulsive cytokines, including TNFα, IL-1β, IL-6, and CCL2, compared with WT mice. Administration of DPI following LPS injection significantly attenuated the increased susceptibility to PTZ-induced seizures and reduced both microglia activation and brain proconvulsive cytokine concentrations compared with vehicle-treated controls. DPI also inhibited the upregulation of $gp91^{phox}$ transcripts following LPS injection.

Conclusions: Our results indicate that NADPH oxidases contribute to the development of increased seizure susceptibility in mice after sepsis. Pharmacologic inhibition of NOX may be a promising therapeutic approach to reducing sepsis-associated neuroinflammation, neuronal hyperexcitability, and seizures.

Keywords: NADPH oxidase, Diphenyleneiodonium, Lipopolysaccharide, Seizure, Cytokine, Neuroninflammation

* Correspondence: richard@mail.ncku.edu.tw; 18288@cch.org.tw
[1]Institute of Basic Medical Sciences, College of Medicine, National Cheng Kung University, Tainan, Taiwan
[3]Inflammation Research & Drug Development Center, Changhua Christian Hospital, Changhua, Taiwan
Full list of author information is available at the end of the article

Background

Seizure is a common acute complication of sepsis and ensuing systemic inflammation, particularly in neonates and infants [1, 2]. Seizures are caused by genetic factors or acquired clinical pathologies that disrupt the excitatory/inhibitory balance within brain circuits. During inflammation, it is believed that hyperexcitation of neurons, resulting from the release of signaling factors such as cytokines and reactive oxygen species (ROS), leads to enhanced seizure predisposition [3–5] and subsequent neuroplastic changes and neurodegeneration, which may eventually induce a chronic seizure syndrome [6, 7].

Growing evidence indicates that transient systemic inflammation can alter neuronal properties and behavior, particularly during critical periods of brain development, resulting in programmed neuron death in adulthood. For instance, a single intraperitoneal (i.p.) injection of the potent immune system activator lipopolysaccharide (LPS) administered to postnatal rats can cause increased seizure susceptibility [7] and alter NMDA receptor subunit mRNA expression in the adult brain [8]. Qin and colleagues also reported that a single systemic LPS injection to adult mice induced chronically persistent activation of microglia and progressive loss of dopaminergic neurons in the substantia nigra [6]. Although brief peripheral inflammation usually does not damage the mature brain, it can induce transient functional deficits in behavior and an acute inflammatory response in the brain similar in some respects to that in the periphery, including elevation of the same proinflammatory cytokines [9, 10]. This induced neuroinflammation can be transient or long-lasting depending on the age at insult [6, 7, 11–13]. Collectively, such studies indicate that both immature and mature brains can be permanently modified after a single brief episode of systemic inflammation, resulting in increased neuronal excitability and behavior changes.

Microglia, the resident macrophage-like immune cells of the central nervous system (CNS), sense local pathological changes, induce and amplify the inflammatory response, and exert additional neuromodulatory effects through dynamic regulation of astroglial activity [14]. In response to systemic inflammation, microglia become activated and may then damage neurons through excessive production and release of neurotoxic factors, including proinflammatory cytokines and ROS. Both clinical reports and experimental studies in vivo and in vitro suggest that these cytokines may increase neuronal excitability and seizure susceptibility [15]. Riazi and colleagues reported that microglia-derived TNFα contributes to neuronal hyperexcitability and exacerbates pentylenetetrazole (PTZ)-induced seizures following peripheral inflammation [4]. Conversely, inhibition of action of the cytokine interleukin (IL)-1β in the brain by application of an exogenous IL-1 receptor antagonist (IL-1ra) or by enhancing endogenous IL-1ra expression can suppress seizure induction or reduce seizure severity in animal models [16–18]. In addition to tumor necrosis factor alpha (TNFα) and IL-1, cytokines reported to modulate neuronal excitability and seizure susceptibility include IL-6 [19, 20], monocyte chemoattractant protein-1 (MCP-1/CCL2) [5], IL-10 [21], and IL-12 [21].

NADPH oxidase 2 (NOX2), also called phagocytic NADPH oxidase (PHOX), is a member of the NADPH oxidase (NOX) family of enzymes implicated in phagocytic bactericidal and fungicidal activities through ROS production. NOX enzymes, principally NOX2, are also involved in microglia activation. When microglial NOX2 is activated, several ROS including superoxide anion ($O_2^{\cdot-}$), hydroxyl radical ($OH^{\cdot-}$), lipid hydroperoxides, and byproducts (e.g., H_2O_2), are generated that can directly damage neurons through extracellular pathways as well as induce further ROS generation and the expression of proinflammatory genes such as IL-1β, TNFα, and inducible nitric oxide synthase (iNOS) [22, 23].

We hypothesized that phagocytic NADPH oxidase (NOX2) within the brain, mainly expressed in microglia, plays an essential role in increased neuronal excitability following systemic inflammation. While targeting inflammation has long been proposed as a potential therapeutic strategy for prevention of neuroinflammation-associated seizures [18, 24–26], there are few studies showing that this is an effective approach. Therefore, the main purpose of this study was to investigate whether NOX2 plays a critical role in seizure susceptibility after systemic inflammation and whether post-treatment with the widely used and long-acting NOX2 inhibitor, diphenyleneiodonium (DPI) [27], can attenuate the enhanced seizure susceptibility induced by systemic inflammation. By comparing seizure susceptibility among mice genetically deficient in NOX2 complex subunits gp91^{phox} and p47^{phox}, DPI-treated mice, and wild types (WT), we demonstrate that NOX2-derived ROS contribute to neuronal hyperexcitability and the increased seizure susceptibility following LPS-induced inflammation. Thus, pharmacological NOX2 blockade is a potential therapeutic strategy for prevention of sepsis-associated seizures.

Methods

Animals and lipopolysaccharide-induced sepsis model

Male C57BL/6J mice (8–9 weeks old, 25–30 g) were purchased from the National Lab Animal Center (Taiwan). The NOX2 subunit knockout mice B6.129S6-Cybbtm1Din/J mice (gp91$^{phox-/-}$, JAX stock 002365) and B6(Cg)-Ncf1<m1J>/J mice (p47$^{phox-/-}$, JAX Stock 004742) were obtained from The Jackson Laboratory (Bar Harbor, ME, USA). The PHOX$^{-/-}$ mutation is maintained on a C57BL/6J background; therefore, C57BL/6J (PHOX$^{+/+}$) mice were used as control animals for this study. The animals were housed in a specific pathogen-free room at 21 °C under a 12-h/12-h artificial light/dark cycle with free access to feed. Experiments were performed using age- and weight-matched male animals. All procedures were approved by the Animal Care and Use Committee of Changhua Christian Hospital. The mouse model of sepsis was induced by intraperitoneal (i.p.) injection of 4 mg/kg lipopolysaccharide (LPS), modified from a previous study in mice [28]. In total, 352 of mice were used in this study, including 248 of WT mice, 52 of p47$^{phox-/-}$ mice, and 52 of gp91$^{phox-/-}$ mice.

Diphenyleneiodonium treatment
Diphenyleneiodonium (DPI) (Sigma-Aldrich, St. Louis, MO, USA) is a pharmacological inhibitor of NADPH oxidase. In the present study, we assessed the efficacy of DPI against PTZ-induced seizure susceptibility in LPS-treated mice. Diphenyleneiodonium was injected i.p. at a dose of 0.01, 0.1, or 1 mg/kg at indicated time points after LPS injection.

Determination of seizure susceptibility to pentylenetetrazol
To assess seizure susceptibility, mice were injected i.p. with 60 mg/kg pentylenetetrazole (PTZ) 48 h after LPS or vehicle treatment (Sigma, St. Louis, MO, USA). Pentylenetetrazole may have multiple mechanisms of action in neurons, one of which is strongly correlated with its affinity for the picrotoxin binding site on the GABA$_A$ receptor complex [29, 30]. Seizure activity was video recorded during an observation period of 2 h after PTZ injection. Behavioral seizures were scored every 5 min according to a previously defined scale [31, 32] as follows: stage 1 (exploring, sniffing, and grooming ceased and immobility); stage 2 (forelimb and/or tail extension, appearance of a rigid posture); stage 3 (isolated myoclonic jerks, with brief twitching movements); stage 4 (forelimb clonus and partial rearing); stage 5 (forelimb clonus, rearing, and falling); and stage 6 (generalized tonic-clonic activity with loss of postural tone, often resulting in death).

Plasma levels of TNFα after peritoneal LPS administration
To assess the acute effects of LPS on systemic inflammation, blood samples were obtained from the cheek of the wild-type and NOX2 knockout mice 1 h after LPS injection (4 mg/kg, i.p.). The plasma samples were stored at −80°C until they were assayed for TNFα concentration according to the manufacturer's instructions (Duo set kit; R&D Systems, Minneapolis, MN, USA).

Microglia-enriched cultures
Primary enriched-microglial cultures were prepared from WT, gp91$^{phox-/-}$, and p47$^{phox-/-}$ pups using a previously described protocol [28, 33]. Briefly, the whole brain obtained from a 0–1-day-old mouse pup was carefully removed, and the olfactory bulbs, cerebellum, brain stem, meninges, and blood vessels were separated. The remaining brain tissue was triturated into a single-cell suspension, which was then centrifuged at 500×g for 6 min at 4 °C. The pellet was resuspended in the warm mixed glial culture maintenance medium. The cells were cultured with a seeding density of five brains per 175-cm^2 flask. The culture medium was refreshed every 3 days. Approximately 14–16 days later, microglia were shaken out at 180 rpm for 30 min to 1 h at 37 °C. After centrifugation, the resuspended microglia were seeded in a 24-well plate at a density of 7.5×10^4/well. After storage overnight, cells were treated with LPS (5 ng/ml), TNFα (500 pg/ml), or IL-1β (500 pg/ml). The purity of microglia was > 98%, confirmed by staining with F4/80 antibody.

Western blotting analysis
For protein lysate extraction, dissected mouse brain tissue (e.g., hippocampus) was homogenized and lysed in ice-cold modified radioimmunoprecipitation assay (RIPA) buffer containing 50 mM Tris-HCl (pH 7.4), 1% Nonidet P-40, 150 mM NaCl, 1 mM EDTA, 1 mM phenylmethylsulfonyl fluoride, 10 μg/ml each of aprotinin, leupeptin, and pepstatin, 1 mM Na$_3$VO$_4$, and 1 mM NaF. Immunobloting analysis was performed as described [28, 33]. Briefly, total proteins from each sample were fractionated by SDS-PAGE and then transferred to polyvinylidene difluoride (PVDF) membranes. Membranes were probed with antibodies against the proteins including gp91 (Cat# sc-5827) and β-actin(Cat# sc-47,778) (the gen loading control) from Santa Cruz Biotechnology (Dallas, TX), Cruz, iba-1(Cat# GTX100042), GFAP(Cat# GTX85454) and BDNF(GTX62495) from GeneTex Biotechnology (Irvine, CA), and hsp 90 (Cat# 4877) (the gel loading control) from Cell Signaling Technology (Danvers, MA) at 1/1000 dilution. Immunoblotted membranes were then washed for 10 min in 0.1% Tris-buffered saline-Tween 20 (TBST), incubated in horseradish peroxidase (HRP)-conjugated secondary antibody (1/10,000 dilution) for 1 h, and washed again in TBST. Signals were visualized and quantified using the GeneGnome chemiluminescence imaging system (Syngene, Maryland).

Measurement of cytokines in brain supernatant
Total brain proteins were extracted using a protocol modified from previous studies on cytokine/chemokine panels [10, 34]. Briefly, temporal lobe tissue was weighed and homogenized with a bench top homogenizer (Kinematica, Switzerland) in a 5× volume of extraction buffer containing 20 mM Tris HCl, 0.15 M NaCl, 2 mM EDTA, 1 mM EGTA, and Protease Inhibitor Cocktail

(Sigma, St. Louis, MO). Samples were centrifuged at $1000\times g$ for 10 min at 4 °C, and the supernatants were centrifuged again at $20,000\times g$ for 40 min at 4 °C to remove any remaining debris. Protein concentration was measured using a BCA Protein Assay Kit (Pierce Biotechnology, Rockford, IL). All cytokine and chemokine measurements were performed using MERCK Millipore Presents MILLIPLEX® MAP multiplex Assays (St. Charles, MO, USA) by the procedures reported previously [10, 34]. Concentrations of TNFα, IL-1β, IL-6, CCL2, IL-10, and IL-12 were simultaneously determined in brain samples using a LINCOplexTM mouse cytokine kit and a Luminex 200 reader (Luminex Corp., Austin, TX, USA). Concentrations were calculated by generating a calibration curve using recombinant cytokines diluted in brain sample extraction buffer and StatLIAs software (Brendan Scientific Corp., Carlsbad, CA, USA). Cytokine and chemokine concentrations were then normalized to total protein for each sample.

Real-time RT-PCR analysis

To assess the expression of proinflammatory factors TNFα, IL-1β, IL-6, CCL2, IL-10, and IL-12, and gp91 in response to LPS-induced systemic inflammation, mouse brains were prepared at the indicated time points following LPS treatment. Total RNA was prepared from temporal lobe tissues using the RNeasy micro kit (Qiagen, Valencia, CA, USA) and reverse transcribed into cDNA using the Super Script-III First-strand Synthesis System kit (Invitrogen, Carlsbad, CA, USA). Real-time PCR was performed using the Rotor-Gene Q cycler (Qiagen, Valencia, CA, USA) according to the manufacturer's protocol. All experiments were conducted in triplicate using TaqMan Gene Expression Master mix (Applied Biosystems) and TaqMan Gene Expression Assays, with optimized primer and TaqMan MGB probe sets (Applied Biosystems, Foster City, CA, USA). The PCR primer pairs and TaqMan MGB probes (assay-IDs) (Applied Biosystems) were as follows: Mm00443260_gl (TNFα), Mm00434228_ml (IL-1β), Mm00446190_ml (IL-6), Mm00441242_ml (CCL2), Mm01288386_ml (IL-10), Mm00434174_ml (IL-12b), and Mm00607939Msl (β-actin). A total of 40 cycles of PCR was performed as follows: activation of AmpliTaq Gold Enzyme (10 min at 95°C), denaturation (15 s at 95 °C), and annealing/extension (1 min at 60 °C). Relative expression levels were calculated using the comparative threshold cycle (Ct value) method and normalized to the ΔCt of *β-actin*.

Immunofluorescence staining

To assess the effects of LPS-induced systemic inflammation on CNS glia, mouse brain sections were prepared for immunostaining. Mice were deeply anesthetized and perfused with 4% paraformaldehyde (PFA) 24 h after vehicle or LPS treatment. The brain was dissected and post-fixed overnight in 4% PFA at 4 °C. Coronal frozen sections (30 μm thick) through hippocampi were prepared as described [28]. Brain sections were permeabilized with 1% Triton X-100 in PBS for 10 min and then blocked in 1% bovine serum albumin in PBST for 1 h. To identify microglia, slices were incubated overnight at 4 °C in blocking buffer containing an antibody against ionized calcium binding adaptor molecule 1 protein (iba-1) (Cat# GTX100042) from GeneTex Biotechnology (Irvine, CA), at 1/200 dilution. The brain sections were then also incubated with donkey anti-rabbit-FITC antibody (1200) at room temperature for 1 h. Sections were then counterstained with 4′, 6-diamidino-2-phenylindole (DAPI) for 5 min at room temperature and observed by fluorescence microscopy. Microglial activation was determined by morphology changes from round and small (resting state) to rod- and/or amoeboid shaped with a significant enlargement of cell size (activated state). We used a stereological approach to count the number of resting and activated microglia from three sections of the hippocampus per mouse ($n = 3$ mice/group), including dentate gyrus (DG) and CA3 subregions on a ZEISS-Axio Observer Z1, HAL 100 microscope (ZEISS, Germany) under bright-field optics [33, 35]. Briefly, images were taken from DG and CA3 subregions at − 2.18 to − 2.54 mm from the bregma. Coordinates for the DG were taken centered from 1.4 to 1.7 mm medial and 1.7 to 1.9 mm ventral. Coordinates for the CA3 were from 2.1 to 2.4 mm medial and from 1.8 to 2.1 mm ventral. Activated microglia were distinguished from resting microglia by the presence of shorter, less-ramified processes and rod-and/or amoeboid appearance. Quantification of microglia was done by a single experimenter who was blind to each animal's treatment, by counting the total number of iba-1 positive cells at 200× magnification in a rectangular region of interest (300×400 μm^2). Results are presented as means ± standard error of the mean (SEM) in the counted area.

Statistical analysis

Values are presented as mean ± SEM. Paired group means were compared by Student's *t* test. The efficacy of *NOX2* deletion or DPI treatment against PTZ-induced seizure severity was assessed by two-way repeated measures ANOVA, adjusted by Bonferroni tests. Multiple group means were compared by one-way ANOVA, followed by Bonferroni post hoc tests. All analyses were conducted using the software GraphPad Prism 7 (La Jolla, CA). Differences were considered significant at $p < 0.05$.

Results

NOX2 deletion reduces the increased seizure susceptibility to pentylenetetrazole following LPS-induced systemic inflammation

To elucidate the role of NOX2 in seizure incidence following systemic inflammation, we induced systemic inflammation in adult (8–9-week-old) wild-type, gp91$^{phox-/-}$, and p47$^{phox-/-}$ mice with a single dose of LPS via i.p. injection and subsequently determined PTZ-induced (60 mg/kg, i.p.) seizure susceptibility by scoring the severity and duration of the PTZ-induced seizure every 5 min for 2 h (Fig. 1a). The latency to initial seizure onset (clonic with/without tonic convulsion) after PTZ administration was significantly decreased in LPS-treated gp91$^{phox-/-}$ and p47$^{phox-/-}$ groups, compared with the LPS-treated WT group (Fig. 1b). In addition, the seizure susceptibility to PTZ of all three genotype groups treated with LPS was significantly increased, compared with the vehicle-treated (saline) control group (all p values < 0.0001 by two-way repeated-measures ANOVA). The main effect for LPS-treated WT, gp91$^{phox-/-}$, and p47$^{phox-/-}$ groups yielded an F ratio of F(2,432) = 34.12, p < 0.0001, indicating a significant difference between these three groups in susceptibility to PTZ-induced seizure. The Bonferroni test further revealed a significant difference between the WT group and gp91$^{phox-/-}$ (F(1,288) = 42.63; p < 0.0001) and between WT and p47$^{phox-/-}$ (F(1,288) = 54.86; p < 0.0001), but no difference between p47$^{phox-/-}$ and gp91$^{phox-/-}$ groups ((F(1,288) = 1.16; p = 0.282). The results indicate that both LPS-treated gp91$^{phox-/-}$ and

p47^{phox} groups exhibited significantly attenuated the increased seizure susceptibility, compared with the LPS-treated WT group (Fig. 1c). We measured the duration of stage 4–6 seizures among the mice receiving LPS or vehicle control. The results showed that the seizure duration was 2.14 ± 0.73 (mean ± SEM), 18.00 ± 2.67, 8.14 ± 1.44, and 8.43 ± 1.36 mins, for the vehicle-treated WT, LPS-treated WT, LPS-treated gp91$^{phox-/-}$, and LPS-treated p47$^{phox-/-}$ groups, respectively (Fig. 1d). Notably, there was no difference between gp91$^{phox-/-}$ and p47$^{phox-/-}$ mice following LPS injection (p > 0.05). These results strongly suggested that NOX2 was a critical component of the elevation in seizure susceptibility following systemic inflammation.

NOX2 deletion attenuated microglial activation and the upregulation of proconvulsive cytokines following LPS injection

To further elucidate how systemic inflammation increased seizure susceptibility, we examined the effect of NOX2 knockout on inflammation in the peripheral and central nervous systems. Peripheral TNFα has been shown as an important mediator of seizure susceptibility following LPS-induced systemic inflammation [4].

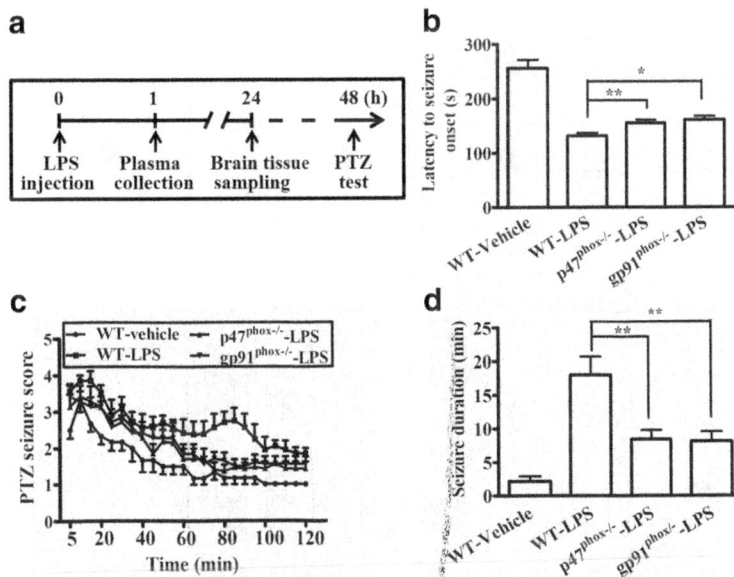

Fig. 1 NADPH oxidase deletion reduced the increased pentylenetetrazole (PTZ)-induced seizure susceptibility following lipopolysaccharide (LPS) stimulation. **a** The experiment protocol is schematized. Wild-type (WT), gp91$^{phox-/-}$, and p47$^{phox-/-}$ mice were injected intraperitoneally (i.p.) with 4 mg/kg lipopolysaccharide (LPS). Plasma samples were collected 1 h later for TNFα quantification and some mice were sacrificed 24 h later for the preparation of brain sections and transcript assays. Two days later, seizure susceptibility to 60 mg/kg PTZ (i.p.) was evaluated (n = 6 or 7 mice per genotype). **b** The latency to initial seizure onset (clonic with/without tonic convulsion) after PTZ administration. Data are presented as mean ± SEM. Bonferroni post hoc test vs. LPS-treated WT group; *p < 0.05, **p < 0.01. **c** Seizure susceptibility of gp91$^{phox-/-}$, and p47$^{phox-/-}$ and WT mice scored once every 5 min over the 2-h period following PTZ injection. Two-way repeated measures ANOVA revealed that the main effect for LPS-treated WT, gp91$^{phox-/-}$, and p47$^{phox-/-}$ groups yielded an F ratio of F(2, 432) = 34.12, p < 0.0001, Bonferroni post-test analysis further revealed significant difference between the WT group and gp91$^{phox-/-}$ (F(1,288) = 42.63; p < 0.0001) and between WT and p47$^{phox-/-}$ (F(1,288) = 54.86; p < 0.0001), but no difference between p47$^{phox-/-}$ and gp91$^{phox-/-}$ groups ((F(1,288) = 1.16; p = 0.282). **d** The total duration (min) of seizure behavior ≥ stage 4. Data are presented as mean ± SEM. Bonferroni post hoc test vs. vehicle-treated or LPS-treated WT group; **p < 0.01, ***p < 0.001

Therefore, we first compared TNFα levels in the plasma collected from these WT, gp91$^{phox-/-}$, and p47$^{phox-/-}$ groups of mice 1 h after LPS or vehicle injection. Our data showed that there was no difference in the basal levels of TNFα among the groups and that LPS increased plasma TNFα levels in those three groups with indistinguishable potency (Fig. 2a). We also examined the basal levels of PTZ-seizure susceptibility, the microglial protein marker iba-1, the astrocytic marker glial fibrillary acidic protein (GFAP), and the brain-derived neurotrophic factor (BDNF), a marker related to neuronal excitability [36] in the brains of the wild-type and NOX2-knockout mice without LPS injection. We found no difference in the PTZ-induced seizure susceptibility, including latency to seizure onset and the duration of seizures (stage 4–6) between the WT and NOX2-knockout mice (see Additional file 1). We also found no differences in the expression of these glial and neuronal markers among these groups (see Additional file 1). In addition, they had similar characteristics to those of resting microglia, composed of long branching processes and a small cellular body (see Additional file 1).

In response to systemic inflammation, microglia are rapidly activated and undergo morphological changes, consisting of the cell body increasing in size and becoming irregular in shape with thicker and shorter processes (Fig. 2b). Following LPS stimulation, the proportion of activated microglia was significantly lower in the brains (including the hippocampus) of gp91^{phox} and p47^{phox} knockout mice compared with WT mice (Fig. 2b,c). Next, we determined the levels of cytokines that have been shown as contributors to seizure occurrence, including TNFα, IL-1β, CCL2, IL-6, and IL-12, and the anti-inflammatory cytokine IL-10, which may protect against seizure activity. We measured the expression of these cytokines in the brains of the wild-type and NOX2-knockout mice 1.5 h after LPS injection. RT-qPCR analyses showed that these six cytokines were significantly elevated in all genotypes, but the increases of TNFα, IL-1β, IL-6, and CCL2 were significantly attenuated, and the increase of IL-10 was enhanced in NOX2-knockout mice compared with WT mice (Fig. 3). Collectively, these data suggest that NOX2-dependent microglial activation and the ensuing production of

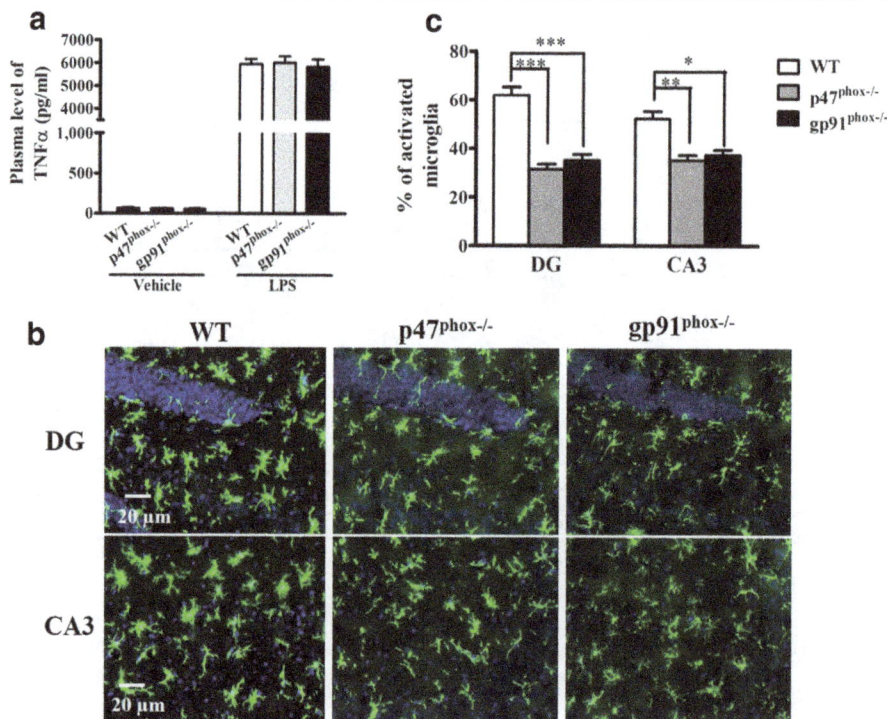

Fig. 2 Effects of NADPH oxidase subunit deletion on plasma TNFα levels and microglial activation after LPS injection. a The plasma TNFα levels were not affected by NOX2 subunit knockout (gp91$^{phox-/-}$ and P47$^{phox-/-}$) 1 h after LPS. Data are presented as mean ± SEM; n = 5/group. Bonferroni post hoc test vs. vehicle-treated or LPS-treated wild-type (WT) group; p > 0.05. b WT, gp91$^{phox-/-}$, and P47$^{phox-/-}$ mice were sacrificed 24 h after 4 mg/kg LPS injection (i.p.). Brain sections were immunostained for the microglial marker Iba-1. Representative images of the stained microglia in the dentate gyrus (DG) and CA3 regions of mouse hippocampus (n = 3 mice per genotype) are shown. c Activated microglia were identified by increased cell size and irregular shape. The proportions of activated microglia in hippocampus were estimated. Data are mean ± SEM of values from three animals per genotype. Bonferroni post hoc test vs. LPS-treated WT mouse group; *p < 0.05, **p < 0.01, ***p < 0.001

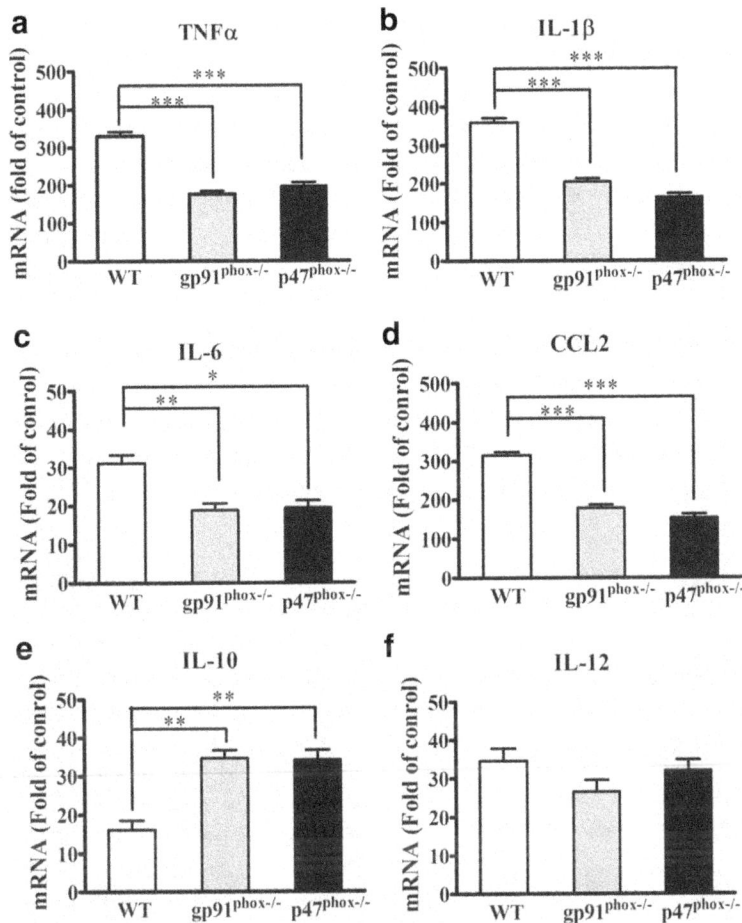

Fig. 3 NADPH oxidase deletion attenuated the upregulation of proconvulsive cytokines in mouse brain following LPS stimulation. Wild-type (WT), gp91$^{phox-/-}$ and P47$^{phox-/-}$ mice were treated with saline (vehicle) or 4 mg/kg LPS (i.p.). Mouse brains (n = 5 per genotype) were harvested 1.5 h after LPS injection. The mRNA levels of TNFα, IL-1β, CCL2, IL-6, IL-10, and IL-12 was determined by RT-qPCR (**a-f**). Cytokine mRNA expression was normalized to β-actin mRNA expression (internal control). Fold change was calculated by comparing the expression of each cytokine of the LPS-treated mice to that of the genotype-matched saline-treated mice. Data present the mean ± SEM. Bonferroni post hoc test vs. corresponding WT control; *$p < 0.05$, **$p < 0.01$, ***$p < 0.001$

proinflammatory cytokines play a key role in the systemic inflammation-elicited increase in seizure susceptibility.

Primary cultured microglia from NOX2-deleted mice showed reduced proconvulsive factor expression after LPS, TNFα, and IL-1β stimulation

In this scenario of systemic inflammation and ensuing neuroinflammation, many factors, including LPS and cytokines, may contribute to microglial activation, which in turn produce many proinflammatory factors [37, 38]. To investigate the role of microglial NOX2 in these events, we prepared primary enriched-microglial cultures from the WT and NOX2-knockout mice, and treated these cultures with 5 ng/ml LPS, 500 pg/ml TNFα, or 500 pg/ml IL-1β for 1 h. TNFα and IL-1β are two main important proconvulsive cytokines in the periphery and in the CNS following LPS administration

[4, 9, 37]. RT-qPCR analyses showed that LPS treatment significantly enhanced the expression of TNFα, IL-1β, and CCL2 in primary microglia from all three groups of mice, but the induction in NOX2-knockout microglia was approximately 50% lower than that in the WT (Fig. 4a). TNFα significantly enhanced levels of TNFα, IL-1β, and CCL2 transcripts, but the increased levels of TNFα and IL-1β were significantly attenuated in p47$^{phox-/-}$ and gp$^{91phox-/-}$ microglia compared with those of WT microglia (Fig. 4b). Similarly, IL1β stimulation upregulated TNFα mRNA levels in all genotypes, but the levels were significantly lower in p47$^{phox-/-}$ and gp$^{91phox-/-}$ microglia than in WT microglia (Fig. 4c). These results suggested that following LPS (i.p.) stimulation, microglial NOX2 played a critical role in the local production of pro-convulsive cytokines such as TNFα and IL-1β, which in turn enhanced neuronal excitability and seizure susceptibility.

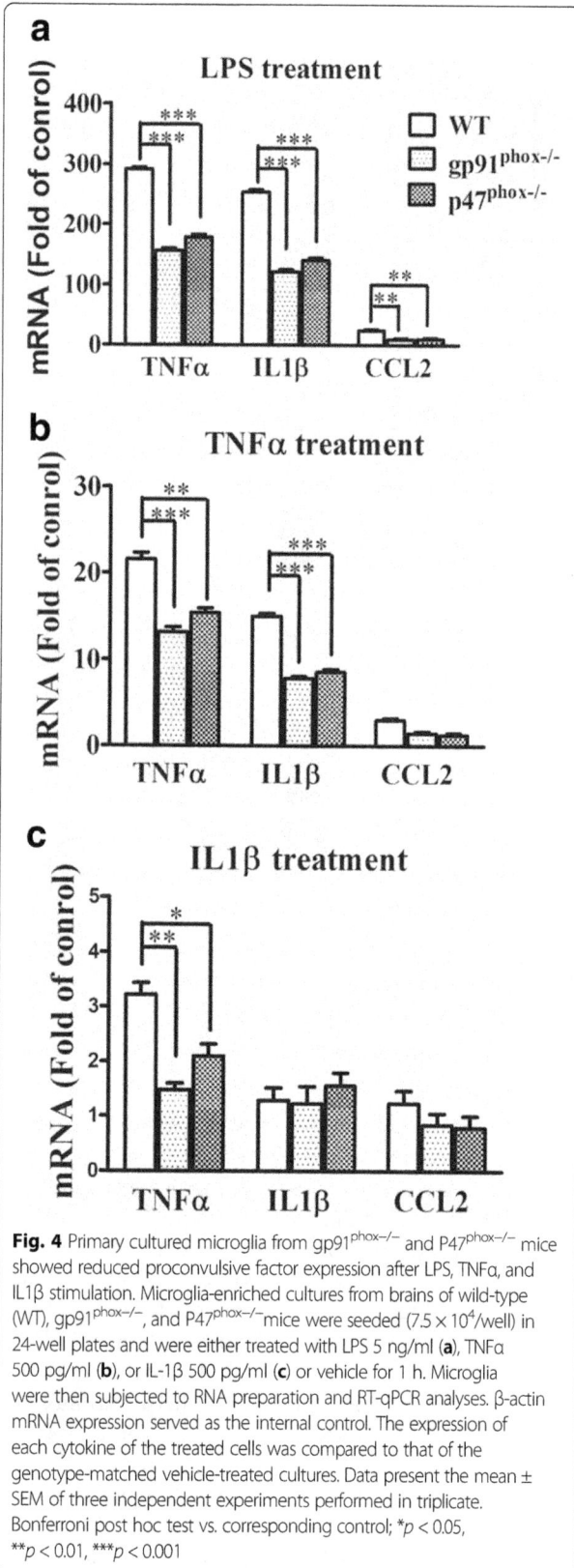

Fig. 4 Primary cultured microglia from gp91$^{phox-/-}$ and P47$^{phox-/-}$ mice showed reduced proconvulsive factor expression after LPS, TNFα, and IL1β stimulation. Microglia-enriched cultures from brains of wild-type (WT), gp91$^{phox-/-}$, and P47$^{phox-/-}$ mice were seeded (7.5 × 10^4/well) in 24-well plates and were either treated with LPS 5 ng/ml (**a**), TNFα 500 pg/ml (**b**), or IL-1β 500 pg/ml (**c**) or vehicle for 1 h. Microglia were then subjected to RNA preparation and RT-qPCR analyses. β-actin mRNA expression served as the internal control. The expression of each cytokine of the treated cells was compared to that of the genotype-matched vehicle-treated cultures. Data present the mean ± SEM of three independent experiments performed in triplicate. Bonferroni post hoc test vs. corresponding control; *$p < 0.05$, **$p < 0.01$, ***$p < 0.001$

DPI post-treatment attenuated the increased seizure susceptibility following systemic inflammation

Based on the findings, we propose that NADPH oxidase is a potential pharmacological target to prevent the development of increased seizure susceptibility following systemic inflammation. We therefore investigated the anticonvulsant efficacy of the NADPH oxidase inhibitor DPI in the mouse sepsis model. Wild-type mice were treated with 0.01, 0.1, or 1 mg/kg (i.p.) DPI or vehicle (0.025% DMSO) 30 min and 24 h after LPS administration, and blood samples were collected to measure plasma TNFα 1 h after LPS, and subsequently determined PTZ-induced (60 mg/kg, i.p.) seizure susceptibility (Fig. 5a). As shown in Fig. 5b, 1 mg/kg of DPI significantly decreased plasma TNFα compared with vehicle treatment. The latency to initial seizure onset after PTZ administration was significantly increased in 1 mg/kg DPI-treated WT group, compared with vehicle-treated WT group 48 h after LPS injection (Fig. 5c). In addition, two-way repeated measures ANOVA revealed that the main effect for LPS-injected vehicle-treated and LPS-injected DPI-treated groups yielded an F ratio of $F(3,576) = 18.06$, $p < 0.0001$, indicating a significant difference between these four groups to PTZ-induced seizure. Further analysis revealed that there is significant difference between the LPS-injected vehicle-treated group and LPS-injected 1 mg/kg DPI-treated group ($F(1,288) = 41.05$; $p < 0.0001$). The results indicate that 1 mg/kg DPI treatment significantly attenuated the PTZ-induced seizures susceptibility following LPS injection (Fig. 5d). The duration of PTZ-induced seizure (stage 4–6) was also significantly decreased by 1 mg/kg DPI treatment (Bonferroni post hoc test; $p < 0.01$) (Fig. 5e). These results indicated that DPI could attenuate peripheral TNFα levels as well as PTZ-induced seizure susceptibility in LPS-treated mice.

DPI post-treatment attenuated microglia activation and pro-convulsive cytokine expression in brains after LPS injection

Subsequent examinations of microglia morphology showed that post-treatment with DPI also decreased the proportion of activated microglia in the mouse CNS following systemic inflammation (Fig. 6a). While LPS induced an approximately 60 and 53% increase of activated microglia in the DG and CA3 regions, respectively, DPI as low as 0.1 mg/kg was able to significantly attenuate microglia activation (Fig. 6b). Post-treatment with 1 mg/kg DPI significantly decreased the upregulation of TNFα, IL-1β, IL-6, and CCL2 mRNA in mouse brain 1.5 h after LPS treatment (Fig. 7a–d). The protein concentrations of these cytokines were measured in brain tissues 24 h after LPS injection using multiplex cytokine assays. DPI at 1 mg/kg, but not at 0.01 or 0.1 mg/kg, significantly

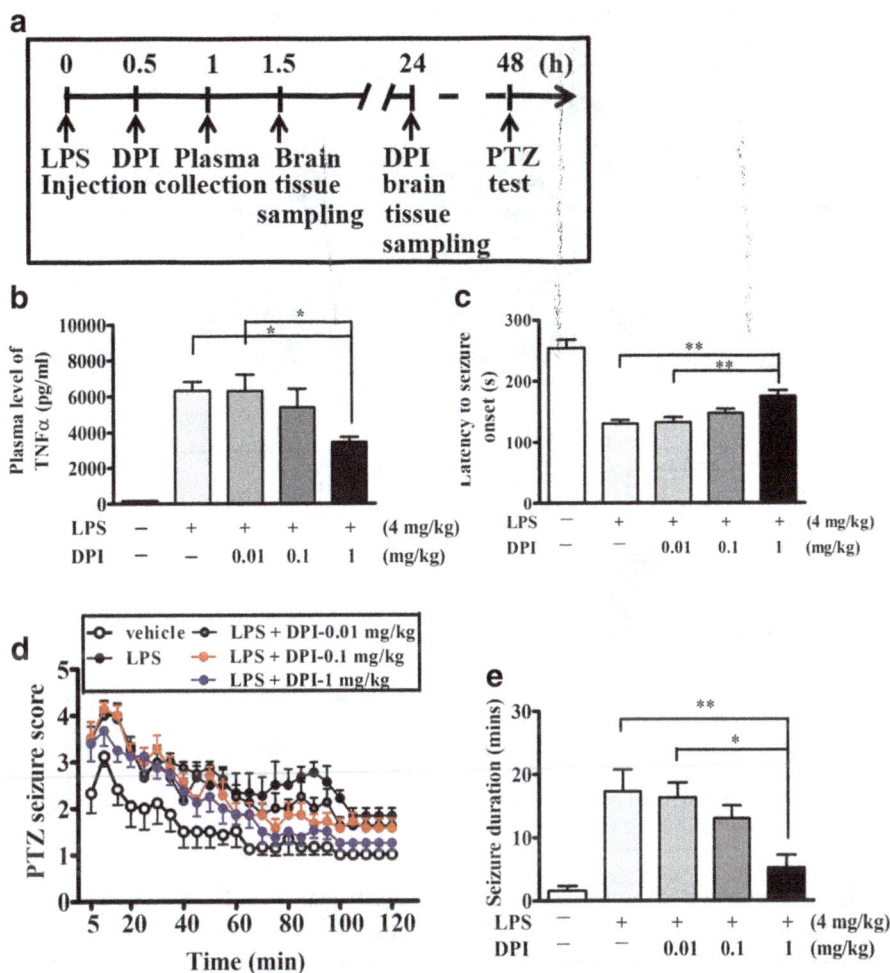

Fig. 5 DPI post-treatment attenuated the increased seizure susceptibility following systemic inflammation. **a** The protocol for DPI post-treatment experiments is schematized. Wild-type (WT) mice were either injected intraperitoneally (i.p.) with 4 mg/kg LPS or with vehicle (saline). Then, the mice were treated with 0, 0.01, 0.1, or 1 mg/kg DPI or vehicle (0.025% DMSO) 30 min and 24 h after LPS injection. 48 h later, all the mice received PTZ (60 mg/kg, i.p.) treatment ($n = 6$ or 7 mice/group). **b** Plasma samples were collected 1 h after LPS injection, and the levels of TNFα were determined and compared with that of the vehicle-treated mice. Data present the mean ± SEM; $n = 5$ for each treatment. Bonferroni post hoc test vs. LPS-vehicle-treated group; $*p < 0.05$. **c** The latency to initial seizure onset (clonic with/without tonic convulsion) after PTZ administration. Data are presented as mean ± SEM. Bonferroni post hoc test vs. LPS-injected vehicle-treated group; $**p < 0.01$. **d** Seizure susceptibility scored once every 5 min for 2 h after PTZ injection. Two-way repeated measures ANOVA revealed that the main effect for LPS-injectee vehicle-treated and LPS-DPI-treated groups yielded an F ratio of $F_{(3,576)} = 18.06$, $p < 0.0001$. Bonferroni test analysis further revealed significant difference between the LPS-injected vehicle-treated group LPS-injected 1 mg/kg DPI-treated group ($F_{(1,288)} = 41.05$; $p < 0.0001$). **e** The total duration (min) of seizure behavior ≥ stage 4. Data present the mean ± SEM. Bonferroni post hoc t-test vs. LPS-injected vehicle treatment; $*p < 0.05$, $**p < 0.01$

attenuated the upregulation of TNFα, IL-1β, IL-6, and CCL2 proteins compared with vehicle treatment (Fig. 7e–h), whereas 0.1 mg/kg DPI was also high enough to decrease IL-6 expression (Fig. 7g). However, there was no difference in the expression of IL-10 and IL-12 between vehicle-treated and DPI-treated mice following LPS injection (see Additional file 2). These results indicated that post-treatment with DPI could inhibit upregulation of proconvulsive cytokines (TNFα, IL-1β, IL-6, and CCL2) at both the mRNA and protein levels in mouse brain following systemic inflammation.

DPI post-treatment attenuated upregulation of gp91 in brain after LPS stimulation

We further examined whether DPI post-treatment affected NOX expression in mouse brain following LPS injection. RT-qPCR analyses showed that the expression of the gp91 transcript in brain was persistently upregulated for at least 1 day following LPS injection (Fig. 8a). We treated the mice with 0.01, 0.1, or 1 mg/kg DPI 30 min after LPS injection and harvested brains 24 h after LPS injection for RT-qPCR and western blot analyses. The data showed that DPI post-treatment dose-

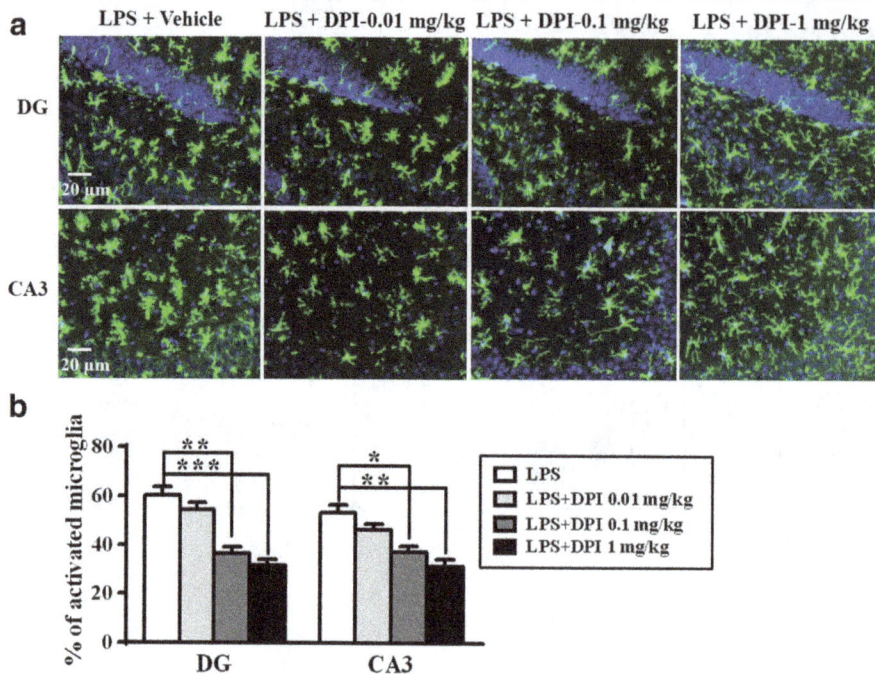

Fig. 6 DPI post-treatment attenuated microglia activation in brain after LPS injection. **a** Wild-type mice were treated with a single dose of 0.01, 0.1, or 1 mg/kg DPI or vehicle (0.025% DMSO) 30 min after 4 mg/kg LPS injection (i.p.), and then sacrificed 24 h after LPS. Brain sections were prepared and immunostained for the microglial marker iba-1. Representative images of the stained microglia in the dentate gyrus (DG) and CA3 regions of mouse hippocampus are shown. **b** Activated microglia were identified by increased cell size and irregular shape. The proportions of activated microglia in hippocampus were estimated. Data represent the mean ± SEM of values from three animals per treatment. Bonferroni post hoc test vs. vehicle-treated mouse group; *$p < 0.05$, **$p < 0.01$, ***$p < 0.001$

dependently reduced the expression of gp91 transcript (Fig. 8b) and gp91 protein (Fig. 8c,d). In comparison, NOX1 levels were not affected by DPI (see Additional file 3). These results further indicated that DPI post-treatment could also inhibit the deleterious neuroinflammatory response by attenuating the upregulation of NOX2 expression in the mouse brain following LPS stimulation.

Discussion

In the present study, we demonstrate that the increased seizure susceptibility following LPS-induced systemic inflammation strongly depends on activation of NOX2 in activated microglia. Our findings suggest that NOX2 activation and proinflammatory cytokine generation by microglia sustains the local neuroinflammatory response and increases neuronal excitability, which in turn reduces the threshold for seizure initiation, exacerbating seizure severity. Indeed, mice with NOX2 subunit knockout exhibited reduced microglial activation, attenuated production of the proconvulsive cytokines IL-1β, TNFα, IL-6, and CCL2, and lower seizure susceptibility to PTZ than wild-type mice following LPS-induced inflammation. Similarly, post-treatment with the NADPH oxidase inhibitor DPI following LPS also attenuated microglia activation and the expression of these proconvulsive cytokines in mouse brain. These results strongly

suggest that like NOX2 deletion, DPI post-treatment suppresses sepsis-associated neuroinflammation and associated neuronal hyperexcitability, thereby reducing the probability of seizure induction.

The NOX family is comprised of seven members including NOX1-5 and DOUX1-2 [39]. Each isoform is composed of distinct NOX and regulatory subunits but all generate superoxide by transferring electrons across biological membranes. Both NOX1 and NOX2 are co-expressed in microglia but may have distinct functions in microglia activation [40, 41]. In the present study, we clearly demonstrate that NOX2-derived ROS is critical for increasing seizure susceptibility following systemic inflammation via promotion of proconvulsive cytokine expression, although we cannot eliminate a contribution by NOX1. NOX2 is initially found in phagocytic cells (e.g., neutrophils) mediating host defense against microorganisms and also identified in non-phagocytic cells such as astroglia and neurons [42, 43]. NOX-derived ROS levels in non-phagocytic cells are typically much lower than in phagocytic cells since they are not generated to host defense, but as second messengers molecules in response to physiological stimuli (e.g., insulin) [44]. A study using LPS as a stimulus of microglial activation showed that only NOX2 from microglia, and not astrocytes and neurons, caused NADPH oxidase-mediated neuron damage

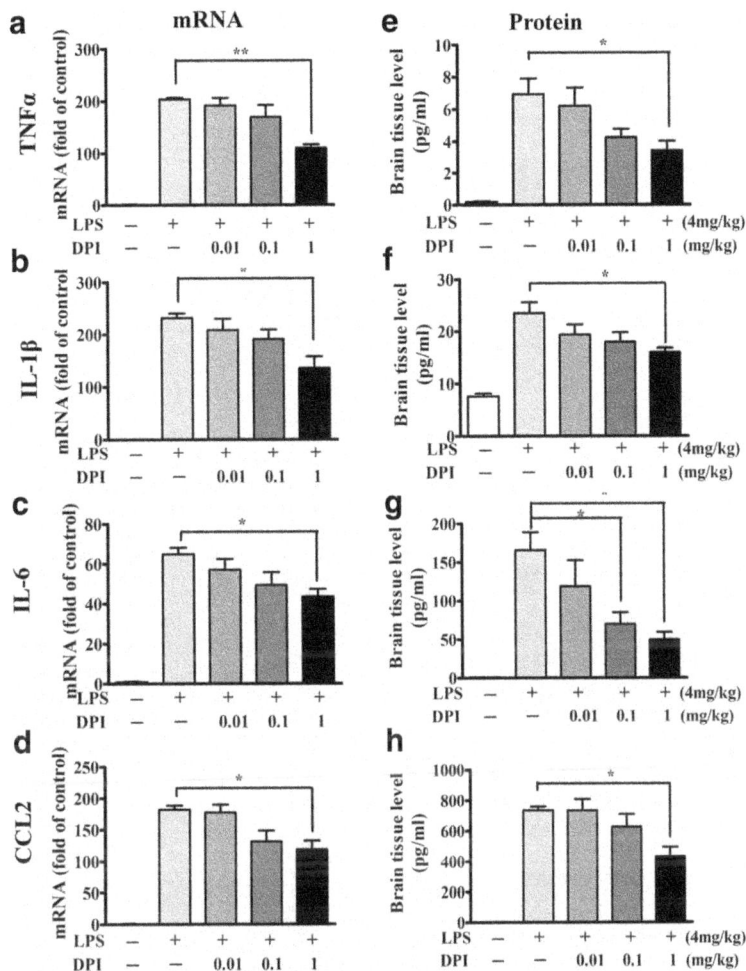

Fig. 7 DPI post-treatment attenuated pro-convulsive cytokine expression in brain after LPS injection. Wild-type mice were treated with a single dose of vehicle or DPI at 0.01, 0.1, or 1 mg/kg 30 min after LPS injection. The brains were harvested for assessment of the transcript expression ($n = 5$/group) of several cytokines using RT-qPCR (**a–d**) 1.5 h after LPS injection, and the protein levels ($n = 3$/group) using multiplex assay 24 h after LPS injection (**e–h**), respectively. β-actin expression served as the internal control. The expression of each cytokine of the DPI-treated mice was compared with that of the LPS-injected vehicle-treated control. Data present the mean ± SEM. Bonferroni post hoc test vs. LPS-injected vehicle-treated group; $*p < 0.05$, $**p < 0.01$

[42]. Another study also showed that immunoreactivity to gp91[phox] (NOX2 catalytic subunit) was mainly co-localized to activated microglia but co-localized to a few astrocytes and neurons in traumatic brain injury [43]. These studies suggest that even though NADPH oxidase can be activated in cells from the non-myeloid lineage, the resulting production of ROS is significantly lower than in microglia and in innate immunity (e.g., macrophages and neutrophils). Thus, microglia are likely the predominant source of NOX2-derived ROS in brain and thus a more effective target for prevention of neuronal hyperexcitability and seizure induction following sepsis.

Accumulating evidence indicates that systemic inflammation is accompanied by a similar inflammatory response in the CNS resulting from microglial activation and local synthesis of proinflammatory cytokines [4, 6,

15, 45]. Although the precise mechanisms responsible for the initial synthesis of cytokines in the brain are not entirely clear, peripheral TNFα may be a critical trigger by promoting leukocyte-endothelial interactions, microglial activation, and subsequent recruitment of monocytes [46]. We found that greater plasma TNFα concentrations (induced by higher LPS doses, i.e., 4 mg/kg vs. 0.5 mg/kg i.p.) evoked more severe neuroinflammation through enhanced brain accumulation of proinflammatory factors such as TNFα, IL-6, and IL-1β (see Additional file 4). Interestingly, LPS-induced plasma TNFα levels did not differ among gp91[phox–/–], p47[phox–/–], and WT mice, either in the current study (Fig. 2a) or in a previous study [47]. However, post-treatment with higher doses of DPI decreased plasma TNFα concentrations in mice following LPS stimulation. One possibility is that DPI, which is a

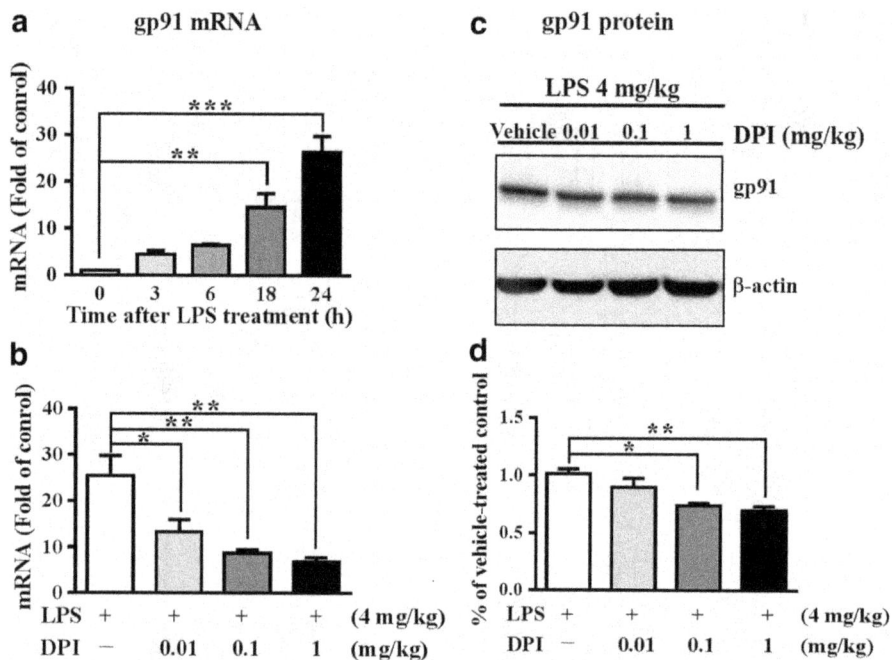

Fig. 8 DPI post-treatment attenuated gp91 expression in brain after LPS stimulation in mice. **a** Wild-type mice (*n* = 3/group) were treated with LPS and were sacrificed 0, 3, 6, 18, and 24 h after LPS and the brains were harvested. The transcript levels of gp91 were determined by RT-qPCR analyses and compared with that of the vehicle-treated control (to which a value of 1 was assigned). Data present the mean ± SEM. Bonferroni post hoc test vs. LPS-injected vehicle-treated group; **$p < 0.01$, ***$p < 0.001$. **b** The mice were treated with a single dose of vehicle or DPI (0.01, 0.1, or 1 mg/kg) 30 min after LPS injection and then were sacrificed 24 h after LPS. The transcript levels of gp91 were determined by RT-qPCR analyses and compared with that of the LPS-injected vehicle-treated control (to which a value of 1 was assigned). Data present the mean ± SEM. Bonferroni post hoc test vs. LPS-injected vehicle-treated group; *$p < 0.05$, **$p < 0.01$. **c** The brains as described in **b** were analyzed by western blot analyses to determine the levels of gp91 protein. Representative blots are shown. **d** The gp91 signals were quantitated and normalized to the internal control. All the normalized values were compared to the LPS-injected vehicle-treated group (to which a value of 1 was assigned). Data represent the mean ± SEM of the results generated from three animals for each group. Bonferroni post hoc test vs. LPS-injected vehicle-treated group; *$p < 0.05$, **$p < 0.01$

general flavoprotein inhibitor, blocks other NOX isoforms as well as xanthine oxidase [48, 49]. Although it remains unclear whether genetic deletion of NOX2 subunits and DPI administration have distinct effects on other NOX enzymes (e.g., through compensatory changes in NOX isoform expression and non-selective pharmacological inhibition), our results suggest that DPI has additional protective benefits against neuroinflammation by inhibiting the production of peripheral inflammatory factors (e.g., TNFα).

There is compelling evidence that proinflammatory cytokines can induce neuronal hyperexcitability and thus contribute to the development of epilepsy [7, 15]. It is believed that these effects are mediated by direct and indirect upregulation of excitatory glutamatergic transmission and downregulation of inhibitory GABAergic transmission [50, 51]. NOX2 is one of the major sources of ROS for cellular signaling. The present study demonstrates that both genetic deletion of NOX2 subunits and DPI post-treatment can strongly inhibit proconvulsive cytokine gene expression in response to systemic inflammation (Figs. 3 and 7) and that microglia are a major source of these cytokines (Fig. 4). In addition, DPI

attenuated NOX2 upregulation following sepsis (Fig. 8b, c), but had no effect on NOX1 expression (Additional file 3). These results support the hypothesis that DPI attenuates neuronal hyperexcitability by inhibiting NOX2 overexpression and NOX2-derived ROS signaling pathways linked to proconvulsive cytokine release.

Given the potential role of proconvulsive cytokines in mediating neuronal hyperexcitability following systemic inflammation, targeting these factors is considered a potential therapeutic strategy for suppressing the development of post-sepsis epilepsy [7, 52]. Moreover, targeting the early stages of neuroinflammation following systemic inflammation may prevent both inflammation- and seizure-associated brain damage due to oxidative stress and excitotoxicity. Based on the underlying molecular mechanism of these proconvulsive cytokines and their signaling pathways, several new immunotherapeutic approaches such as IL-1β-converting enzyme inhibitors and suppression of NF-kB are currently in the experimental phase of development for drug-resistant epilepsy [52–54]. However, it still has not been established whether a single proconvulsive cytokine inhibitor such as a TNFα blocker is sufficient to prevent neuroinflammation-mediated neuronal hyperexcitability. In fact, following sepsis, multiple cytotoxic factors such as cytokines/chemokines, ROS, and NOS are released by activated microglia and can both damage neurons directly and induce hyperexcitability. Consequently, a self-sustaining cycle is created through interactions between damaged neurons and dysregulated microglia, which may eventually result in chronic neuroinflammation, epilepsy development, and progressive neurodegeneration [6, 7, 55]. NOX2 complexes that drive ROS signaling pathways are essential mediators of this process [24]. It is thus reasonable to speculate that inhibiting NADPH oxidases can reduce the accumulation of neurotoxic factors (e.g., cytokines, and ROS) and disrupt the development of this vicious pathogenic cycle [24, 55]. Our findings indicated that NOX2 subunit deletion and pharmacological NOX2 inhibition reduced the upregulation of a broad spectrum of proconvulsive cytokines following LPS injection and attenuated subsequent increased seizure susceptibility.

A few studies have examined the therapeutic potential of preventing neuronal hyperexcitability associated with neuroinflammation. Hernandes and colleagues reported that pretreatment with the NOX2 inhibitor apocynin was effective in preventing the development of long-term cognitive impairment from sepsis-associated neuroinflammation [56]. Suppression of COX2-mediated inflammation is also a potential strategy for reducing neuronal hyperexcitability since COX-2 mRNA expression and PGE2 production are widely induced in rodent brain following sepsis [57]. In fact, a COX-2 inhibitor ameliorated the increase in KA-induced seizure susceptibility following sepsis via inhibition of NOX2 signaling [57, 58]. Wang and colleagues reported that post-treatment with ultra-low doses of DPI (10 ng/kg/day) for 2 weeks prevented dopaminergic neurodegeneration and motor deficits in Parkinson's disease models through inhibition of chronic neuroinflammation [59]. In the present study, a single dose of 0.01 mg/kg DPI significantly reduced the expression of proconvulsive cytokine mRNA and gp91^{phox} mRNA within 24 h after LPS injection, but only higher doses (1 mg/kg) attenuated seizure susceptibility. Collectively, these findings suggest that pharmacological NOX2 inhibitors may suppress the sepsis-associated increase in seizure susceptibility and resulting neurodegeneration by preventing microglial activation and downstream neuroinflammatory signaling.

Conclusions

In conclusion, this study shows that NOX2 contributes to neuronal hyperexcitability and increased seizure susceptibility in the LPS animal model of sepsis. Our data strongly suggest that pharmacological inhibition of NOX2-derived ROS may be an effective strategy to prevent sepsis-associated neuroinflammation, neuronal hyperexcitability, and seizures.

Additional file

Additional file 1: Basal seizure susceptibility, molecular levels of cell populations, and morphology of microglia in wild-type and NADPH-oxidase knockout mice. (A) The latency to initial seizure onset (clonic with/without tonic convulsion) after PTZ administration. Data are presented as mean ± SEM. Bonferroni post hoc test vs. LPS-treated WT group; $p > 0.05$. (B) Basal seizure susceptibility scored once every 5 min over the 2-h period to 60 mg/kg PTZ (i.p.) in wild-type (WT), gp91$^{phox-/-}$, and P47$^{phox-/-}$ mice ($n = 6$ or 7 per genotype). (C) The total duration (min) of seizure behavior ≥ stage 4 in gp91$^{phox-/-}$, P47$^{phox-/-}$, and WT mice. Data represent the mean ± SEM. Bonferroni post hoc test vs. WT mouse group. (D) Representative immunoblots showing the basal protein levels of Iba-1 (microglia marker), GFAP (astroglia marker), and BDNF (neuronal marker) in brains of WT, gp91$^{phox-/-}$ and P47$^{phox-/-}$ mice ($n = 3$ per genotype). Bonferroni post hoc test vs. WT mouse group. (E) Photomicrograph of iba1-staining microglia from the dentate gyrus regions (DG) and CA3 regions of each genotype mice (n = 3 per genotype). Resting microglia are composed of a small cellular body and long branching processes (arrow).

Additional file 2: DPI post-treatment had no effect to attenuate IL10on attenuating IL-10 and IL-12 expression in brain after LPS injection. Wild-type mice were treated with a single dose of vehicle or DPI at 0.01, 0.1, or 1 mg/kg 30 min after LPS injection. At 1.5 and 24 h after LPS injection, mice were sacrificed and brain extracts prepared for analysis of cytokine transcript ($n = 5$/group) and protein expression ($n = 3$/group) by real-time PCR and multiplex assay, respectively. The transcript levels of IL-10 (A), and IL-12 (B) at 1.5 h after LPS injection. Data are presented as mean ± SEM. Bonferroni post hoc test vs. LPS-injected vehicle-treated group, $p > 0.05$. The protein levels of IL-10 (C), and IL-12 (D) in brain at 24 h after LPS injection. Values are presented as mean ± SEM. Bonferroni post hoc test vs. LPS-injected vehicle-treated control.

Additional file 3: DPI post-treatment after LPS stimulation had no significant effect on NOX1 expression. C57BL/6 mice were treated with a single dose of vehicle or DPI 30 min after LPS injection (4 mg/kg; i.p.) and sacrificed 24 h after LPS injection. Representative immunoblots showing the levels of NADPH oxidase 1 (NOX1) protein in vehicle- or DPI-treated mouse brain are shown (A). Quantitative analysis indicated that NOX1 protein expression was not significantly changed by DPI post-treatment (B). Data represent the mean ± SEM of three animals per treatment group. Bonferroni post hoc test vs. LPS-injected vehicle-treated group; $p > 0.05$.

Additional file 4: Dose response of LPS on plasma TNFα levels and cytokine gene expression in mouse brain. Male C57BL/6J mice were treated with a lower dose (0.5 mg/kg) or a higher dose (4 mg/kg) of LPS. (A) Plasma levels of TNF-α 1 h after LPS stimulation. Student's t-test; n = 5/group; ***$p < 0.001$. (B) The levels of TNFα, IL-1β, and IL-6 transcripts in brain 1.5 h after LPS stimulation (n = 3/group). The mRNA levels were calculated relative to expression in matched saline-treated mice. β-actin mRNA was the internal control. Data present the mean ± SEM. Student's t-test; ***$p < 0.001$.

Abbreviations
BDNF: Brain-derived neurotrophic factor; CCL2: C-C motif chemokine ligand 2; DPI: Diphenyleneiodonium; GFAP: Glial fibrillary acidic protein; Iba-1: Ionized calcium binding adaptor molecule 1; IL-12: Interleukin 12; IL-1β: Interleukin 1β; IL-6: Interleukin 6; LPS: Lipopolysaccharide; NOX2: NADPH oxidase 2; PTZ: Pentylenetetrazol; ROS: Reactive oxygen species; TNFα: Tumor necrosis factor-alpha

Acknowledgements
We thank Chew-Teng Kor PhD. Department of Internal Medicine, Changhua Christian Hospital for her valuable help in data analysis.

Funding
The study was funded by grant NSC100–2314-B-371-004 and NSC 101–2314-B-371-006-MY3 from Ministry of Science and Technology, Taiwan.

Authors' contributions
SL, HYX, TYC, and YPC performed the experiments. HMW and KSH designed the study, and WYH analyzed the data and wrote the manuscript. All authors read and approved the final manuscript.

Competing interests
The authors declare that they have no competing interests.

Author details
[1]Institute of Basic Medical Sciences, College of Medicine, National Cheng Kung University, Tainan, Taiwan. [2]Pediatrics of Kung-Ten General Hospital, Taichung City, Taiwan. [3]Inflammation Research & Drug Development Center, Changhua Christian Hospital, Changhua, Taiwan. [4]Department of Neurology, Changhua Christian Hospital, Changhua City, Taiwan. [5]Institute of Acupuncture, School of Chinese Medicine, China Medical University, Taichung City, Taiwan.

References
1. Sonneville R, Verdonk F, Rauturier C, Klein IF, Wolff M, Annane D, et al. Understanding brain dysfunction in sepsis. Ann Intensive Care. 2013;3:15.
2. Idro R, Gwer S, Kahindi M, Gatakaa H, Kazungu T, Ndiritu M, et al. The incidence, aetiology and outcome of acute seizures in children admitted to a rural Kenyan district hospital. BMC Pediatr. 2008;8:5.
3. Riazi K, Galic MA, Pittman QJ. Contributions of peripheral inflammation to seizure susceptibility: cytokines and brain excitability. Epilepsy Res. 2010;89:34–42.
4. Riazi K, Galic MA, Kuzmiski JB, Ho W, Sharkey KA, Pittman QJ. Microglial activation and TNFalpha production mediate altered CNS excitability following peripheral inflammation. Proc Natl Acad Sci U S A. 2008;105:17151–6.
5. Cerri C, Genovesi S, Allegra M, Pistillo F, Puntener U, Guglielmotti A, et al. The chemokine CCL2 mediates the seizure-enhancing effects of systemic inflammation. J Neurosci. 2016;36:3777–88.
6. Qin L, Wu X, Block ML, Liu Y, Breese GR, Hong JS, et al. Systemic LPS causes chronic neuroinflammation and progressive neurodegeneration. Glia. 2007;55:453–62.
7. Galic MA, Riazi K, Heida JG, Mouihate A, Fournier NM, Spencer SJ, et al. Postnatal inflammation increases seizure susceptibility in adult rats. J Neurosci. 2008;28:6904–13.
8. Harre EM, Galic MA, Mouihate A, Noorbakhsh F, Pittman QJ. Neonatal inflammation produces selective behavioural deficits and alters N-methyl-D-aspartate receptor subunit mRNA in the adult rat brain. Eur J Neurosci. 2008;27:644–53.
9. Skelly DT, Hennessy E, Dansereau MA, Cunningham C. A systematic analysis of the peripheral and CNS effects of systemic LPS, IL-1beta, TNF-alpha and IL-6 challenges in C57BL/6 mice. PLoS One. 2013;8:e69123.
10. Erickson MA, Banks WA. Cytokine and chemokine responses in serum and brain after single and repeated injections of lipopolysaccharide: multiplex quantification with path analysis. Brain Behav Immun. 2011;25:1637–48.
11. Eklind S, Mallard C, Arvidsson P, Hagberg H. Lipopolysaccharide induces both a primary and a secondary phase of sensitization in the developing rat brain. Pediatr Res. 2005;58:112–6.
12. Hagberg H, Mallard C. Effect of inflammation on central nervous system development and vulnerability. Curr Opin Neurol. 2005;18:117–23.
13. Godbout JP, Johnson RW. Age and neuroinflammation: a lifetime of psychoneuroimmune consequences. Imunol Allergy Clin North Am. 2006;24:521–38.
14. Pascual O, Ben Achour S, Rostaing P, Triller A, Bessis A. Microglia activation triggers astrocyte-mediated modulation of excitatory neurotransmission. Proc Natl Acad Sci U S A. 2012;109:197–205.
15. Galic MA, Riazi K, Pittman QJ. Cytokines and brain excitability. Front Neuroendocrinol. 2012;33:116–25.
16. Heida JG, Pittman QJ. Causal links between brain cytokines and experimental febrile convulsions in the rat. Epilepsia. 2005;46:1906–13.
17. Rodgers KM, Hutchinson MR, Northcutt A, Maier SF, Watkins LR, Barth DS. The cortical innate immune response increases local neuronal excitability leading to seizures. Brain. 2009;132:2478–86.

18. Vezzani A, Moneta D, Richichi C, Aliprandi M, Burrows SJ, Ravizza T, et al. Functional role of inflammatory cytokines and antiinflammatory molecules in seizures and epileptogenesis. Epilepsia. 2002;43(s5):30–5.
19. Gruol DL. IL-6 regulation of synaptic function in the CNS. Neuropharmacology. 2015;96:42–54.
20. Vezzani A, Ravizza T, Balosso S, Aronica E. Glia as a source of cytokines: implications for neuronal excitability and survival. Epilepsia. 2008;49(s2):24–32.
21. Li G, Bauer S, Nowak M, Norwood B, Tackenberg B, Rosenow F, et al. Cytokines and epilepsy. Seizure. 2011;20:249–56.
22. Wilkinson BL, Landreth GE. The microglial NADPH oxidase complex as a source of oxidative stress in Alzheimer's disease. J Neuroinflammation. 2006;3:30.
23. Block ML, Zecca L, Hong JS. Microglia-mediated neurotoxicity: uncovering the molecular mechanisms. Nat Rev Neurosci. 2007;8:57–69.
24. Vezzani A, French J, Bartfai T, Baram TZ. The role of inflammation in epilepsy. Nat Rev Neurol. 2011;7:31–40.
25. Iori V, Frigerio F, Vezzani A. Modulation of neuronal excitability by immune mediators in epilepsy. Curr Opin Pharmacol. 2016;26:118–23.
26. Somera-Molina KC, Robin B, Somera CA, Anderson C, Stine C, Koh S, et al. Glial activation links early-life seizures and long-term neurologic dysfunction: evidence using a small molecule inhibitor of proinflammatory cytokine upregulation. Epilepsia. 2007;48:1785–800.
27. Doussiere J, Gaillard J, Vignais PV. The heme component of the neutrophil NADPH oxidase complex is a target for aryliodonium compounds. Biochemistry. 1999;38:3694–703.
28. Qian L, Wu HM, Chen SH, Zhang D, Ali SF, Peterson L, et al. β2-adrenergic receptor activation prevents rodent dopaminergic neurotoxicity by inhibiting microglia via a novel signaling pathway. J Immunol. 2011;186:4443–54.
29. Dhir A. Pentylenetetrazol (PTZ) kindling model of epilepsy. Curr Protoc Neurosci. 2012;9:9–37.
30. Corda MG, Orlandi M, Lecca D, Carboni G, Frau V, Giorgi O. Pentylenetetrazol-induced kindling in rats: effect of GABA function inhibitors. Pharmacol Biochem Behav. 1991;40:329–33.
31. Liu H, Cao Y, Basbaum AI, Mazarati AM, Sankar R, Wasterlain CG. Resistance to excitotoxin-induced seizures and neuronal death in mice lacking the preprotachykinin A gene. Proc Natl Acad Sci U S A. 1999;96:12096–101.
32. Morrison RS, Wenzel HJ, Kinoshita Y, Robbins CA, Donehower LA, Schwartzkroin PA. Loss of the p53 tumor suppressor gene protects neurons from kainate-induced cell death. J Neurosci. 1996;16:1337–45.
33. Wu HM, Tzeng NS, Qian L, Wei SJ, Hu X, Chen SH, et al. Novel neuroprotective mechanisms of memantine: increase in neurotrophic factor release from astroglia and anti-inflammation by preventing microglial activation. Neuropsychopharmacology. 2009;34:2344–57.
34. Fox C, Dingman A, Derugin N, Wendland MF, Manabat C, Ji S, et al. Minocycline confers early but transient protection in the immature brain following focal cerebral ischemia-reperfusion. J Cereb Blood Flow Metab. 2005;25:1138–49.
35. Mirrione MM, Konomos DK, Gravanis I, Dewey SL, Aguzzi A, Heppner FL, et al. Microglial ablation and lipopolysaccharide preconditioning affects pilocarpine-induced seizures in mice. Neurobiol Dis. 2010;39:85–97.
36. Binder DK, Croll SD, Gall CM, Scharfman HE. BDNF and epilepsy: too much of a good thing? Trends Neurosci. 2001;24:47–53.
37. Thomson CA, McColl A, Cavanagh J, Graham GJ. Peripheral inflammation is associated with remote global gene expression changes in the brain. J Neuroinflammation. 2014;11:73.
38. Hanisch UK. Microglia as a source and target of cytokines. Glia. 2002;40:140–55.
39. Bedard K, Krause KH. The NOX family of ROS-generating NADPH oxidases: physiology and pathophysiology. Physiol Rev. 2007;87:245–313.
40. Brown DI, Griendling KK. Nox proteins in signal transduction. Free Radic Biol Med. 2009;47:1239–53.
41. Chéret C, Gervais A, Lelli A, Colin C, Amar L, Ravassard P, Mallet J, Cumano A, Krause KH, Mallat M. Neurotoxic activation of microglia is promoted by a nox1-dependent NADPH oxidase. J Neurosci. 2008;28:12039–51.
42. Qin L, Liu Y, Wang T, Wei SJ, Block ML, Wilson B, et al. NADPH oxidase mediates lipopolysaccharide-induced neurotoxicity and proinflammatory gene expression in activated microglia. J Biol Chem. 2004;279:1415–21.
43. Dohi K, Ohtaki H, Nakamachi T, Yofu S, Satoh K, Miyamoto K, et al. Gp91phox (NOX2) in classically activated microglia exacerbates traumatic brain injury. J Neuroinflammation. 2010;7:41.

44. Angeloni C, Prata C, Dalla Sega FV, Piperno R, Hrelia S. Traumatic brain injury and NADPH oxidase: a deep relationship. Oxid Med Cell Longev. 2015;2015:370312. https://doi.org/10.1155/2015/370312.

45. Pyter LM, Pineros V, Galang JA, McClintock MK, Prendergast BJ. Peripheral tumors induce depressive-like behaviors and cytokine production and alter hypothalamic-pituitary-adrenal axis regulation. Proc Natl Acad Sci U S A. 2009;106:9069–74.

46. D'Mello C, Le T, Swain MG. Cerebral microglia recruit monocytes into the brain in response to tumor necrosis factoralpha signaling during peripheral organ inflammation. J Neurosci. 2009;29:2089–102.

47. Zhang WJ, Wei H, Frei B. Genetic deficiency of NADPH oxidase does not diminish, but rather enhances, LPS-induced acute inflammatory responses in vivo. Free Radic Biol Med. 2009;46:791–8.

48. Maraldi T. Natural compounds as modulators of NADPH oxidases. Oxidative Med Cell Longev. 2013;2013:271602.

49. Wind S, Beuerlein K, Eucker T, Müller H, Scheurer P, Armitage ME, et al. Comparative pharmacology of chemically distinct NADPH oxidase inhibitors. Br J Pharmacol. 2010;161:885–98.

50. Zhou Y, Tang H, Liu J, Dong J, Xiong H. Chemokine CCL2 modulation of neuronal excitability and synaptic transmission in rat hippocampal slices. J Neurochem. 2011;116:406–14.

51. Zhu G, Okada M, Yoshida S, Mori F, Ueno S, Wakabayashi K, et al. Effects of interleukin-1beta on hippocampal glutamate and GABA releases associated with Ca2+-induced Ca2+-releasing systems. Epilepsy Res. 2006;71:107–16.

52. Matin N, Tabatabaie O, Falsaperla R, Lubrano R, Pavone P, Mahmood F, et al. Epilepsy and innate immune system: a possible immunogenic predisposition and related therapeutic implications. Hum Vaccin Immunother. 2015;11:2021–9.

53. Ravizza T, Noe F, Zardoni D, Vaghi V, Sifringer M, Vezzani A. Interleukin converting enzyme inhibition impairs kindling epileptogenesis in rats by blocking astrocytic IL-1b production. Neurobiol Dis. 2008;31:327–33.

54. Youn HS, Lee JY, Fitzgerald KA, Young HA, Akira S, Hwang DH. Specific inhibition of MyD88-independent signaling pathways of TLR3 and TLR4 by resveratrol: molecular targets are TBK1 and RIP1 in TRIF complex. J Immunol. 2005;175:3339–46.

55. Gao HM, Hong JS. Why neurodegenerative diseases are progressive: uncontrolled inflammation drives disease progression. Trends Immunol. 2008;29:357–65.

56. Hernandes MS, D'Avila JC, Trevelin SC, Reis PA, Kinjo ER, Lopes LR, Castro-Faria-Neto HC, Cunha FQ, Britto LR, Bozza FA. The role of Nox2-derived ROS in the development of cognitive impairment after sepsis. J Neuroinflammation. 2014;11:36.

57. Akarsu ES, Ozdayi S, Algan E, Ulupinar F. The neuronal excitability time-dependently changes after lipopolysaccharide administration in mice: possible role of cyclooxygenase-2 induction. Epilepsy Res. 2006;71:181–7.

58. Ho YH, Lin YT, Wu CW, Chao YM, Chang AY, Chan JY. Peripheral inflammation increases seizure susceptibility via the induction of neuroinflammation and oxidative stress in the hippocampus. J Biomed Sci. 2015;22:46.

59. Wang Q, Qian L, Chen SH, Chu CH, Wilson B, Oyarzabal E, et al. Post-treatment with an ultra-low dose of NADPH oxidase inhibitor diphenyleneiodonium attenuates disease progression in multiple Parkinson's disease models. Brain. 2015;138:1247–62.

Disruption of the blood–brain barrier after generalized tonic-clonic seizures correlates with cerebrospinal fluid MMP-9 levels

Ya-Jun Li[1*], Zheng-Hai Wang[2], Bei Zhang[1], Xiao Zhe[1], Ming-Jue Wang[1], Shao-Ting Shi[1], Jing Bai[1], Tao Lin[1], Chang-Jiang Guo[1], Shi-Jun Zhang[1], Xiang-Li Kong[1], Xing Zuo[1] and Hang Zhao[1]

Abstract

Background: Increasing evidence suggests seizures cause blood–brain barrier (BBB) dysfunction including decreased seizure threshold and higher onset potential of future seizures. However, the mechanisms underlying BBB damage in seizures remains poorly understood. Evidence in human and animal models shows BBB disruption is associated with activation of matrix metalloproteinase-9 (MMP-9) after cerebral ischemia and inflammation. The objective of this study was to determine whether MMP-9 concentrations in cerebral spinal fluid (CSF) are associated with BBB disruption in patients after epileptic seizures.

Methods: Thirty-one patients with generalized tonic-clonic (GTC) seizures were included in the study: 20 had recurrent GTC seizures (RS), and 11 had a single GTC seizure (SS) episode. Twenty-five adult non-seizure patients were used as controls. CSF samples were collected by lumbar puncture within 24 h after seizure cessation (range: 3–15 h, mean 6.2 h). CSF MMP-9 levels were determined by an enzyme-linked immunosorbent assay (ELISA). MMP enzyme activity was measured by gelatin zymography. The CSF/serum albumin ratio (albumin quotient, QAlb) was used as a measure of blood–brain barrier permeability.

Results: We found significantly higher CSF MMP-9 concentrations in seizure patients compared with controls ($P < 0.001$). CSF MMP-9 levels and QAlb values were higher in RS patients compared with SS and controls. Moreover, CSF MMP-9 concentration showed strong correlation between QAlb values ($r = 0.76$, $P < 0.0001$) and between CSF leukocyte counts ($r = 0.77$, $P < 0.0001$) in patients after seizures. Gelatin zymography showed MMP-9 proteolytic activity only in GTC seizure patients.

Conclusions: Our results suggest MMP-9 plays a role in BBB dysfunction, characterized by invasion of leukocytes into the CSF during seizures.

Keywords: Cerebrospinal fluid, Seizure, BBB, Metalloproteinase-9, Leukocytes

Background

The blood–brain barrier (BBB) is the most important vascular barrier of the central nervous system (CNS). Due to its unique structure, the BBB limits penetration of a variety of harmful substances from the blood into the brain, while also supplying the brain with nutrients required for proper function. In recent years, animal models and human clinical data have described a central role for vascular integrity, specifically the permeability of the BBB, as an important mediator of brain damage, including the delayed appearance of neuronal dysfunction and death [1-4]. Studies show BBB dysfunction is common following traumatic, ischemic or infectious brain insults, and it may last from several days to weeks and even years after the acute event [5,6]. Recently, clinical and experimental data have correlated primary BBB lesions with seizures and epileptogenesis. Experimental studies have demonstrated a rapid increase in BBB permeability in animals experiencing long-lasting seizures, especially status epilepticus (SE). Studies in human

* Correspondence: liyajun9@hotmail.com
[1]Department of Neurology, The Affiliated Hospital of Xi'an Medical University, No. 48, West Fenghao Road, Xi'an 710077, Shaanxi Province, China

Disruption of the blood–brain barrier after generalized tonic-clonic seizures correlates with cerebrospinal...

29

epileptic patients are consistent with the animal data, showing an increase in BBB permeability during seizures [7,8]. Pentylenetetrazole-induced seizures cause BBB disruption, allowing permeation of blood-borne large molecules, such as albumin, into the CNS [9,10]. BBB disruption decreases the seizure threshold and facilitates the onset of seizures, and it is independent of the fact that such disruption is associated with or a result of the seizure itself [11]. The mechanisms underlying the BBB disruption in seizures and epileptogenesis are not entirely clear. There is evidence in human and animal stroke models that BBB disruption is associated with activation of matrix metalloproteinases (MMPs) [12-14].

MMPs are a family of zinc-dependent endopeptidases that are subdivided according to their substrate affinities for different components of the extracellular matrix. Among the various MMPs, metalloproteinase-9 (MMP-9), also known as gelatinase B, is thought to play an important role in BBB disruption after cerebral ischemia and inflammation [12,15-17]. MMP-9 degrades collagen IV, a major component of the basement membrane of the cerebral epithelium that is responsible for the integrity of BBB. The activity of MMP-9 is further controlled by the specific tissue inhibitor TIMP-1. However, the link between CSF MMP-9 levels and the presence of BBB disruption in patients after seizures has not yet been investigated in humans. Our study aimed to determine whether MMP-9 can be measured in CSF of patients after epileptic seizures and whether there is a correlation between CSF MMP-9 levels and QAlb values in patients after epileptic seizures.

Methods

Patient recruitment
The study was performed at the Department of Neurology of the Affiliated Hospital of Xi'an Medical University. Thirty-one patients with either tonic-clonic or partial secondarily generalized seizures were included in the study: 20 had recurrent GTC seizures (RS), and 11 had a single GTC seizure (SS) episode confirmed by an eyewitness that occurred within 3 h before admission. On admission to the emergency ward, all seizure patients received standard intravenous treatment with diazepam (dose range 10–20 mg) to stop seizure activity. Then patients were admitted to a neurologic ward for further evaluation. All patients underwent a standard diagnostic workup including neurologic examination and blood biochemical assessment. Ten patients presented the first-ever epileptic seizure and underwent further examinations including electroencephalography (EEG) and either a computed tomography (CT) or magnetic resonance imaging (MRI) scan, and the final diagnosis of epilepsy was confirmed (8 with cryptogenic localization-related epilepsy and 2 with idiopathic generalized epilepsy). Twenty-one patients already had an epilepsy diagnosis: 6 with cryptogenic localization-related

epilepsy and 15 with symptomatic localization-related epilepsy with secondary generalization. Those patients presenting apparent symptomatic etiology of seizures, that is, electrolyte disturbances, defined metabolic causes, drug intoxication, infections, trauma or abnormal CT or MRI suggestive of acute brain diseases were excluded. All patients were studied within 24 h after the seizure. Epilepsy was diagnosed and classified according to the criteria proposed by the International League Against Epilepsy in 2011 [18]. Seizures and epileptic syndromes were classified according to the ILAE diagnostic criteria.

The control samples were obtained from 25 adult patients (mean age 39 ±13.6 years; range 16–56 years) by lumbar puncture and examined to exclude those with neurological disease, including nonspecific symptoms without diagnosed organic neurologic disease ($n = 7$), peripheral nervous system disorders ($n = 4$), acute headache ($n = 5$), spontaneous intracranial hypotension ($n = 3$), compressive radiculopathy ($n = 4$) and primary dementia ($n = 2$). All controls had normal neurological examination and normal CSF results on routine analysis.

All epileptic patients and controls were fully informed of the risks and potential benefits of the CSF examination as part of the diagnostic workup. Informed consent to participate in the study was obtained from each subject (or from the next of kin if the patient was incapable). Five patients were considered for the study but did not agree to undergo lumbar puncture and were not included in the study. The study protocol was approved by the Ethics Committee of the Affiliated Hospital of Xi'an Medical University, and all investigations were done in accordance with the criteria of the Declaration of Helsinki.

CSF/serum sampling and biochemical analysis
CSF samples were taken between 10 a.m. and 5 p.m. by lumbar puncture from the L3/L4 or L4/L5 intervertebral space. Lumbar puncture was performed within 24 h after seizure cessation (range: 3–15 h, mean 6.2 h). CSF samples that were not clear or initially contained blood with gradual clearing were excluded from analysis. The first 2 ml of CSF was used for routine clinical tests and the subsequent 0.5 ml for our study. The CSF white blood cell (WBC) count, differential leukocyte count, total protein concentration, glucose (Glu) and chloride (CL) values were determined by standard methods immediately after lumbar puncture. Cytology of CSF cells was also performed. CSF and peripheral blood samples were collected simultaneously and centrifuged for 10 min at 2,500 g; 500 μl of the cell-free samples was immediately frozen and stored at –80°C until analysis. Concentrations of MMP-9 were measured by commercial enzyme-linked immunosorbent assay (ELISA) kits (R & D Systems, Minneapolis, MN) performed according

to the manufacturer's instructions. Optical density values were determined with a microplate reader set to 450 nm.

Measurement of the QAlb value

Quantitative determination of albumin in the CSF and serum of all specimens were measured by a commercial kit (BioAssay Systems, Hayward, CA). The CSF/serum albumin ratio (albumin quotient, QAlb) was used as a measure of blood–brain barrier permeability. QAlb was calculated using the formula: $QAlb = CSFAlb/serum Alb \times 10^3$.

Gelatin zymography

Activity of MMP-2 and MMP-9 enzymes in CSF samples was determined by gelatin zymography as previously described [16]. Briefly, activity of MMPs was analyzed by modified sodium dodecyl sulfate-polyacrylamide gel electrophoresis. Stacking gels contained 4% polyacrylamide, and separating gels contained 12.5% polyacrylamide and 0.1% gelatin. The 2 ml CSF was centrifuged at $10,000 \times g$ for 15 min at 4°C to remove debris. Protein contents of supernatants were then mixed with an equal volume of 2× non-reducing sample buffer, and 25 μl was loaded per well. The gels underwent electrophoresis at 90 V and 4°C in running buffer (25 mM Tris, 250 mM glycine, 0.1% sodium dodecyl sulfate) until the bromophenol blue marker dye reached the bottom of the gel. After electrophoresis, the gel was transferred into a 2.5% Triton X-100 wash for 1 h at room temperature. After decanting the washing solution, the gel was equilibrated with developing buffer (50 mM Tris–HCl, pH 7.5, 200 mM NaCl, 5 mM CaCl2, 0.02% Brij-35, 0.01% NaN3) for 30 min at room temperature with gentle agitation. The gel was then placed in fresh developing buffer and incubated at 37°C for 18 h. The gel was stained for 1 h with 0.25% Coomassie Brilliant Blue R-250 (Sigma, St. Louis, MO) and was destained in 15% methanol/7.5% acetic acid. MMP activity was detected as white bands of lysis against the Coomassie blue-stained gel. The CSF zymography experiments were performed in triplicate. The gels were digitalized and the integrated density of the bands expressed as arbitrary units. The intensities of the gelatinolytic bands corresponding to MMP-9 and MMP-2 were calculated using the open-access software Image J 1.46r (National Institutes of Health, Bethesda, MD, USA; http://rsb.info.nih.gov/ij).

Statistical analysis

Data are presented as mean ± SD for normally distributed and non-parametric data. Student's t-test and Mann–Whitney U-test were used for comparison of normally distributed and non-parametric data, respectively, between groups. ANOVA and Kruskal-Wallis test were used for comparison of normally distributed and non-parametric data, respectively, between multiple groups. Spearman's correlation coefficient was used to correlate variables in the groups studied. The calculations were performed with GraphPadInStat version 3.05 software (GraphPad Software, Inc., San Diego, CA, USA). For all tests, $P < 0.05$ was considered significant.

Results

Demographics of study participants

Demographic details of patients with epilepsy and controls are presented in Table 1. Thirty-one seizure patients and 25 controls provided data for the study. The mean age of the seizure patients was 42.5 (range, 20–68) years, and 16 (44%) were women. Among the controls, mean age was 38.7 (range, 22–71) years, and 12 (48%) were women. There were no differences between the two groups for these demographics. Twelve patients were receiving monotherapy, 9 polytherapy (the mean number of medications 2.3) and 10 patients no medication.

MMP-9 concentrations and QAlb values are higher in seizure patients

We measured significantly higher MMP-9 concentrations (Table 2 and Figure 1A; $P < 0.001$) and QAlb values (Table 2 and Figure 2A) in seizure patients compared with

Table 1 Clinical characteristics of seizure patients and control subjects

Variable	Patient	Control	P value
Number (n)	31	25	
Current age (years)	42.5 (15.1)	38.7 (17.6)	P > 0.05
Age at onset of epilepsy (years)	23.3 (14.8)		
Gender (M:F), n	20/16	13/12	P > 0.05
Red blood cells (10^{12}/l)	4.3	4.5	P > 0.05
White blood cells (10^9/l)	5.9	6.2	P > 0.05
Focus of seizure			
Temporal, n (%)	13 (41.9)		
Extratemporal, n (%)	18 (58.1)		
Type of seizure			
Single GTC seizure, n (%)	11 (35.5)		
Repetitive GTC seizure, n (%)	20 (64.5)		
Epilepsy duration (years)	6.3 (1–18)		
Frequency of seizures (month)	1.5 (1–5)		
Number of seizures	3.3 (1–10)		
Total duration of seizure (min)	8.3 (2–13)		
Time to sampling (h)	6.2 (3–15)		
Anti-epileptic drugs used	21 (67.7)		
No treatment	10 (32.3)		

Mann–Whitney U-test for continuous variables; cross tabulations and chi-square-test for categorical variables.

Table 2 The mean concentrations of CSF MMP-9, CSF cell count and albumin, and serum albumin from patients with GTC seizures and controls

Variable	Patient (mean ± SD)	Control (mean ± SD)	P
CSF leukocytes (10^6/l)	8.2 ± 2.3	2.0036 ± 1.4	<0.05
CSF erythrocytes (10^6/l)	19.6 ± 30.5	14.4 ± 21.8	>0.05
CSF albumin (g/l)	278.6 ± 35.5 ($\times 10^{-3}$)	198.2 ± 48.7 ($\times 10^{-3}$)	<0.05
Serum albumin (g/l)	41.6 ± 1.3	42.3 ± 1.5	>0.05
QAlb	8.35 ± 2.6 ($\times 10^{-3}$)	4.7 ± 1.4 ($\times 10^{-3}$)	<0.001
MMP-9 (ng /ml)	7.0 ± 2.4	1.80 ± 0.63	<0.001

Patient compared to control by Mann–Whitney test.

controls. We found significantly higher concentrations of MMP-9 (Figure 1B) and QAlb values (Figure 2B) in RS patients compared with SS and controls (Figure 1B). Analysis of temporal epilepsy and extra-temporal epilepsy showed no significant difference in CSF MMP-9 (Figure 1C) or QAlb values (Figure 2C). In addition, when considering use of anti-epileptic drugs (AEDs), we found no difference in MMP-9 levels (Figure 1D) or QAlb values (Figure 2D).

All seizure patients had normal serum protein and albumin concentrations. These data suggest that the CSF albumin increase was regulated by the increased permeability of the damaged BBB.

MMP-9 concentrations and QAlb values are correlated
To determine if the increased MMP-9 levels and higher QAlb values were related, we performed correlation

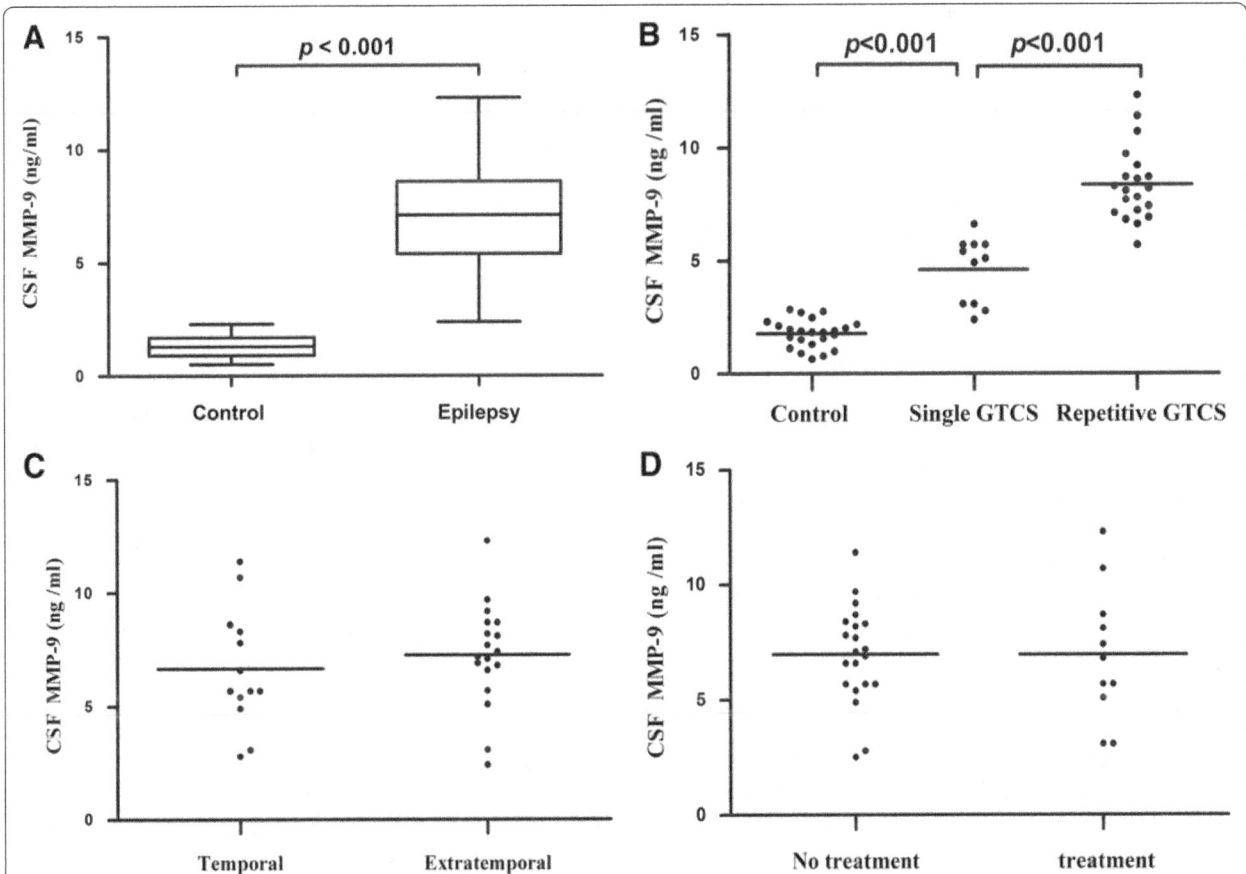

Figure 1 CSF MMP-9 levels in seizure patients and controls. (**A**) Boxplot representing the distribution (median and interquartile range) of CSF MMP-9 concentrations for control subjects (Control) and seizure patients (Epilepsy). Significantly higher MMP-9 levels in seizure patients compared with controls are shown. (**B**) Patients with repetitive generalized tonic-clonic seizures tended to have higher CSF MMP-9 levels compared with those who had single generalized tonic-clonic seizure and controls. (**C**) No significant difference found between temporal and extratemporal epilepsy (P > 0.05). (**D**) No significant difference between AEDs treatment groups (P > 0.05). Horizontal line indicates median. Significant change at P < 0.001 using Mann–Whitney U tests.

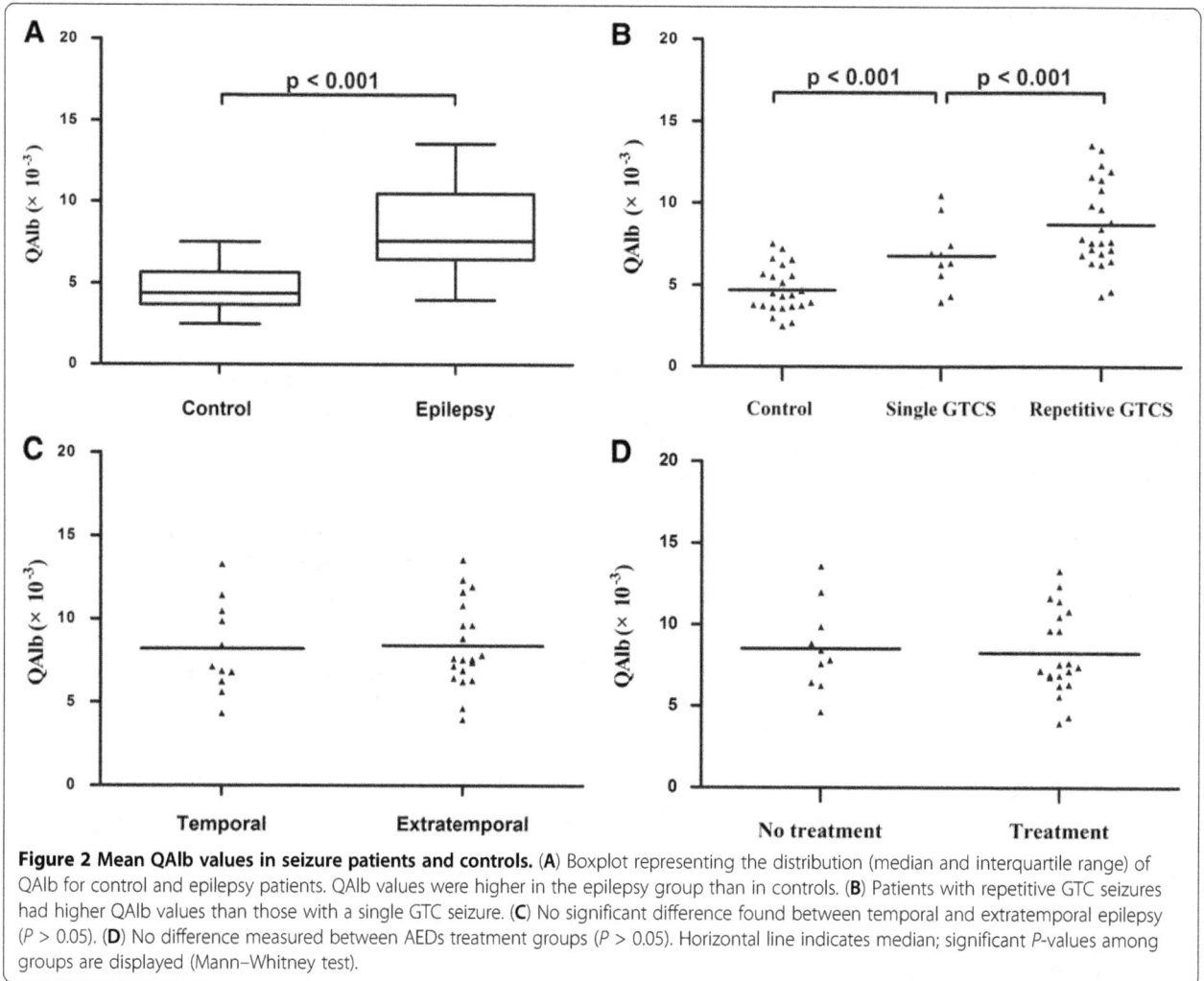

Figure 2 Mean QAlb values in seizure patients and controls. (**A**) Boxplot representing the distribution (median and interquartile range) of QAlb for control and epilepsy patients. QAlb values were higher in the epilepsy group than in controls. (**B**) Patients with repetitive GTC seizures had higher QAlb values than those with a single GTC seizure. (**C**) No significant difference found between temporal and extratemporal epilepsy ($P > 0.05$). (**D**) No difference measured between AEDs treatment groups ($P > 0.05$). Horizontal line indicates median; significant P-values among groups are displayed (Mann–Whitney test).

analysis. We found a strong correlation between MMP-9 concentration and QAlb values in patients after GTC seizures (Figure 3A, $r = 0.76$, $P < 0.001$). We also found a correlation between CSF MMP-9 concentration and leukocyte counts in patients after GTC seizures (Figure 3B, $r = 0.77$, $P < 0.001$). In fact, our data show the greater number of leukocytes in the CSF aligned with higher MMP-9 concentrations. These results suggest leukocytes are the source of increased MMP-9 levels in CSF after seizure.

We also looked at the correlation between CSF MMP-9 levels and seizure frequency and correlation between QAlb values and seizure frequency. We found that neither CSF MMP-9 levels nor QAlb values correlated with seizure frequency (Figure 3C-D).

MMP-9 enzyme activity detected in seizure samples
We randomly selected CSF specimens from two patients and two controls for enzyme activity analysis by gelatin zymography. As shown in Figure 4, all CSF specimens from patients and controls show a band at molecular

mass 72 kD, representing MMP-2. However, only CSF specimens from patients after seizure showed MMP-9 activity. We found that RS and SS samples had a higher ratio of active/inactive MMP-9 activity, supporting the argument that higher MMP-9 levels and the severity of BBB damage are dependent on the number of seizure insults but not MMP-2. Interestingly, polymorphonuclear neutrophils were present in 42% of patient CSF samples. This confirms a transient influx of neutrophils into the CSF of patients after epileptic seizure.

Discussion
Many questions are unanswered regarding how BBB integrity changes during epileptic seizures. And it is unclear whether elevated CSF MMP-9 contributes to alterations in BBB permeability. Our study addresses these questions by demonstrating, in vivo, a marked dysfunction of the BBB with significantly higher MMP-9 in CSF after epileptic seizures. To our knowledge, this is the first prospective study of the link between CSF MMP-9 and BBB dysfunction in patients after epileptic seizure.

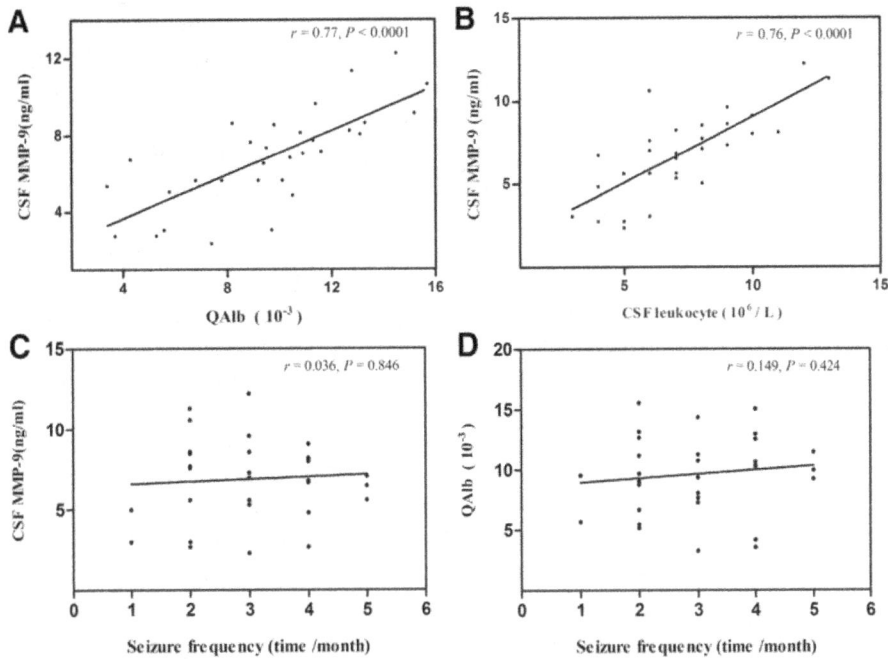

Figure 3 Correlation analysis of CSF MMP-9 levels in seizure patients. (A) Significant correlation between CSF MMP-9 levels and QAlb value ($P < 0.0001$, $r = 0.77$). **(B)** Significant correlation between CSF MMP-9 levels and CSF leukocyte count ($P < 0.0001$, $r = 0.76$). **(C)** No significant correlation between CSF MMP-9 levels and seizure frequency ($P = 0.846$, $r = 0.036$). **(D)** No significant correlation between QAlb value and seizure frequency ($P = 0.424$, $r = 0.149$). Correlation analysis performed with Spearman's rank correlation coefficient.

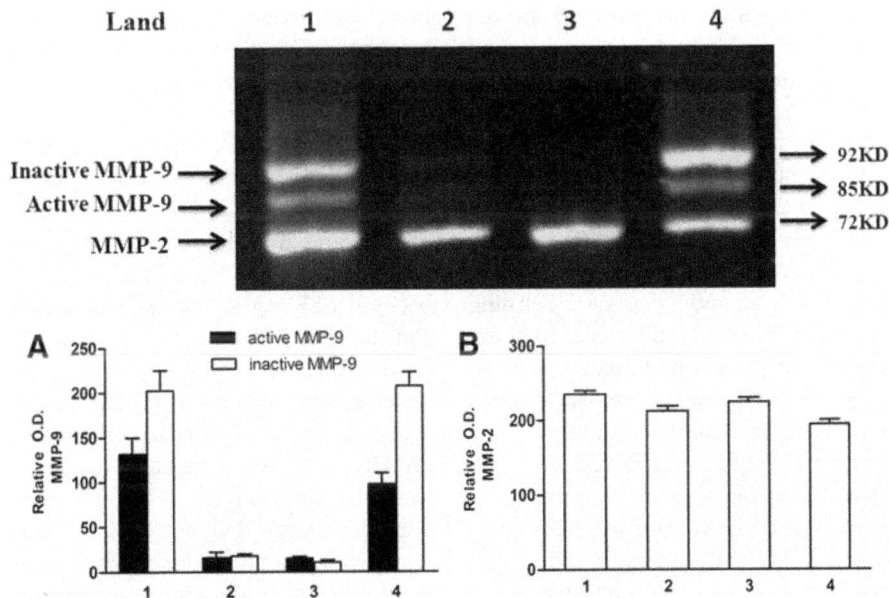

Figure 4 MMP enzyme activity of CSF samples. Top panel: Gelatin zymography gel results. Lane 1: GTC seizure sample; lanes 2 and 3 are controls; lane 4: single GTC seizure sample. Note that only seizure samples had positive MMP activity. **(A)** The relative optical density of MMP-9. **(B)** The relative optical density of MMP-2.

A dysfunctional BBB leads to increased permeability, allowing increased CSF marker passage. Therefore, CSF protein levels are a reliable way to monitor BBB integrity without using invasive methods. A common and well-established assessment of BBB function measures the level of albumin, a blood-specific protein in CSF and serum, reported as the CSF/serum albumin ratio (QAlb) [19,20]. An increase in QAlb reflects the serum albumin leakage in CSF due to BBB dysfunction, especially blood-CSF barrier dysfunction [21-23]. Previous studies have shown increased QAlb is correlated with status epilepticus [7]. In our study, we found the QAlb value was significantly increased in patients after seizure, suggesting BBB dysfunction after epileptic seizure. This finding is consistent with histological studies showing albumin accumulation in human epileptic brains [24,25]. Ultrastructural studies on human resected epileptic tissue also show clear BBB abnormalities, including increased micropinocytosis and the presence of abnormal tight junctions [26,27].

Accumulating experimental evidence indicates BBB dysfunction and inflammatory mediators decrease the threshold for individual seizures and contribute to epileptogenesis. Thus, BBB breakdown is regarded as an important pathophysiological event in seizures and epileptogenesis. Therefore, understanding the mechanisms controlling BBB disruption is critical to the understanding of epileptogenesis and may lead to new therapeutic targets for the prevention and treatment of epilepsy.

Matrix metallopeptidases (MMPs) represent a family of extracellular soluble or membrane bound neutral proteases having complex functions in normal and pathological conditions. Among MMPs, MMP-2 and MMP-9 are the only two gelatinases in humans. MMP-2 is normally found in brain and CSF [28]. In our study we found MMP-2 in the control CSF and in the patient CSF, indicating that expression of CSF MMP-2 in patients was not a result of seizure. MMP-9 is most abundantly expressed in the developing brain and is produced mainly by neurons and, to some extent, by glial cells in the CNS [29-31]. Under normal physiological conditions, MMP-9 is involved in dendritic spine remodeling, synaptic plasticity, learning and memory formation [32-35]. Increasing evidence in experimental animal models of epilepsy and human epileptic brains shows that MMP-9 plays a role in the pathogenesis of epilepsy by contributing to neuronal death, aberrant synaptic plasticity and neuroinflammation [36-39]. One study found that MMP-9 participates in the occurrence of seizures by converting pro-BDNF to mature BDNF in the hippocampus [38]. BDNF contributes to epilepsy in many ways. The roles of BDNF are not only important in acute seizures and epileptogenesis, but are also likely to be important in chronic epilepsy. Increased levels of BDNF exert functional effects that are consistent with a

pro-convulsant action. Animal model studies suggest intrahippocampal infusion of BDNF, and transgenic overexpression of BDNF significantly increases seizure susceptibility and severity [40-43]. Other studies have reported MMP-9-induced cell death is closely linked with the pathogenesis of epilepsy after SE [34,44]. In particular, MMP-9 knockout mice were less susceptible to seizure-induced brain injury, and MMP-9 inhibition ameliorated cell death following pilocarpine-induced seizures in infant rats [34]. Further, MMP-9 plays an important role in epileptogeness mainly due to MMP-9-related synaptic plasticity changes rather than neuronal death [45]. However, the relationship between CSF MMP-9 and BBB dysfunction in patients after epileptic seizures remains unclear.

A growing body of experimental and clinical evidence shows MMP-9 plays a major role in BBB disruption in a variety of pathological conditions including CNS infections [46-48], stroke [12,15,49,50], multiple sclerosis [51] and traumatic brain injury [52]. MMP-9 cleaves type IV collagen, a major component of the basement membrane of the cerebral epithelium that is responsible for the integrity of the BBB. MMP-9 also degrades a number of other extracellular matrix molecules including type V and XI collagens, laminin and aggrecan core protein [29,53,54]. Our study confirms a strong correlation between CSF MMP-9 levels and BBB dysfunction in patients after GTC seizures and argues MMP-9, not MMP-2, plays a role in BBB disruption during seizures.

Here, we also confirmed a transient influx of granulocytes into CSF of patients after epileptic seizure. Neutrophils in CSF samples are commonly considered a pathological feature. The migration of leukocytes from the bloodstream into the CNS is a key event in the pathogenesis of inflammatory neurological diseases. Recent data suggest that leukocyte-endothelial interaction and brain infiltration by leukocytes plays an important role in the pathogenesis of epilepsy [55-57]. In our study, we also found that elevated MMP-9 levels in CSF are primarily related to the number of immigrated leukocytes, with positive correlation between CSF MMP-9 levels and CSF leukocytes as well as between CSF MMP-9 levels and QAlb values. Leukocytes contribute to seizure pathogenesis acutely through affects on the BBB and chronically through several mechanisms including generation of oxygen free radicals, release of cytotoxic enzymes, vascular alterations and increase in cytokine and chemoattractant release [58]. Thus, we confirm that increased CSF MMP-9 represents the accumulation of activated leukocytes. It is reasonable to suspect that leukocytes are major producers of MMP-9. Furthermore, it has been demonstrated that injured neuronal and glial cells are major sources of MMP-9, supporting the neuroinflammatory response by releasing cytokines during epileptic seizures [36,37,53]. Indeed, we observed MMP-9 activity in CSF specimens from patients with seizures only.

We also analyzed effects of antiepileptic drugs (AEDs) on CSF MMP-9 concentrations and found no significant MMP-9 changes in patients with seizure. It is important to note several other reports show AEDs inhibit MMP-9 production and protect BBB function in epileptic patients and cerebral ischemic rats [59,60]. It has been proposed that MMP-9 is involved in aberrant synaptic formation in hippocampi of patients with temporal lobe epilepsy [39]. Therefore, we also analyzed temporal and extra-temporal seizures. Our findings show no differences in CSF MMP-9 levels between patients with temporal seizures and patients with extra-temporal seizures. In general, our findings argue MMP-9 overexpression is associated with activation of leukocytes, most likely polymorphonuclear, that serve as a key cellular source of MMP-9 in CSF. In turn, this promotes leukocyte recruitment, causing BBB breakdown, microvascular basal lamina proteolysis, and ultimately contributes to neuronal injury after epileptic seizure.

Conclusions

In this study, we found a significant correlation between CSF MMP-9 concentrations and CSF leukocyte counts, leading to BBB dysfunction. We suggest increased concentrations of MMP-9 in CSF were partly derived from leukocytes. These results demonstrate that seizure is characterized by invasion of leukocytes into the CSF and increased CSF MMP-9 levels are associated with BBB dysfunction in patients with seizures.

Competing interests
The authors declared that they have no competing interest.

Authors' contributions
YJL designed the research, ZHW reviewed and helped in analyzing data, BZ, XZ, MJW and STS processed serum and CSF from the patients and controls, JB, TL, CJG, SJZ, XLK, XZ and HZ performed the research, and YJL and ZHW wrote the paper. All authors read and approved the final manuscript.

Acknowledgments
This work was supported by grants from Natural Science Foundation of Shaanxi Province (no. 2009JM4035) and Science and Technology Plan Projects of the Shaanxi Provincial Department of Education (no. 07JK372), and from Science and Technology Project of Xi'an Lianhu District (no. K2011-024). We thank Dr. Austin Cape for careful reading and insightful feedback.

Author details
[1]Department of Neurology, The Affiliated Hospital of Xi'an Medical University, No. 48, West Fenghao Road, Xi'an 710077, Shaanxi Province, China. [2]Department of Neurology, The General Hospital of Ningxia Medical University, Ningxia, China.

References
1. Abbott NJ, Ronnback L, Hansson E: Astrocyte-endothelial interactions at the blood–brain barrier. Nat Rev Neurosci 2006, 7:41–53.
2. Hawkins BT, Davis TP: The blood–brain barrier/neurovascular unit in health and disease. Pharmacol Rev 2005, 57:173–185.
3. Tomkins O, Shelef I, Kaizerman I, Eliushin A, Afawi Z, Misk A, Gidon M, Cohen A, Zumsteg D, Friedman A: Blood–brain barrier disruption in post-traumatic epilepsy. J Neurol Neurosurg Psychiatry 2008, 79:774–777.
4. van Vliet EA, da Costa AS, Redeker S, van Schaik R, Aronica E, Gorter JA: Blood–brain barrier leakage may lead to progression of temporal lobe epilepsy. Brain 2007, 130:521–534.
5. Korn A, Golan H, Melamed I, Pascual-Marqui R, Friedman A: Focal cortical dysfunction and blood–brain barrier disruption in patients with postconcussion syndrome. J Clin Neurophysiol 2005, 22:1–9.
6. Strbian D, Durukan A, Pitkonen M, Marinkovic I, Tatlisumak E, Pedrono E, Abo-Ramadan U, Tatlisumak T: The blood–brain barrier is continuously open for several weeks following transient focal cerebral ischemia. Neuroscience 2008, 153:175–181.
7. Correale J, Rabinowicz AL, Heck CN, Smith TD, Loskota WJ, DeGiorgio CM: Status epilepticus increases CSF levels of neuron-specific enolase and alters the blood–brain barrier. Neurology 1998, 50:1388–1391.
8. Friedman A: Blood–brain barrier dysfunction, status epilepticus, seizures, and epilepsy: a puzzle of a chicken and egg? Epilepsia 2011, 52(Suppl 8):19–20.
9. Sahin D, Ilbay G, Ates N: Changes in the blood–brain barrier permeability and in the brain tissue trace element concentrations after single and repeated pentylenetetrazole-induced seizures in rats. Pharmacol Res 2003, 48:69–73.
10. Marchi N, Angelov L, Masaryk T, Fazio V, Granata T, Hernandez N, Hallene K, Diglaw T, Franic L, Najm I, Janigro D: Seizure-promoting effect of blood–brain barrier disruption. Epilepsia 2007, 48:732–742.
11. Marchi N, Tierney W, Alexopoulos AV, Puvenna V, Granata T, Janigro D: The etiological role of blood–brain barrier dysfunction in seizure disorders. Cardiovasc Psychiatry Neurol 2011, 2011:482415.
12. Barr TL, Latour LL, Lee KY, Schaewe TJ, Luby M, Chang GS, El-Zammar Z, Alam S, Hallenbeck JM, Kidwell CS, Warach S: Blood–brain barrier disruption in humans is independently associated with increased matrix metalloproteinase-9. Stroke 2010, 41:e123–e128.
13. Aoki T, Sumii T, Mori T, Wang X, Lo EH: Blood–brain barrier disruption and matrix metalloproteinase-9 expression during reperfusion injury: mechanical versus embolic focal ischemia in spontaneously hypertensive rats. Stroke 2002, 33:2711–2717.
14. Jin R, Yang G, Li G: Molecular insights and therapeutic targets for blood–brain barrier disruption in ischemic stroke: critical role of matrix metalloproteinases and tissue-type plasminogen activator. Neurobiol Dis 2010, 38:376–385.
15. Gidday JM, Gasche YG, Copin JC, Shah AR, Perez RS, Shapiro SD, Chan PH, Park TS: Leukocyte-derived matrix metalloproteinase-9 mediates blood–brain barrier breakdown and is proinflammatory after transient focal cerebral ischemia. Am J Physiol Heart Circ Physiol 2005, 289:H558–H568.
16. Tsai HC, Chung LY, Chen ER, Liu YC, Lee SS, Chen YS, Sy CL, Wann SR, Yen CM: Association of matrix metalloproteinase-9 and tissue inhibitors of metalloproteinase-4 in cerebrospinal fluid with blood–brain barrier dysfunction in patients with eosinophilic meningitis caused by Angiostrongylus cantonensis. Am J Trop Med Hyg 2008, 78:20–27.
17. Fernandez-Lopez D, Faustino J, Daneman R, Zhou L, Lee SY, Derugin N, Wendland MF, Vexler ZS: Blood–brain barrier permeability is increased after acute adult stroke but not neonatal stroke in the rat. J Neurosci 2012, 32:9588–9600.
18. Berg AT, Scheffer IE: New concepts in classification of the epilepsies: entering the 21st century. Epilepsia 2011, 52:1058–1062.
19. Tibbling G, Link H, Ohman S: Principles of albumin and IgG analyses in neurological disorders. I. Establishment of reference values. Scand J Clin Lab Invest 1977, 37:385–390.
20. Ganrot K, Laurell CB: Measurement of IgG and albumin content of cerebrospinal fluid, and its interpretation. Clin Chem 1974, 20:571–573.
21. Chalbot S, Zetterberg H, Blennow K, Fladby T, Andreasen N, Grundke-Iqbal I, Iqbal K: Blood-cerebrospinal fluid barrier permeability in Alzheimer's disease. J Alzheimers Dis 2011, 25:505–515.
22. Sindic CJ, Van Antwerpen MP, Goffette S: The intrathecal humoral immune response: laboratory analysis and clinical relevance. Clin Chem Lab Med 2001, 39:333–340.
23. Reiber H, Padilla-Docal B, Jensenius JC, Dorta-Contreras AJ: Mannan-binding lectin in cerebrospinal fluid: a leptomeningeal protein. Fluids Barriers CNS 2012, 9:17.

24. Raabe A, Schmitz AK, Pernhorst K, Grote A, von der Brelie C, Urbach H, Friedman A, Becker AJ, Elger CE, Niehusmann P: Cliniconeuropathologic correlations show astroglial albumin storage as a common factor in epileptogenic vascular lesions. *Epilepsia* 2012, 53:539–548.

25. Marchi N, Teng Q, Ghosh C, Fan Q, Nguyen MT, Desai NK, Bawa H, Rasmussen P, Masaryk TK, Janigro D: Blood–brain barrier damage, but not parenchymal white blood cells, is a hallmark of seizure activity. *Brain Res* 2010, 1353:176–186.

26. Cornford EM: Epilepsy and the blood–brain barrier: endothelial cell responses to seizures. *Adv Neurol* 1999, 79:845–862.

27. Heinemann U, Kaufer D, Friedman A: Blood–brain barrier dysfunction, TGFbeta signaling, and astrocyte dysfunction in epilepsy. *Glia* 2012, 60:1251–1257.

28. Grossetete M, Phelps J, Arko L, Yonas H, Rosenberg GA: Elevation of matrix metalloproteinases 3 and 9 in cerebrospinal fluid and blood in patients with severe traumatic brain injury. *Neurosurgery* 2009, 65:702–708.

29. Dong X, Song YN, Liu WG, Guo XL: Mmp-9, a potential target for cerebral ischemic treatment. *Curr Neuropharmacol* 2009, 7:269–275.

30. Michaluk P, Kaczmarek L: Matrix metalloproteinase-9 in glutamate-dependent adult brain function and dysfunction. *Cell Death Differ* 2007, 14:1255–1258.

31. Szklarczyk A, Lapinska J, Rylski M, McKay RD, Kaczmarek L: Matrix metalloproteinase-9 undergoes expression and activation during dendritic remodeling in adult hippocampus. *J Neurosci* 2002, 22:920–930.

32. Michaluk P, Wawrzyniak M, Alot P, Szczot M, Wyrembek P, Mercik K, Medvedev N, Wilczek E, De Roo M, Zuschratter W, et al: Influence of matrix metalloproteinase MMP-9 on dendritic spine morphology. *J Cell Sci* 2011, 124:3369–3380.

33. Wang XB, Bozdagi O, Nikitczuk JS, Zhai ZW, Zhou Q, Huntley GW: Extracellular proteolysis by matrix metalloproteinase-9 drives dendritic spine enlargement and long-term potentiation coordinately. *Proc Natl Acad Sci U S A* 2008, 105:19520–19525.

34. Hoehna Y, Uckermann O, Luksch H, Stefovska V, Marzahn J, Theil M, Gorkiewicz T, Gawlak M, Wilczynski GM, Kaczmarek L, Ikonomidou C: Matrix metalloproteinase 9 regulates cell death following pilocarpine-induced seizures in the developing brain. *Neurobiol Dis* 2012, 48:339–347.

35. Nagy V, Bozdagi O, Matynia A, Balcerzyk M, Okulski P, Dzwonek J, Costa RM, Silva AJ, Kaczmarek L, Huntley GW: Matrix metalloproteinase-9 is required for hippocampal late-phase long-term potentiation and memory. *J Neurosci* 2006, 26:1923–1934.

36. Konopka A, Grajkowska W, Ziemianska K, Roszkowski M, Daszkiewicz P, Rysz A, Marchel A, Koperski L, Wilczynski GM, Dzwonek J: Matrix metalloproteinase-9 (MMP-9) in human intractable epilepsy caused by focal cortical dysplasia. *Epilepsy Res* 2013, 104:45–58.

37. Li S, Yu S, Zhang C, Shu H, Liu S, An N, Yang M, Yin Q, Yang H: Increased expression of matrix metalloproteinase 9 in cortical lesions from patients with focal cortical dysplasia type IIb and tuberous sclerosis complex. *Brain Res* 2012, 1453:46–55.

38. Mizoguchi H, Nakade J, Tachibana M, Ibi D, Someya E, Koike H, Kamei H, Nabeshima T, Itohara S, Takuma K, et al: Matrix metalloproteinase-9 contributes to kindled seizure development in pentylenetetrazole-treated mice by converting pro-BDNF to mature BDNF in the hippocampus. *J Neurosci* 2011, 31:12963–12971.

39. Wilczynski GM, Konopacki FA, Wilczek E, Lasiecka Z, Gorlewicz A, Michaluk P, Wawrzyniak M, Malinowska M, Okulski P, Kolodziej LR, et al: Important role of matrix metalloproteinase 9 in epileptogenesis. *J Cell Biol* 2008, 180:1021–1035.

40. Lahteinen S, Pitkanen A, Koponen E, Saarelainen T, Castren E: Exacerbated status epilepticus and acute cell loss, but no changes in epileptogenesis, in mice with increased brain-derived neurotrophic factor signaling. *Neuroscience* 2003, 122:1081–1092.

41. Scharfman HE, Goodman JH, Sollas AL, Croll SD: Spontaneous limbic seizures after intrahippocampal infusion of brain-derived neurotrophic factor. *Exp Neurol* 2002, 174:201–214.

42. Croll SD, Suri C, Compton DL, Simmons MV, Yancopoulos GD, Lindsay RM, Wiegand SJ, Rudge JS, Scharfman HE: Brain-derived neurotrophic factor transgenic mice exhibit passive avoidance deficits, increased seizure severity and in vitro hyperexcitability in the hippocampus and entorhinal cortex. *Neuroscience* 1999, 93:1491–1506.

43. Xu B, Michalski B, Racine RJ, Fahnestock M: The effects of brain-derived neurotrophic factor (BDNF) administration on kindling induction, Trk

44. Kim GW, Kim HJ, Cho KJ, Kim HW, Cho YJ, Lee BI: The role of MMP-9 in integrin-mediated hippocampal cell death after pilocarpine-induced status epilepticus. *Neurobiol Dis* 2009, 36:169–180.

45. Takacs E, Nyilas R, Szepesi Z, Baracskay P, Karlsen B, Rosvold T, Bjorkum AA, Czurko A, Kovacs Z, Kekesi AK, Juhasz G: Matrix metalloproteinase-9 activity increased by two different types of epileptic seizures that do not induce neuronal death: a possible role in homeostatic synaptic plasticity. *Neurochem Int* 2010, 56:799–809.

46. Paul R, Lorenzl S, Koedel U, Sporer B, Vogel U, Frosch M, Pfister HW: Matrix metalloproteinases contribute to the blood–brain barrier disruption during bacterial meningitis. *Ann Neurol* 1998, 44:592–600.

47. Matsuura E, Umehara F, Hashiguchi T, Fujimoto N, Okada Y, Osame M: Marked increase of matrix metalloproteinase 9 in cerebrospinal fluid of patients with fungal or tuberculous meningoencephalitis. *J Neurol Sci* 2000, 173:45–52.

48. Brown HC, Chau TT, Mai NT, Day NP, Sinh DX, White NJ, Hien TT, Farrar J, Turner GD: Blood–brain barrier function in cerebral malaria and CNS infections in Vietnam. *Neurology* 2000, 55:104–111.

49. Guo M, Cox B, Mahale S, Davis W, Carranza A, Hayes K, Sprague S, Jimenez D, Ding Y: Pre-ischemic exercise reduces matrix metalloproteinase-9 expression and ameliorates blood–brain barrier dysfunction in stroke. *Neuroscience* 2008, 151:340–351.

50. Wang Z, Meng CJ, Shen XM, Shu Z, Ma C, Zhu GQ, Liu HX, He WC, Sun XB, Huo L, et al: Potential contribution of hypoxia-inducible factor-1alpha, aquaporin-4, and matrix metalloproteinase-9 to blood–brain barrier disruption and brain edema after experimental subarachnoid hemorrhage. *J Mol Neurosci* 2012, 48:273–280.

51. Fainardi E, Castellazzi M, Bellini T, Manfrinato MC, Baldi E, Casetta I, Paolino E, Granieri E, Dallocchio F: Cerebrospinal fluid and serum levels and intrathecal production of active matrix metalloproteinase-9 (MMP-9) as markers of disease activity in patients with multiple sclerosis. *Mult Scler* 2006, 12:294–301.

52. Higashida T, Kreipke CW, Rafols JA, Peng C, Schafer S, Schafer P, Ding JY, Dornbos D 3rd, Li X, Guthikonda M, et al: The role of hypoxia-inducible factor-1alpha, aquaporin-4, and matrix metalloproteinase-9 in blood–brain barrier disruption and brain edema after traumatic brain injury. *J Neurosurg* 2011, 114:92–101.

53. Yin P, Yang L, Zhou HY, Sun RP: Matrix metalloproteinase-9 may be a potential therapeutic target in epilepsy. *Med Hypotheses* 2011, 76:184–186.

54. Ralay Ranaivo H, Hodge JN, Choi N, Wainwright MS: Albumin induces upregulation of matrix metalloproteinase-9 in astrocytes via MAPK and reactive oxygen species-dependent pathways. *J Neuroinflammation* 2012, 9:68.

55. Silverberg J, Ginsburg D, Orman R, Amassian V, Durkin HG, Stewart M: Lymphocyte infiltration of neocortex and hippocampus after a single brief seizure in mice. *Brain Behav Immun* 2010, 24:263–272.

56. Zattoni M, Mura ML, Deprez F, Schwendener RA, Engelhardt B, Frei K, Fritschy JM: Brain infiltration of leukocytes contributes to the pathophysiology of temporal lobe epilepsy. *J Neurosci* 2011, 31:4037–4050.

57. Fabene PF, Navarro Mora G, Martinello M, Rossi B, Merigo F, Ottoboni L, Bach S, Angiari S, Benati D, Chakir A, et al: A role for leukocyte-endothelial adhesion mechanisms in epilepsy. *Nat Med* 2008, 14:1377–1383.

58. Fabene PF, Laudanna C, Constantin G: Leukocyte trafficking mechanisms in epilepsy. *Mol Immunol* 2013, 55:100–104.

59. Takahashi Y, Imai K, Ikeda H, Kubota Y, Yamazaki E, Susa F: Open study of pranlukast add-on therapy in intractable partial epilepsy. *Brain Dev* 2013, 35:236–244.

60. Wang Z, Leng Y, Tsai LK, Leeds P, Chuang DM: Valproic acid attenuates blood–brain barrier disruption in a rat model of transient focal cerebral ischemia: the roles of HDAC and MMP-9 inhibition. *J Cereb Blood Flow Metab* 2011, 31:52–57.

4

Brain region and epilepsy-associated differences in inflammatory mediator levels in medically refractory mesial temporal lobe epilepsy

Kenneth I. Strauss[1*] and Kost V. Elisevich[2,3]

Abstract

Background: Epilepsy patients have distinct immune/inflammatory cell profiles and inflammatory mediator levels in the blood. Although the neural origin of inflammatory cells and mediators has been implied, few studies have measured these inflammatory components in the human brain itself. This study examines the brain levels of chemokines (8), cytokines (14), and vascular injury mediators (3) suspected of being altered in epilepsy.

Methods: Soluble protein extracts of fresh frozen resected hippocampus, entorhinal cortex, and temporal cortex from 58 medically refractory mesial temporal lobe epilepsy subjects and 4 nonepileptic neurosurgical subjects were assayed for 25 inflammation-related mediators using ultrasensitive low-density arrays.

Results: Brain mediator levels were compared between regions and between epileptic and nonepileptic cases, showing a number of regional and possible epilepsy-associated differences. Eotaxin, interferon-γ, interleukin (IL)-2, IL-4, IL-12 p70, IL-17A, tumor necrosis factor-α, and intercellular adhesion molecule (ICAM)-1 levels were highest in the hippocampus, the presumptive site of epileptogenesis. Surprisingly, IL-1β and IL-1α were lowest in the hippocampus, compared to cortical regions. In the temporal cortex, IL-1β, IL-8, and MIP-1α levels were highest, compared to the entorhinal cortex and the hippocampus.

The most pronounced epilepsy-associated differences were decreased levels of eotaxin, IL-1β, C-reactive protein, and vascular cell adhesion molecule (VCAM)-1 and increased IL-12 p70 levels. Caution must be used in interpreting these results, however, because nonepileptic subjects were emergent neurosurgical cases, not a control group. Correlation analyses of each mediator in each brain region yielded valuable insights into the regulation of these mediator levels in the brain. Over 70 % of the associations identified were between different mediators in a single brain region, providing support for local control of mediator levels. Correlations of different mediators in different brain regions suggested more distributed control mechanisms, particularly in the hippocampus. Interestingly, only four mediators showed robust correlations between the brain regions, yet levels in three of these were significantly different between regions, indicating both global and local controls for these mediators.

Conclusions: Both brain region-specific and epilepsy-associated changes in inflammation-related mediators were detected. Correlations in mediator levels within and between brain regions indicated local and global regulation, respectively. The hippocampus showed the majority of interregional associations, suggesting a focus of inflammatory control between these regions.

Keywords: Neuroinflammation, Clinical study, Medically refractory epilepsy, Hippocampus, Entorhinal cortex, Temporal cortex, Brain cytokine levels, Brain chemokine levels, Brain vascular mediator levels

* Correspondence: kenneth.strauss@hc.msu.edu
[1]College of Human Medicine, Michigan State University, 333 Bostwick Ave NE, Grand Rapids, MI, USA
Full list of author information is available at the end of the article

Background

Over sixty-five million people worldwide and three million people in the USA have epilepsy [1], 15–20 % of whom are medically refractory [2]. Of these, mesial temporal lobe epilepsy (mTLE) defines the majority, accounting for 60–75 % of epilepsy patients undergoing surgery [3]. No consensus has been reached regarding the mechanisms underlying epileptogenicity, although over the past decade, increasing evidence has supported the contribution of inflammatory processes in promoting its occurrence [4–6].

Little is known regarding the postulated neuroinflammatory mechanisms in epilepsy; however, inflammation-related mediators have been implicated in a number of studies. Preclinical models of epilepsy have revealed changes in a few brain inflammatory mediators [7–9]; however, only recently have clinical investigations focused on peripheral markers of inflammation [10–17]. Findings of elevated blood cytokine levels in epilepsy patients have stimulated interest in brain tissue levels of inflammation-related mediators [10, 12]. Importantly, one study showed that neurosurgical resection of a small epileptic focus significantly reduced elevated blood levels of interleukin (IL)-1β, tumor necrosis factor (TNF)-α, and macrophage inflammatory protein (MIP)-1α but not IL-6 or TGF-β that were also elevated in mTLE [11]. Thus, it is likely that the source of these mediators was, at least in part, within the central nervous system.

Cells of both peripheral (e.g., leukocytes) and brain (e.g., microglia, astrocytes, neurons) origin produce a plethora of inflammation-related mediators. Cytokines, chemokines, and certain vascular-related mediators regulate the inflammatory state locally and communicate this to other tissues. In the brain, such mediators activate microglia and astrocytes, alter cerebrovascular function, act as chemoattractants, affect the infiltration of peripheral inflammatory cells, and/or promote cellular proliferation, survival, or death. They can also affect ionic fluxes, neurotransmission, and neural cell-cell communications through a variety of mechanisms [18].

Local inflammatory responses may be an important factor in chronic epilepsies, mediating secondary tissue damage and increasing the likelihood of seizures and their recurrence. For example, in epilepsy patients, several studies have identified fluctuations in circulating inflammatory cells [13, 19–21], as well as the infiltration of peripheral blood cells within injured and epileptic brain [21–26]. Regions of neuronal death and dysfunction in epileptogenic tissues have been associated with increased leukocyte numbers and altered blood levels of inflammatory mediators [11, 13, 27–29]. Moreover, the chemokine CCL21, produced by neurons after insult or injury, can be packaged into vesicles for transport along axons; its release activates microglia via their CXCR3 receptors, which may account for remote microglial activation [30]. Areas of highly concentrated afferent input, such as the entorhinal cortex with its reciprocal connection with the hippocampus, may be particularly vulnerable under such conditions producing a site of epileptogenicity remote from the site of the original injury [31].

Inflammatory mediators, produced by either blood or brain cells, can uniquely instigate brain inflammation, with little or no effect on the extracranial environment [23]. Thus, the neuroinflammatory milieu at the site of epileptogenesis is likely related to seizure onset, recurrence, and/or resistance to antiepileptic drug (AED) treatments.

Characterization of inflammation-related mediator levels at the epileptic focus will aid in further understanding these phenomena as well as better defining the set of relevant targets for novel epilepsy therapies. Moreover, although epilepsy-associated alterations in inflammation-related mediators at the site of epileptogenesis may not be directly reflected in the systemic circulation, these changes could indirectly affect circulating inflammatory mediators and cells in such a way that permits minimally invasive detection (i.e., in the blood or cerebral spinal fluid (CSF)).

Unfortunately, there have been few investigations of *local* alterations in inflammatory mediators *within or around* the site of epileptogenesis, particularly in freshly resected human brain tissue [18]. In the present study, brain levels of 25 cytokines, chemokines, and vasoactive proteins were quantified in soluble protein extracts of fresh frozen, surgically resected temporal cortex, entorhinal cortex, and hippocampus from 58 epileptic and 4 nonepileptic patients. To our knowledge, direct, simultaneous quantification of multiple inflammation-related mediators (e.g., pro- and anti-inflammatory, immune, and vascular effectors) in resected human epileptic and nonepileptic brain tissue has not previously been accomplished.

Methods

Participants

This study was undertaken through an institutional review board approved process at the Henry Ford Health System (Detroit, MI, USA) where the harvest of the tissues took place between 2002 and 2008. Subsequent analyses took place at the Spectrum Health System and Michigan State University (Grand Rapids, MI, USA). Inflammation-related mediator brain levels were determined in a series of 62 neurosurgical cases (Tables 1 and 2; Additional file 1 (Patient_Data_Repository.xlsx, available online)), 58 of which were focal epilepsy patients undergoing surgical resection for medically resistant epilepsy. Four nonepileptic cases were included in the study, involving (1) intratumoral (glioblastoma) hemorrhage with herniation; (2) putaminal hypertensive hemorrhage with middle cerebral

Table 1 Study enrollee demographics by Engel classification. Enrollees were operated for mTLE by a single surgeon (KE) and followed for more than 18 months postsurgically. Individual case details can be found in the Additional file 1, available online

Total enrolled	Side resected		Gender		Mean age
(N) 62	Right, 32	Left, 30	Female, 24	Male, 38	(Y), 39 ± 1
Engel classification	Modified class	(n)	% Total		
1A	"1"	39	63 %		38 ± 1
1D	"1D"	7	11 %		45 ± 3
2A	"2"	1	2 %		37 ± 2
2B	"2"	4	6 %		
2D	"2"	1	2 %		
3A	"3"	5	8 %		41 ± 2
Unclassified	–	1	2 %		–
Nonepileptic	"Ø"	4	6 %		65 ± 3

artery infarction and herniation; (3) middle cerebral artery aneurysm hemorrhage with herniation; and (4) acute subdural hematoma with temporal contusion and herniation.

Clinical specimens

The hippocampus, entorhinal cortex, and temporal cortex specimens were flash frozen in liquid nitrogen immediately upon resection and stored in polyethylene screw-cap tubes below –70 °C. Each specimen was homogenized at the same tissue concentration in order to improve comparisons. Brain pieces were dissected (100–200 mg, avoiding blood and white matter as much as possible) and pulverized on dry ice, transferred to pre-weighed polyethylene tubes on dry ice, weighed, and immediately sonicated in 5 vol. ice cold buffer H (100 mM potassium phosphate (pH 7.4), 10 mM ethylenediaminetetraacetic

Table 2 Established epilepsy risk factors and clinical variables. Individual case details can be found in the Additional file 1, available online

Epilepsy risk factor	(n)	Mean age	Brain side (R/L)	Family history of seizures
Closed head Injury	15	40.13	7/8	3/12
Febrile	11	32.91	8/3	4/7
Infection	5	38.00	2/3	0/5
Developmental	4	42.50	0/4	1/3
Hypoxic Injury	4	37.00	1/3	1/3
Mild head injury	4	40.75	2/2	2/2
Lesional	3	32.33	2/1	0/3
Not Known	12	38.83	7/5	3/9
Nonepileptic	4	63.50	3/1	0/4

acid (EDTA), 1 mM dithiothreitol containing Cømplete® Protease Inhibitor (Roche)), then centrifuged at 15K×g for 20 min at 4 °C. A small portion of each supernatant was assayed for total protein (microplate Bradford assay), and the remainder of the soluble protein extracts split into several aliquots that were stored frozen below –70 °C.

Measurements

For assays, tissue extracts were thawed on ice, differentially diluted for the various VPLEX® assay sets (Additional file 2: Table S1A) in Buffer H, and assayed in duplicates. This study utilized ultrasensitive (fg/mL range) multiplex enzyme immunoassays (custom-designed nine-plex human array plates, Meso Scale Discovery (MSD), Gaithersburg, MD). The multiplex assay plates were processed according to the manufacturer's instructions and read on the MSD Sector 6000 electrochemiluminescence plate scanner (MSD). Each VPLEX® set was accompanied by sets of mixed calibrator standards provided by the manufacturer, with seven serial dilutions in duplicates on each plate, to serve as a standard curve for the analytes measured. Prior studies (K. Strauss, unpublished data) established the appropriate dilution of protein extracts to minimize signal suppression and yield reproducible standard curves. Blanks containing the diluent only (i.e., no tissue) were also included in each study set. Analyte concentrations were extrapolated only from within the ranges for each standard curve, with coefficient of correlation, $R^2 \geq 0.98$. Lower limits of detection (LLOD) and quantification (LLOQ) were determined from these curves. LLOD was the mean background from blanks plus 6 standard deviations above the mean background value. LLOQ was designated as the point on each standard curve above which the coefficient of variation (i.e., standard deviation/mean) of calibrator concentrations was less than 15 %. None of the brain extract values approached the upper limits of any assay. Values below the LLOD were assigned a value of zero. For values between the LLOQ and LLOD, a value of half the LLOQ was assigned for analysis. Mass concentrations in the original specimen were calculated by accounting for assay volume, dilution at homogenization, differential dilution at assay (depending on the VPLEX® set), and normalization to tissue wet weight (picogram analyte per gram tissue). These concentrations approximate tissue concentrations when the specific gravity of the brain tissue is close to 1 g/mL [32].

Statistics

To determine which inflammation-related mediators might be germane to recurrent seizure disorders, two primary hypotheses were addressed in this study. These were as follows: (1) inflammatory mediator levels would be greater in brain regions proximal vs. distal to the epileptogenic focus in epilepsy cases and (2) mediators important in a recurrent seizure disorder would show different levels in epilepsy vs. nonepilepsy cases. Hypothesis (1) was tested using multiple analyses of variance (MANOVA) with brain region repeated measures, and hypothesis (2) tested using two-way ANOVA (brain region × epilepsy status). The criterion for rejecting the null hypothesis that there was no difference between group means was $p < 0.05$, unless otherwise noted.

For each mediator, outliers (on the right) were removed based upon the generalized extreme Studentized deviate test ($\alpha < 0.005$, one-sided) [33]. In cases where there were significant main and specific effects, but no significant post hoc result ($p > 0.05$; Tukey's honest significant difference test, the Tukey-Kramer method (Tukey's HSD)), non-parametric analyses (i.e., Wilcoxon rank sum test or Kruskal-Wallis for multiple comparisons) were initiated to mitigate the effects of large interindividual mediator level variability. Statistical analyses were carried out using JMP 11 software (SAS Institute Inc.). Note that full analyses of the data using $\log_{10}$ transformation for normalization yielded virtually identical results to those presented below.

In the figures, individual case data are in red (epileptic) or blue (nonepileptic), the grand mean is indicated by a horizontal line, diamond center lines indicate group means, and diamond upper and lower triangles indicate the 95 % confidence interval.

Secondary analyses compared the mediator levels in all three tissues with each secondary independent variable using two-way ANOVA (brain region × secondary variable). These variables included the following: age at surgery (years); side of the brain (L/R); gender (M/F); epilepsy duration (years); Engel classification (modified to a five-point scale including nonepileptic, 1A, 1D, 2A–C, 3A,B); epilepsy risk factor (nonepileptic, lesional, moderate-to-severe closed head injury (CHI), mild CHI, developmental, febrile, or infection); and pathology/imaging reports (hippocampus-only abnormalities, cortex-only abnormalities, or both).

To determine whether mediator values were linearly correlated, levels in each brain region were compared using multivariate analysis. Due to the large number of simultaneous comparisons (i.e., 25 mediators in three brain regions gives 2775 pairwise comparisons), a high degree of type I error was expected. To achieve acceptable rates of type I and type II errors, a more stringent type I error ($\alpha' = 0.0001$, $df = 73$, $r \geq 0.4340$) was used to select significant correlations; however, all significant comparisons with correlation coefficient 99.9 % confidence intervals that overlapped zero were eliminated.

Results

Soluble protein extracts from fresh frozen surgically resected human hippocampus, entorhinal cortex, and temporal cortex specimens from 58 medically refractory epilepsy and 4 nonepileptic neurosurgical cases (Tables 1 and 2) were assayed for 25 inflammation-related mediators using ultrasensitive multiplex enzyme immunoassay technology (see "Methods" section, Additional file 2: Figures S2A - S2AA). The primary independent variables for the study were the brain region and preoperative epilepsy status.

Variability in mediator measurements

Median mediator values varied over 4 orders of magnitude, and interindividual variability was great, even after outlier removal (Additional file 2: Table S3B). Variability was examined using coefficients of variation (CV) calculated for each mediator, between the brain regions and by the epilepsy status (Additional file 2: Tables S3C–E). The grand mean CV for all mediators was 125 %, with tissue means of 114 % in the hippocampus, 130 % in the entorhinal cortex, and 132 % in the temporal cortex. The highest variability was seen with VEGF (236 %), IL-2 (232 %), IL-6 (195 %), IL-8 (195 %), and IL-10 (183 %) levels. Interestingly, IL-2 and IL-10 had high variability across all tissues independent of epilepsy status, whereas VEGF, IL-6, and IL-8 showed greater variability in epileptic compared to nonepileptic tissues (Additional file 2: Tables S3D, E).

Brain mediator levels

Levels of 23 inflammation-related mediators were detectable in the majority of specimens. The exceptions were granulocyte-macrophage colony-stimulating factor (GM-CSF) (74 % tested negative; see Additional file 2: Tables S3F, G) and IFN-γ (94 % of specimens tested negative).

Most of the brain tissue examined did not exhibit detectable GM-CSF (see Table 3 note 4, Additional file 2: Figure S2H); however, GM-CSF was present in the hippocampus (15/48 epilepsy and 0/3 nonepileptic cases), entorhinal cortex (3/58 epilepsy and 1/4 nonepileptic cases), and temporal cortex (22/55 epilepsy and 3/4 nonepileptic cases). Entorhinal cortical GM-CSF levels were lower overall (Table 3; $p < 0.005$ Tukey's HSD). This was further supported by examining the number of nonzero GM-CSF values in each brain region (Additional file 2: Table S3G(A–C)). There was significant nonhomogeneity between the brain regions ($p < 0.0001$ chi-square, $df = 2$), with entorhinal cortex showing the lowest incidence of GM-CSF-positive cases. In addition, nonhomogeneity was shown between the brain region and epilepsy status groups ($p < 0.001$ chi-square, $df = 5$) (Additional file 2: Figure S2H, Table S3G(C)).

Table 3 Inflammation-related mediators by brain region

Mediator[a] (pg/g tissue)	Hippocampus			Entorhinal cortex			Temporal cortex			MANOVA, brain region P value[b]	Two-way ANOVA, epilepsy (±) × region P value[c]
	Mean	SEM	N	Mean	SEM	N	Mean	SEM	N		
Eotaxin	627****	67	51	404	40	62	307	42	59	<0.0001	<0.0001
IP-10	3597**	453	51	6213	1292	59	7004	1413	59	0.0306	0.0038
MCP-1	8051	1199	51	4551*	465	60	8440	1803	58	0.0045	0.1923
MCP-4	839	89	51	545*	35	62	676	152	57	0.0011	0.3751
MIP-1α	1008	189	51	590	124	62	2187****	361	59	0.0001	<0.0001
MIP-1β	2362	311	51	1636	208	61	3306***	437	59	0.0037	0.0153
TARC	666	111	51	501	49	61	855	205	59	0.1047	0.3991
GM-CSF[d]	3062	710	51	470****	230	62	2579	400	59	<0.0001	0.0009
IFN-γ[d]	33.1****	10.9	51	0	0	62	1.56	1.56	59	0.0143	0.0008
IL-1α	992**	162	51	3616**	372	62	2576**	271	58	<0.0001	<0.0001
IL-1β	13.8**	2.2	51	27.8**	3.9	62	39.7**	5.0	57	<0.0001	0.0002
IL-2[d]	38.3****	7.9	49	4.16	1.83	62	7.97	2.27	59	<0.0001	<0.0001
IL-4	11.7****	1.2	49	7.17	0.40	62	6.45	0.44	59	0.0010	<0.0001
IL-6	33.4	8.2	51	34.8	8.5	60	60.8	15.2	57	0.1409	0.0161
IL-8	570	121	51	933	251	61	1473*	331	57	0.0029	0.0259
IL-10[d]	4.21	0.75	51	1.49**	0.47	61	3.37	0.85	59	0.0225	0.1399
IL-12/23 p40	72.9	14.8	51	97.9	12.8	61	88.2	13.3	58	0.1490	0.1273
IL-12 p70	5.17	0.68	50	2.65***	0.43	62	3.59	0.29	58	0.0494	0.0019
IL-17A	949****	112	49	378	44	62	252	28	59	<0.0001	<0.0001
TNF-α	5.89	0.75	51	3.16	0.67	60	5.26	0.85	57	0.1176	0.0518
TNF-β	3.85	0.89	49	8.52****	0.58	62	4.90	0.56	59	0.0143	<0.0001
VEGF	7716***	1865	49	3553	1199	62	1889	720	59	0.0231	0.0465
CRP	26,540	2222	49	22,069	1435	62	15,624****	1115	59	<0.0001	<0.0001
ICAM-1	12,088**	1110	50	9243	786	62	8291	897	58	0.0035	<0.0001
VCAM-1	21,887	4754	51	21,351	3659	62	14,427	2632	59	0.0103	<0.0001

Abbreviations: Eotaxin (also known as (aka) CCL-11), *IP-10* interferon gamma-induced protein 10 (aka CXCL-10), *MCP-1* monocyte chemoattractant protein 1 (aka CCL-2), *MCP-4* monocyte chemoattractant protein 4 (aka CCL-13), *MIP-1α* macrophage inflammatory protein 1-alpha (aka CCL-3), *MIP-1β* macrophage inflammatory protein 1-beta (aka CCL-4), *TARC* thymus- and activation-regulated chemokine (aka CCL-17), *GM-CSF* granulocyte-macrophage colony-stimulating factor (aka CSF2), *IFN-γ* interferon gamma, *IL* interleukin, *IL-8* (aka CXCL-8), *TNF* tumor necrosis factor, *VEGF* vascular endothelial growth factor, *CRP* C-reactive protein, *ICAM-1* intercellular adhesion molecule 1 (aka CD54) , *VCAM-1* vascular cell adhesion molecule 1 (aka CD106)

*$p \leq 0.01$, Wilcoxon/Kruskal-Wallis; **$p < 0.05$, Tukey's HSD; ***$p < 0.01$, Tukey's HSD; ****$p < 0.001$, Tukey's HSD

[a]Mediator values in pg/g tissue, N is number of observations, SEM = (standard deviation/$N^{1/2}$). The total number of specimens assayed was as follows: hippocampus = 51, entorhinal cortex = 62, temporal cortex = 59; differences from these values indicate outlier removals. Case data, distributions, and summary statistics can be found in Additional file 2: Figures S2A - S2AA, and the complete data set in Additional file 1

[b]Repeated measures MANOVA of mediator levels by brain region, brain region effect. Italicized *P* values indicate significant post hoc comparisons

[c]Two-way ANOVA epilepsy status (±) × brain region, main effect. See Table 4 for post hoc comparisons

[d]GM-CSF and IFN-γ exhibited 74 and 94 % assay values of zero (below the lower limit of detection), and assays for IL-2 and IL-10 had 65 and 59 % zero values, with more than half the zero values in the cortical region specimens

Similarly, most of the brain tissues examined did not exhibit detectable IFN-γ levels (see Table 3, Additional file 2: Figure S2U, Table S3H(A–C)) and no epilepsy-related differences could be discerned. However, IFN-γ was more often detected in the hippocampus (10/51 cases) than in the entorhinal cortex (0/62) or temporal cortex (1/59) ($p = 0.0001$ chi-square, $df = 2$). As with GM-CSF, there was nonhomogeneity between groups with respect to the brain region and epilepsy status ($p = 0.004$ chi-square, $df = 5$).

Chemokines

Eotaxin levels (Table 3) showed brain region-specific differences over all cases using brain region repeated measures (MANOVA; $p < 0.0001$). Hippocampal eotaxin levels were higher than those in the entorhinal and temporal cortices (Fig. 1a, $p < 0.001$ post hoc Tukey's HSD). Epilepsy-related differences in eotaxin were also apparent. Eotaxin levels were higher in nonepileptic cases (Table 4, Fig. 1b) and, specifically in the entorhinal cortex using epilepsy ×

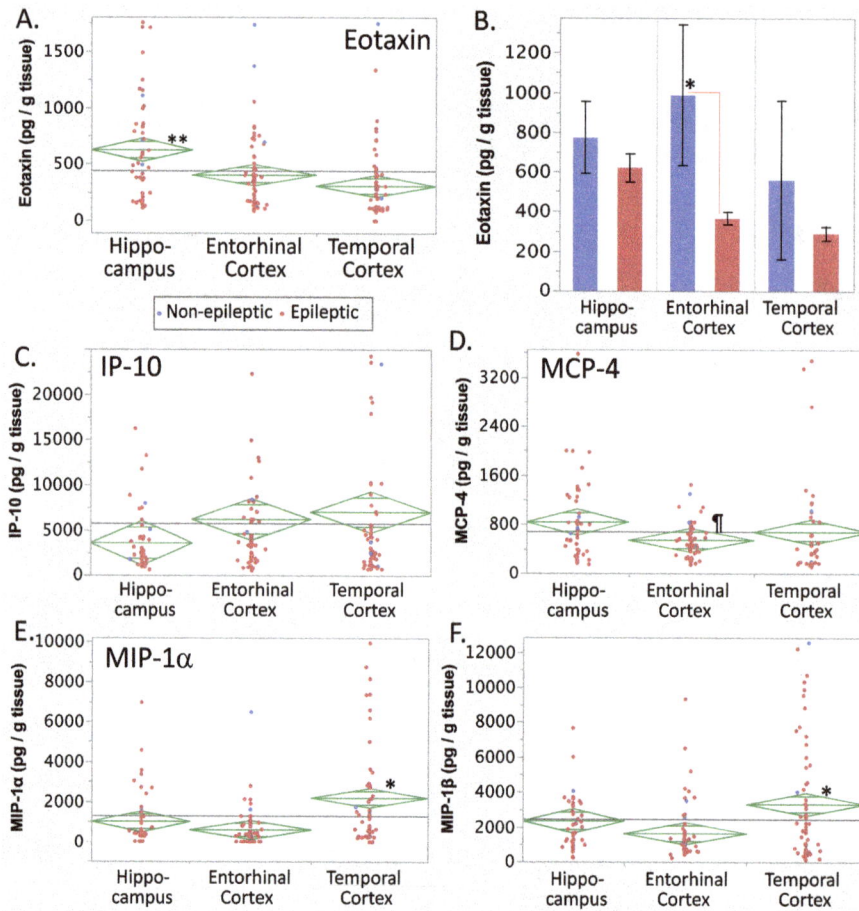

Fig. 1 a Eotaxin levels in human brain specimens. Overall, the hippocampal levels were greater than the entorhinal and temporal cortex. **b** Epilepsy-related eotaxin differences. Brain levels of eotaxin were greater among nonepileptic cases overall, and the nonepileptic entorhinal cortex eotaxin was greater than in the epileptic entorhinal cortex. **c** IP-10 levels were not significantly different between brain regions. **d** MCP-4 levels appeared lower in the entorhinal cortex than the other tissues. **e** MIP-1α and **f** MIP-1β levels in the human brain showed similar regional differences. In all graphs, *blue* = nonepileptic cases, *red* = epileptic cases. Data points are means of duplicate measurements; *diamond graphs* show the grand mean for all cases as a *horizontal line*, *diamond center line* indicates group mean, *upper and lower triangles* indicate the 95 % confidence intervals. *Histograms* show group mean ± standard error; *solid lines* show within epilepsy status, and *dashed lines* show between epilepsy status group differences. Post hoc testing: ****p < 0.001; *p < 0.01; §p < 0.05, Tukey's HSD; ¶p < 0.01, non-parametric Wilcoxon/Kruskal-Wallis, unless otherwise noted

brain region repeated measures (MANOVA; epilepsy effect, $p < 0.01$ Tukey's HSD).

Levels of IP-10 showed no regional differences (Fig. 1c), likely due to the high variance in cortical specimens. Although IP-10 levels were greater in nonepileptic cases overall, and specifically in the entorhinal cortex, when considering the epilepsy effect and epilepsy × brain region interaction (both $p < 0.001$ Tukey's HSD), these effects may have been due to a few extreme nonoutlier values in the cortical specimens (see Additional file 2: Figure S2B).

Monocyte chemoattractant protein (MCP)-1 and MCP-4 levels had brain region-specific but no epilepsy-related differences (Table 3). Nonparametric analyses suggested that entorhinal cortex levels were lower for each than in the hippocampus or temporal cortex (post hoc Wilcoxon/

Kruskal-Wallis, $p = 0.002$ and $p = 0.0005$, respectively). Inspection of the individual case data showed that this was true in 67 % of cases for MCP-1 (Additional file 2: Figure S2C) and in 53 % of cases for MCP-4 levels (Fig. 1d, Additional file 2: Figure S2D).

MIP-1α levels showed brain region-specific differences overall (Fig. 1e, Table 3). Temporal cortical MIP-1α levels were greater than in the entorhinal cortex or hippocampus ($p < 0.01$ Tukey's HSD). MIP-1β levels showed similar region-specific differences overall (Fig. 1f, brain region effect $p = 0.0037$). The temporal cortical MIP-1β levels were higher than in the entorhinal cortex (Table 3, $p = 0.002$ Tukey's HSD) but not different from the hippocampal levels. No epilepsy-related MIP-1α or MIP-1β differences were detected.

Table 4 Epilepsy-related differences in inflammation-related mediator levels

Mediator (pg/g tissue)	Brain region					
	Hippocampus		Entorhinal cortex		Temporal cortex	
	Nonepileptic	Epileptic	Nonepileptic	Epileptic	Nonepileptic	Epileptic
Eotaxin	$772 \pm 180^{a,**}$	618 ± 71	$986 \pm 355^{a,**}$	364 ± 31	$558 \pm 401^{a,**}$	289 ± 36
n	3	48	4	58	4	55
IP-10[c]	4.96 ± 1.79	3.51 ± 0.47	$24.0 \pm 17.4^{b,**}$	5.26 ± 0.97	7.68 ± 5.27	6.96 ± 1.48
n	3	48	3	56	4	55
MIP-1α[d]	698 ± 494	1027 ± 199	2192 ± 1463	480 ± 80	873 ± 437	2283 ± 383
n	3	48	4	58	4	55
IL-1β[d]	$29.1 \pm 15.3^{a,**}$	12.9 ± 2.1	$59.0 \pm 26.4^{a,**}$	25.7 ± 3.7	$49.3 \pm 39.2^{a,**}$	39.0 ± 4.8
n	3	48	4	58	4	53
IL-2	24.6 ± 24.6	39.2 ± 8.3	11.3 ± 6.7	3.67 ± 1.90	$30.1 \pm 30.1^{b,***}$	6.37 ± 1.25
n	3	46	4	58	4	55
IL-6[d]	$149 \pm 38^{a,****}$	26.1 ± 7.2	65.2 ± 47.6	33.2 ± 8.6	61.7 ± 35.2	60.7 ± 16.0
n	3	48	3	57	3	54
IL-12 p70	2.26 ± 2.26	$5.35 \pm 0.71^{a,**}$	1.94 ± 1.94	$2.69 \pm 0.44^{a,**}$	0	$3.79 \pm 0.28^{a,**}$
n	3	47	4	58	3	55
TNF-α[d]	5.04 ± 3.21	5.95 ± 0.77	7.60 ± 4.44	2.93 ± 0.67	0.79 ± 0.79	5.51 ± 0.88
n	3	48	3	57	3	54
CRP[c]	$50.5 \pm 37.4^{a,****}$	25.5 ± 18.8	$39.7 \pm 11.7^{a,****}$	20.9 ± 12.1	$23.8 \pm 7.9^{a,****}$	15.0 ± 1.0
n	2	47	4	58	4	55
ICAM-1[c]	16.0 ± 8.7	11.9 ± 1.1	$19.1 \pm 8.1^{b,****}$	8.57 ± 0.59	6.60 ± 2.26	8.42 ± 0.95
n	2	48	4	58	4	54
VCAM-1[c]	$131 \pm 9^{b,****}$	15.0 ± 2.9	$75.7 \pm 22.5^{b,****}$	17.6 ± 3.1	$49.9 \pm 16.1^{b,****}$	11.9 ± 2.3
n	3	48	4	58	4	55

$**p < 0.05$; $***p < 0.01$; $****p < 0.001$, post hoc Tukey's HSD

[a]Epilepsy effect; overall epileptic vs. nonepileptic cases. Only the greater set of values are marked

[b]Epilepsy × brain region interactions, epileptic vs. nonepileptic cases in individual brain region(s). Only the greater set of values are marked

[c]The units of these mediators are in ng/g tissue

[d]These mediators were elevated in the blood of mTLE patients [11]; neurosurgical resection reduced the blood levels of TNF-α, IL-1β, and MIP-1α, but not IL-6

Brain levels of the thymus- and activation-regulated chemokine (TARC) showed neither brain region- nor epilepsy-related changes. The temporal cortex from epileptic cases had very high TARC levels; however, this was obscured by a high variability of TARC levels in the epileptic temporal cortex (Additional file 2: Figure S2G, Table S3E).

Cytokines

Interleukin (IL-)1α levels showed graded brain region-specific differences overall (Fig. 2a, Table 3) with greatest expression in the entorhinal cortex followed by that in the temporal cortex and, lastly, the hippocampus ($p < 0.03$ post hoc Tukey's HSD). No epilepsy-related differences were discerned. On the other hand, IL-1β levels (Fig. 2b, Table 3) showed both graded brain region-specific differences and epilepsy-related effects. IL-1β levels were greatest in the temporal cortex, intermediary in the entorhinal cortex, and lowest in the hippocampus (Table 3; $p < 0.05$ Tukey's HSD). In addition, nonepileptic brain

regions showed greater IL-1β levels than epileptic brain regions overall (Table 4; epilepsy × brain region ANOVA, epilepsy effect $p < 0.04$, $p < 0.05$ Tukey's HSD).

IL-2 (Fig. 2c) and IL-4 (Fig. 2d) brain levels showed similar patterns of regional differences. IL-2 was elevated in the hippocampus compared to either the entorhinal or temporal cortices (Table 3, $p < 0.005$ Tukey's HSD). A significant epilepsy status × brain region repeated measures interaction ($p < 0.03$) was noted, with IL-2 levels in the nonepileptic temporal cortex exceeding those in the epileptic temporal cortex ($p < 0.01$ Tukey's HSD). Similarly, hippocampal IL-4 levels were elevated compared to other tissues (Table 3, $p < 0.001$ Tukey's HSD), but no epilepsy-related differences were observed.

IL-6 levels were numerically highest in the temporal cortex but variability in both epileptic and nonepileptic cases confounded the analysis (Additional file 2: Figure S2M, Tables S3C–E, H). Although there were no overall differences in IL-6 between brain regions (Fig. 2e), there

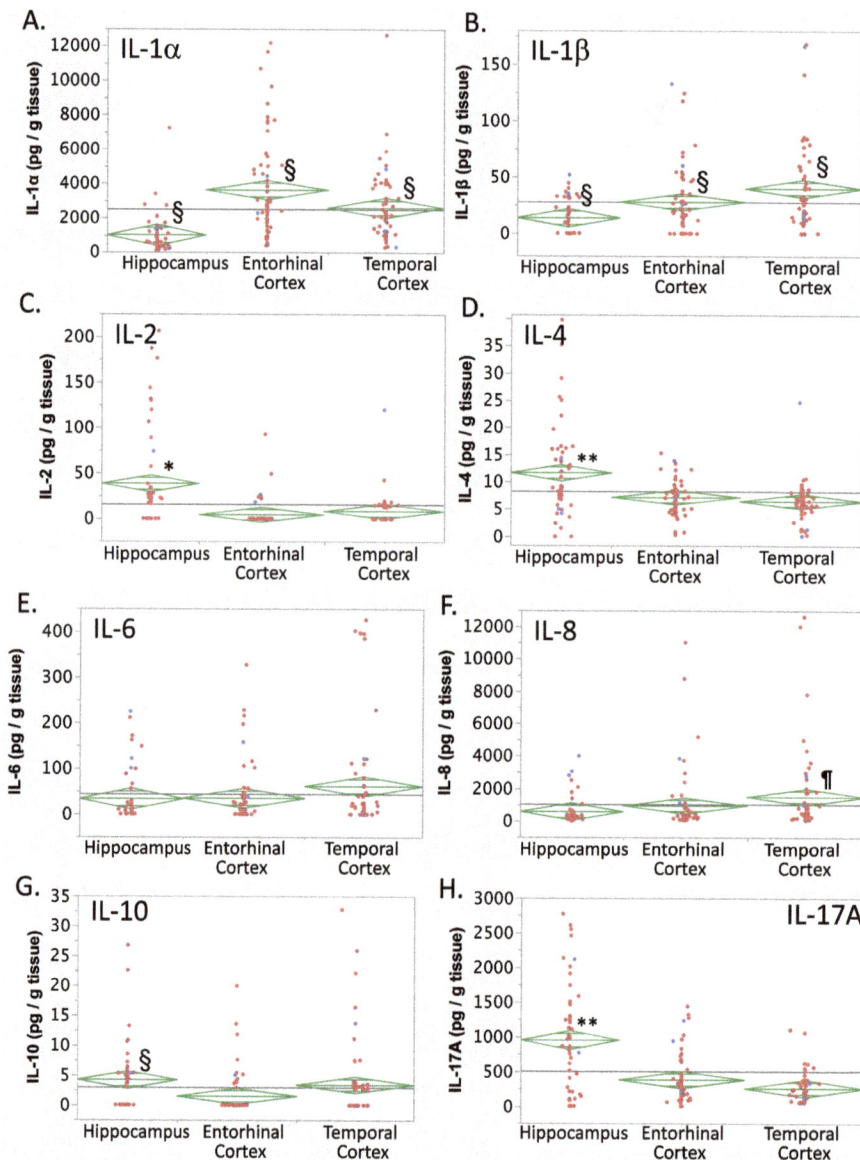

Fig. 2 Brain region differences in interleukin (IL) levels. **a** IL-1α and **b** IL-1β levels differed between all three brain regions. **c** IL-2 and (**d**) IL-4 levels were elevated in the hippocampus. (**e**) IL-6 levels showed high variability without brain region-specific or epilepsy-related differences. **f** IL-8 levels were higher in the temporal cortex than the other brain regions, whereas **g** IL-10 levels were higher in the hippocampus than in the entorhinal cortex, and **h** IL-17A levels were higher in the hippocampus than the entorhinal cortex and temporal cortex. For graphics details, see Fig. 1

was a significant epilepsy × repeated measures brain region interaction ($p < 0.02$). The hippocampal IL-6 levels were greater in nonepileptic compared to epileptic cases (Table 4, $p < 0.001$ Tukey's HSD).

Overall, IL-8 levels in the temporal cortex were greater than in the hippocampus or entorhinal cortex (Table 3, Fig. 2f, $p < 0.008$ post hoc Wilcoxon/Kruskal-Wallis), with the entorhinal cortical levels intermediary to these regions (not significantly different (n.s.d.)). In contrast, IL-10 levels were higher in the hippocampus than in the entorhinal cortex (Fig. 2g, $p < 0.05$ Tukey's HSD), with intermediary levels (n.s.d.) found in the temporal cortex.

IL-17A levels showed brain region-specific differences, with the hippocampal levels higher than both the entorhinal and temporal cortices (Table 3, $p < 0.001$ Tukey's HSD). Neither epilepsy-related differences nor brain region × epilepsy interactions were detected for brain IL-17A levels.

Bioactive IL-12 is a p35:p40 heterodimer-designated IL-12 p70. The p40 subunit also binds with other proteins, such as p17, to form IL-23. Two IL-12-related assays were performed, the IL-12/23 p40 assay that detected p40 in all its forms *except* for IL-12 p70, and the IL-12 p70 assay which detected only intact heterodimers (Paul Grulich, MSD Scientific Support Group, personal communication).

Brain region and epilepsy-associated differences in inflammatory mediator levels in medically refractory...

45

Though IL-12/23 p40 levels showed neither brain region- nor epilepsy-related differences (Fig. 3a), the heterodimer IL-12 p70 exhibited both brain region-specific and epilepsy-related differences. IL-12 p70 was increased in the hippocampus compared to the entorhinal cortex (Fig. 3b, $p < 0.005$ Tukey's HSD). A bimodal distribution might be present for IL-12 p70 but could not be confirmed because most measurable values were close to the lower limit of quantification. Epileptic brain had higher levels of IL-12 p70 than nonepileptic cases (Table 4, epilepsy effect $p < 0.03$, $p < 0.05$ Tukey's HSD).

Brain levels of IL-12/23 p40 were much greater than that of IL-12 p70 (Fig. 3a–d, Additional file 2: Table S3B). Mean p40 to p70 molar ratios (Fig. 3c, Additional file 2: Figure S2AA) were 13 ± 4 in the hippocampus, 23 ± 5 in the entorhinal cortex, and 31 ± 6 in the temporal cortex, suggesting that only a small proportion of the total p40 tissue content was in IL-12 p70. In addition, the mean p40:p70 molar ratio was higher in the temporal cortex than in the hippocampus (Fig. 3c, repeated measures MANOVA $p = 0.0271$, $p < 0.02$ Tukey's HSD). Moreover, the IL-12 p70:p40 molar ratio showed lower values in the entorhinal cortex compared with other tissues (Fig. 3d, Additional file 2: Figure S2Z, repeated measures MANOVA, brain region effect $p = 0.0007$, $p \leq 0.01$ Tukey's HSD). Both of the latter findings were consistent with elevated hippocampal IL-12 p70 levels (Fig. 3b).

TNF-α showed no brain region-specific or epilepsy-related differences (Table 3). Nonetheless, case data showed that the entorhinal cortical levels were lower than those in the hippocampus and temporal cortex in most individuals (69 and 52 %, respectively, Additional file 2: Figure S2S). In contrast, TNF-β brain levels were highest in the entorhinal cortex overall (Fig. 4b, $p < 0.001$ Tukey's HSD). Data showed the entorhinal cortical levels to be higher than in the hippocampus and temporal cortex in 76 and 83 % of cases, respectively (Additional file 2: Figure S2T).

Vascular mediators
Hippocampal VEGF levels were two- and fourfold greater than in the entorhinal and temporal cortical regions, respectively (Table 3, Fig. 4c, $p < 0.01$ Tukey's HSD). Nonparametric analyses suggested graded VEGF levels, with the hippocampus showing the highest levels followed by the entorhinal cortex, and lastly, the temporal cortex ($p < 0.0002$ Wilcoxon/Kruskal-Wallis). No epilepsy-related differences were observed; however, there was increased VEGF variation in epileptic tissue specimens (Additional file 2: Figure S2V, top right) that may have obscured differences between epileptic and nonepileptic VEGF levels (Additional file 2: Tables S3C, E, I).

Brain levels of C-related protein (CRP) were lower in the temporal cortex than in the hippocampus or entorhinal cortex (Fig. 5a, $p < 0.01$ Tukey's HSD). Moreover, two-way ANOVA showed 50, 53, and 63 % lower CRP levels in the

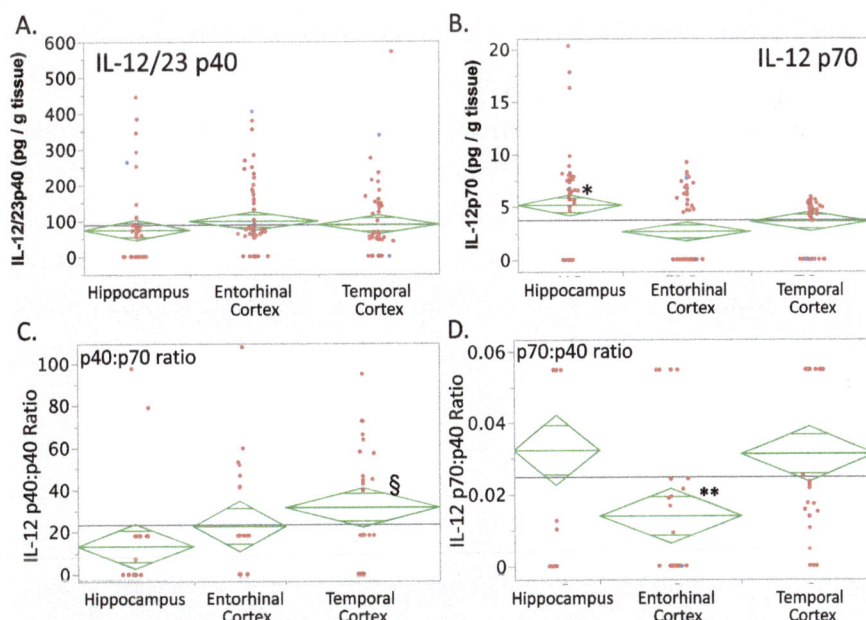

Fig. 3 IL-12 brain levels. **a** IL-12/23 p40 levels did not show brain region-specific differences. **b** The heterodimeric IL-12 p70 showed brain region-specific differences, with higher levels in the hippocampus than in the entorhinal cortex. **c** The molar ratio of IL-12/23 p40 to IL-12 p70 (p40:p70) was elevated in the temporal cortex compared with the hippocampus and entorhinal cortex ($^§p < 0.02$, Tukey's HSD). **d** IL-12 p70:p40 molar ratios were depressed in the entorhinal cortex (compared to the hippocampus and temporal cortex, $**p \leq 0.01$ Tukey's HSD), despite higher p70 levels in the hippocampal specimens. For graphics details, see Fig. 1

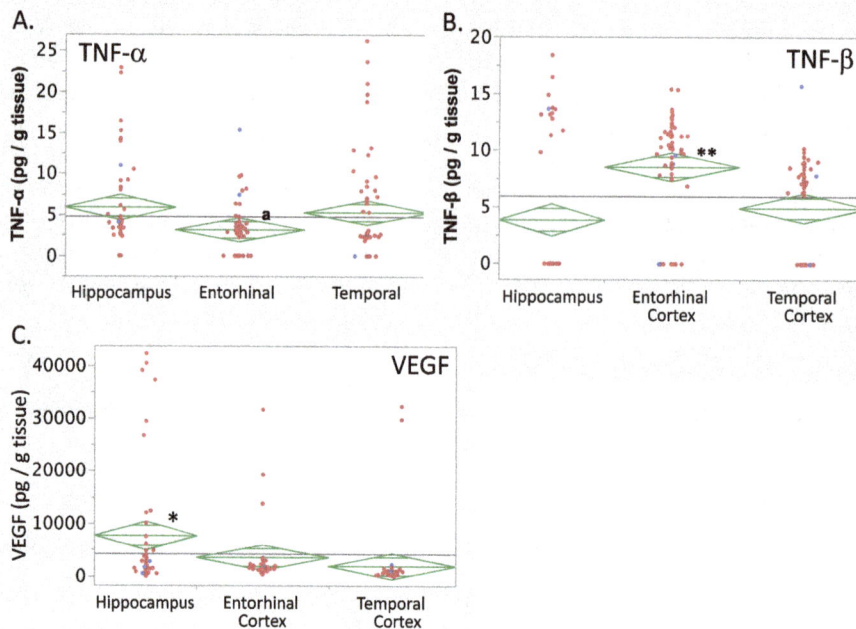

Fig. 4 a TNF-α levels in the human brain did not show region-specific differences by post hoc testing. However, on a case-by-case analysis (*a*), the entorhinal cortex TNF-α levels were lower than in the hippocampus or temporal cortex for 59 % of all individuals. **b** TNF-β brain levels were higher in the entorhinal cortex, and higher than in the hippocampus or temporal cortex for 80 % of all individual cases. **c** VEGF levels were greater in the hippocampus than in the entorhinal or temporal cortex. For graphics details, see Fig. 1

epileptic hippocampus, entorhinal cortex, and temporal cortex, respectively (Fig. 5b, Table 4, epilepsy effect $p < 0.0001$, all p values <0.05 Tukey's HSD).

Intercellular adhesion molecule (ICAM)-1 levels were highest in the hippocampus compared to the cortical regions overall (Table 3, Fig. 6a, $p < 0.03$ Tukey's HSD). While there was no significant epilepsy-related effect, there were significant epilepsy × brain region repeated measures interactions ($p = 0.0008$). ICAM-1 levels in the nonepileptic entorhinal cortex were higher than in the epileptic cases (Fig. 6b, $p < 0.001$ Tukey's HSD).

Vascular cell adhesion molecule (VCAM)-1 levels did not appear different across brain regions overall (Fig. 6c) but showed multiple effects among the nonepileptic cases (Table 4, epilepsy effect $p < 0.0001$, brain region effect $p < 0.0001$, epilepsy × brain region interaction $p < 0.0001$). Specifically, VCAM-1 levels were greater in each of the nonepileptic brain region cases compared to the epileptic cases (Fig. 6d, $p < 0.001$ Tukey's HSD). Also, VCAM-1 levels in the nonepileptic hippocampus were greater than in either the nonepileptic entorhinal cortex or temporal cortex (Fig. 6d, Table 4, $p < 0.05$ Tukey's HSD).

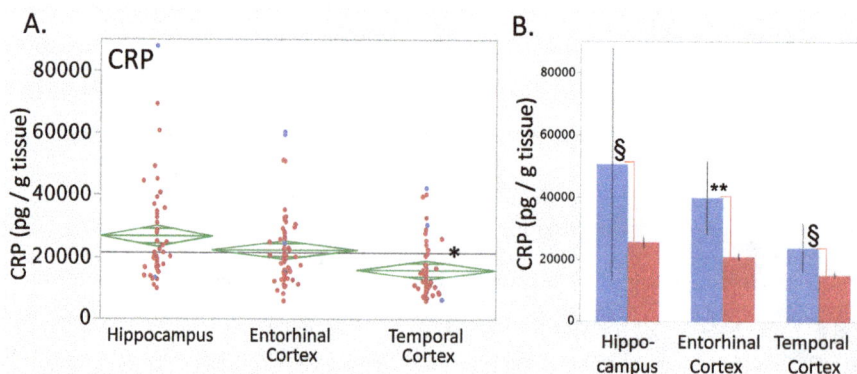

Fig. 5 a CRP (C-reactive protein) levels were the lowest in the temporal cortex compared to the hippocampus and entorhinal cortex. **b** CRP levels were higher in the nonepileptic hippocampus and entorhinal cortex. For graphics details, see Fig. 1

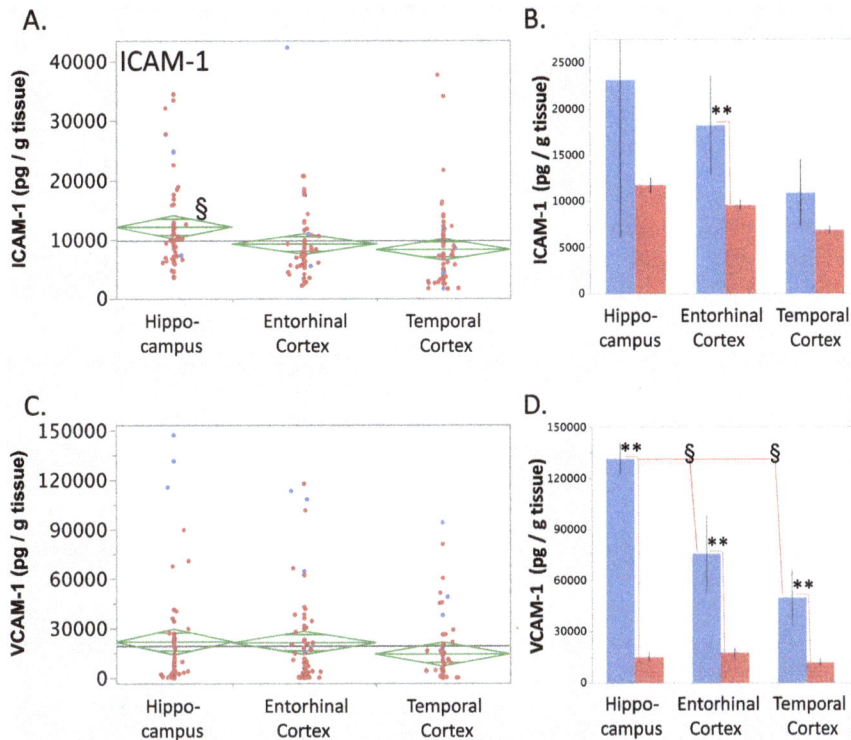

Fig. 6 **a**, **b** ICAM-1 and (**c**, **d**) VCAM-1 levels in the human brain. **a** ICAM-1 levels were higher in the hippocampus than in the entorhinal or temporal cortex (brain region repeated measures MANOVA $p < 0.0007$, $p < 0.03$ Tukey's HSD). **b** In nonepileptic cases, the entorhinal cortex ICAM-1 levels were higher than in the epileptic cases (epilepsy × brain region MANOVA $p < 0.0007$, $p < 0.001$ Tukey's HSD). **c** VCAM-1 levels showed no brain region-specific differences over all cases. **d** VCAM-1 levels were higher in nonepileptic cases in all three regions (*dashed lines*, epilepsy × brain region interaction $p < 0.0001$). In the nonepileptic hippocampus, VCAM-1 levels were elevated compared with other brain regions (*solid lines*, $p < 0.05$ Tukey's HSD). For graphics details, see Fig. 1. **$p < 0.001$, §$p < 0.05$, post hoc Tukey's HSD

Secondary analyses

Secondary independent variables were also considered in the analyses of these brain mediator levels. Differences based upon gender, side of the brain resected, epilepsy duration, age at surgery, presumptive epilepsy risk factors, surgical electrode placement prior to resection ("phase 2"), and Engel outcome classifications were evaluated. Moreover, pathology and imaging findings were also investigated as potential covariates.

Gender, side of brain, and epilepsy duration

None of the mediator levels differed with respect to patient gender, side of the brain affected, or time since seizure onset.

Age at surgery (years)

Age at surgery was a significant predictor only for the hippocampal VCAM-1 (linear regression, $R^2 = 0.340$, $p < 0.02$) and IL-8 ($R^2 = 0.294$, $p < 0.05$), both increasing with age (Additional file 2: Figure S4A).

These findings brought into question the observed brain region- and epilepsy-related differences. For VCAM-1, a difference of 26 years in the mean age between epileptic

and nonepileptic groups yielded a difference of 39,650 pg/g tissue in the hippocampal VCAM-1 levels, according to the predicted VCAM-1 vs. age fit line (Additional file 2: Figure S4A). Nevertheless, the difference in the hippocampal VCAM-1 levels between nonepileptic and epileptic cases was over 200 % of this value (Table 4, Fig. 6d). Brain region × epilepsy × age interactions were significant (three-way ANOVA main effect $p < 0.0001$, triple interaction $p = 0.013$). Thus, age- and epilepsy-related differences were confirmed for the hippocampal VCAM-1 levels. Interestingly, although no other brain region showed a significant correlation between VCAM-1 and age, the entorhinal cortex exhibited ~150 % and the temporal cortex ~95 % of the predicted differences between nonepileptic and epileptic cases according to the hippocampal VCAM-1 vs. age fit line.

The findings for IL-8 differences were also supportive of epilepsy-related differences in the hippocampus. Whereas the nonepileptic hippocampal IL-8 levels were 300 % for those expected by age alone (according to the predicted IL-8 vs. age fit line, Additional file 2: Figure S4A), the entorhinal and temporal cortical levels were closer to predicted age-related levels (88 and –53 %, respectively). Finally, analyses of epilepsy status × age for each brain region showed significant effects for IL-8 levels only in the hippocampus (main effect $p < 0.0001$, epilepsy effect $p = 0.0002$, age effect $p = 0.554$, interaction $p = 0.642$).

Epilepsy risk factors

Previously identified epilepsy risk factor(s), presumed to have contributed to patients' recurrent seizures (Table 2), were analyzed to find associations with inflammation-related mediators in the brain. Other than the expected brain region differences (brain region × epilepsy risk factor ANOVAs), several risk factor associations appeared significant.

Multivariate screening analyses revealed that high VEGF levels in the hippocampus were associated with mild closed head injury (mCHI); elevated IP-10 and IL-12/23 p40 levels in the entorhinal cortex were associated with the infection risk factor (Additional file 2: Figure S4B). No temporal cortical mediator differences showed significant associations with any presumptive epilepsy risk factor(s). Univariate analyses suggested several other associations. Overall IL-1α levels were higher in the infection subgroup compared to CHI or febrile risk factor subgroups; overall IL-6 levels were higher in the CHI subgroup compared to the febrile subgroup; and overall MIP-1β levels were higher in the mCHI subgroup compared to the

developmental, infection, febrile, or lesional risk factor subgroups (Additional file 2: Figure S4B).

Phase 2 electrode placement

Several associations emerged between the mediators assayed and prior placement of intracranial surface electrodes for localization of epileptogenic foci. Cases that had electrode placement prior to resection ($n = 31$) exhibited higher levels of eotaxin, IL-1α, MCP-1, MCP-4, CRP, and ICAM-1 over all brain regions combined and, specifically, in both cortical regions (Additional file 2: Table S4I). There were no mediator level differences noted in the hippocampus, which might suggest that electrode placement had minimal effect on nonadjacent brain structures.

Engel classification

Using a modified Engel classification score (Table 1), several mediators appeared to be associated with Engel outcome subgroups. The majority of associations observed were between the nonepileptic group and the epileptic subgroups; these differences were not described here because they were reported above. Such differences may reflect less on outcome after surgery and more on neurophysiologic differences between nonepileptic and epileptic cases. There were, nonetheless, several instances of differences between Engel subgroups (Fig. 7, brain

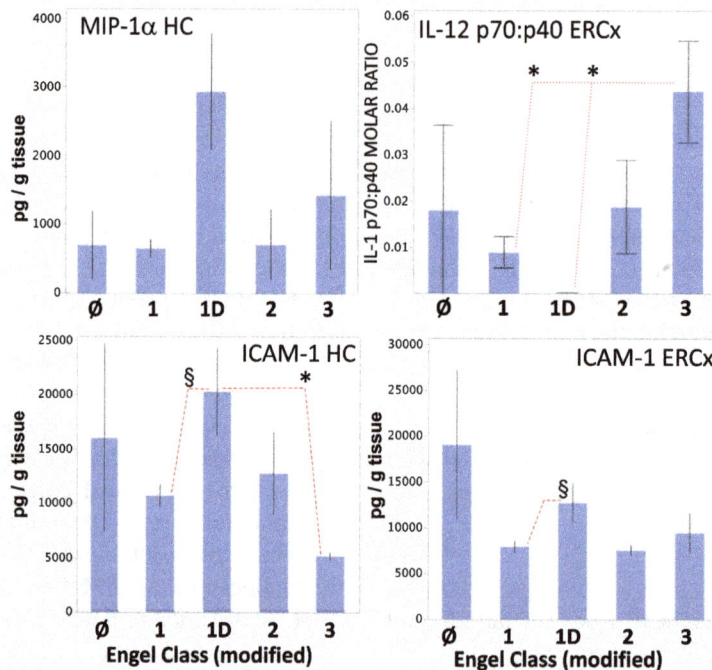

Fig. 7 Differences in selected mediator levels correlated with a modified Engel outcome scale. Engel classifications were simplified to 1A, 1D, "2," and "3" (see Table 1, classifications 1A, 1D, 2A - 2D and 3A, respectively). The nonepileptic group is represented by "Ø". *HC* hippocampus, *ERCx* entorhinal cortex, *TCx* temporal cortex. *Dashed lines* show epileptic subgroup differences, **$p < 0.001$, *$p \leq 0.01$, §$p < 0.05$ Tukey's HSD vs. subgroups indicated

region × modified Engel main effects $p \leq 0.002$). Hippocampal MIP-1α and ICAM-1 levels were greater in the Engel - 1D subgroup than those in the Engel-1A subgroup (Fig. 7, top row; Engel effect $p = 0.0060$ and $p = 0.0412$, respectively, $p \leq 0.02$ Tukey's HSD). The same is held for ICAM-1 in the entorhinal cortex (brain region × modified Engel interaction $p = 0.0213$, $p < 0.05$ Tukey's HSD). In the temporal cortex, MCP-4 levels were increased in the Engel-2 subgroup compared with those in better outcome Engel-1A and -1D subgroups (Fig. 7, bottom row, left; brain region × modified Engel interaction $p = 0.0091$, $p < 0.01$ and $p < 0.04$ Tukey's HSD, respectively). In addition, the molar ratio of IL-12 p70 (bioactive IL-12) to its p40 subunit was increased in the worst outcome (Engel-3) subgroup, compared to those in both the Engel-1A and -1D subgroups (Fig. 7, bottom row, right; brain region × modified Engel interaction $p = 0.0280$, $p < 0.05$ Tukey's HSD).

Pathology and imaging reports
Of the 55 cases with pathology and imaging report data, 84 % had observed hippocampal pathology, with two thirds of these showing hippocampal sclerosis. Of the 55 cases, 44 % showed cortical pathology. Interestingly, 56 % had hippocampal with no cortical findings, but only 15 % had cortical with no hippocampal findings.

An analysis was performed to interrogate differences of inflammatory-related mediator levels with respect to neuropathological findings (hippocampus only, cortex only, or both). The phase 2 status was considered salient to this analysis because half the cases underwent prior surface electrode placement. Phase 2 status was taken into account using two-way ANOVAs. Both pathology and MRI reports were tested separately with the following results. Cases in which both the hippocampal and cortical abnormalities were reported by the pathologist showed significantly ($p < 0.05$ Tukey's HSD) increased levels of MIP-1α (hippocampus), IL-17A (temporal cortex), and ICAM-1 (temporal cortex). MIP-1α and ICAM-1 results were complicated by significant interaction between neuropathologic findings and phase 2 status (phase 2[+] cases had higher levels). The IL-17A finding appeared more robust, as MR imaging showing abnormalities in both regions was also associated with increased IL-17A levels in the temporal cortex. In addition, MR imaging abnormalities in both regions were associated with elevated levels of TARC (entorhinal cortex) and IP-10 (temporal cortex).

Cases in which only the hippocampal abnormalities were reported by the pathologist were associated with increased IL-1α levels (entorhinal cortex), and a trend ($p \approx 0.05$) was noted in the MR imaging-evident hippocampus-only analysis as well. Thus, abnormal findings in both the cortex and hippocampus may be associated with increased proinflammatory mediator levels such as IL-17A and IP-10 in the temporal cortex or IL-1α and TARC in the entorhinal cortex. Involvement of the hippocampus only may be associated with increased IL-1α levels in the entorhinal cortex. Intriguingly, no mediator differences were observed in cases with pathology or MR abnormalities in the cortex only.

Mediator-to-mediator correlations
Another approach to understanding brain inflammatory regulation is to identify groups of mediators with associated expression profiles. Robust mediator-to-mediator associations were observed in 141 pairwise comparisons across the hippocampus, entorhinal cortex, and temporal cortex ($p < 0.0001$, see "Methods" section). These correlations (Additional file 2: Figure S4C) were distributed rather evenly, with each brain region having approximately one third of the associations. Of the 141, 70 % were between different mediators within a single brain region, 24 % were between different mediators in different brain regions, and 6 % were individual mediators between different brain regions. Only two negative correlations were observed between region-specific mediators. The hippocampal CRP and IL-12 p70 levels were inversely associated, and the entorhinal cortex TNF-α levels were inversely associated with hippocampal TNF-β levels.

Of the correlations of different mediators within a single brain region, half were in the temporal cortex and one quarter each were in the hippocampus and entorhinal cortex. For correlations of different mediators in different regions, 57 % were between the hippocampus and temporal cortex, 36 % were between the hippocampus and entorhinal cortex, and 7 % were between the entorhinal and temporal cortices. These proportions may suggest differential control of inflammation-related mediator levels within/between these regions.

Individual mediator levels that correlated between different brain regions were as follows: VCAM-1 levels correlated between all three brain regions; MCP-1, IL-1α, IL-2, and VEGF levels correlated between the entorhinal and temporal cortices; ICAM-1 levels between the hippocampus and entorhinal cortex; as well as IP-10 levels between the hippocampus and temporal cortex. These interregional associations indicate predominantly extrinsic (i.e., cerebral or systemic) control of these brain mediator levels.

Interestingly, of the 141 mediator-to-mediator correlations observed in these three brain regions, the majority (78 %) were accounted for by eight mediators, namely, eotaxin (22), ICAM-1 (17), MCP-1 (16), IL-4 (14), IL-6 (14), IL-8 (11), MIP-1α (9), and VCAM-1 (8). This observation implies a hierarchical dynamic in which mediators with multiple correlations may regulate, directly or indirectly, the levels of other mediators.

Conversely, there were several mediators that had three or fewer correlations with mediators in any other tissue (Additional file 2: Figure S4C, bottom). These included GM-CSF and IFN-γ, for which most tissue values were below the level of detection, IL-1α and VEGF which were self-correlated between the temporal and entorhinal cortices, as well as TNF-β. Moreover, in specific brain regions, a few mediators had zero or one correlation with other mediators.

Blood mediator levels vs. brain tissue content

Although usually considered intravascular mediators, cytokines and chemokines in CSF and, by inference, in the central nervous system (CNS) may be more concentrated than those found in the systemic circulation. For example, during the first 10 days after severe head trauma, patient CSF levels of IL-6 and TNF-α (but not CRP) were greater than in the blood [34]. Also, at least in lupus patients, MCP-1 and GM-CSF were present at much higher levels in neural tissue than in the serum [35]. In epilepsy patients, there were clear transients of leukocyte and mediator changes immediately postictally [19] leaving open the question as to whether there were transient changes in the brain or at the site(s) of epileptogenesis.

In order to rule out brain mediator content in the present study being entirely due to blood levels, brain levels were compared with published blood levels (Additional file 2: Table S4J–K) and potential differences were identified. Not only were median MCP-1 levels in the brain greater than in peripheral blood, but IP-10, MIP-1β, IL-1α, IL-8, IL-17A, VEGF, CRP, and ICAM-1 levels appeared to exceed maximal blood levels by two- to sixfold or more. In contrast, Yoshio et al. [35] found no differences between serum and CSF levels for IP-10 and IL-8 and greater levels in serum than CSF for MIP-1β, IL-17A, and VEGF (IL-1α, CRP, and ICAM-1 were not assayed). These comparisons would seem to reveal the existence of neural-based degradation mechanisms for these mediators.

Discussion
Mediator levels

Human epilepsy disorders exhibit peripheral cytokine changes that may originate at sites of neural dysfunction and contribute to seizure propagation (reviewed in [12]). Sinha et al. [15] analyzed serum IL-1β, IL-2, IL-4, IL-6, IFN-γ, or TNF-α detectability in 100 postictal patients and 100 healthy controls. None of the age- and sex-matched control subjects had detectable levels of any of these cytokines, whereas among epilepsy patients, the overall incidence was 74 %. Of the nine epilepsy patients who had a lumbar puncture, CSF levels of these cytokines were detectable in subject(s) with no serum levels.

Significantly, none of the subjects who were serum-positive for a cytokine were CSF-negative for that cytokine. Serum IL-6, IL-1β, TNF-α, and MIP-1α levels were elevated in AED-resistant epilepsy patients and, in patients undergoing resection of the epileptogenic region, IL-1β, TNF-α, and MIP-1α levels decreased after 8 weeks postoperatively [11]. These results implied that the epileptogenic brain tissue removed was either a direct or indirect source of these mediators. Until now, there has been a paucity of data on human brain tissue inflammation-related mediator levels [10].

In the current study, however, none of these mediators appeared to be elevated proximal to the site of epileptogenesis. In fact, IL-6, IL-1β, and MIP-1α levels were higher in the temporal cortex than in the hippocampus, and TNF-α showed no regional or epilepsy-related differences, though levels in entorhinal cortex may have been lower than either the hippocampus or temporal cortex (see Additional file 2: Figure S2S). If both studies are valid, and the patient samples represent the greater population, then it must be concluded that the resected tissue had been an indirect stimulus for production of these mediators in the blood.

Proinflammatory mediator levels were hypothesized to be higher in the hippocampus at the site of epileptogenesis. This was true for eotaxin, IFN-γ, IL-2, IL-4, IL-12 p70, IL-17A, TNF-α, and ICAM-1. Interestingly, Sinha et al. [15] found that blood levels of most of these were more detectable in epilepsy patients than in age-matched controls. Eotaxin (CCL11) recruits eosinophils by activating their CCR3 receptors. CCL11 transport across the blood-brain barrier (BBB) resulted in region-specific alterations of eotaxin brain levels [36] and age-related increases in humans have been implicated in cognitive decline in a novel mouse model [37]. IFN-γ, an important activator of macrophages and inducer of major histocompatibility class II immune/inflammatory activities, is associated with a number of autoinflammatory and autoimmune diseases. Its brain levels were virtually undetectable except in 10/49 hippocampus specimens exclusively from epileptic cases. IL-17A, also highest in the hippocampus, has synergistic effects with IFN-γ, IL-1, and TNF-α, acting as a proinflammatory mediator not unlike IFN-γ [38]. TNF-α levels were among the lowest measured in this study (Additional file 2: Table S3B). Some variability in the convulsive effect of TNF-α has been noted previously and its relatively reduced levels in the entorhinal cortex may attest to this variability. The proconvulsive effect may be concentration-dependent, as with its role in *Shigella dysenteriae*-related seizures at low concentrations and an anticonvulsive role at high concentrations [39]. Lower picomolar concentrations may preferentially affect the p55 receptor pathway, increasing synaptic activity [40], and promoting epileptogenicity in the longer term. ICAM-1 signaling is proinflammatory via recruitment of macrophages and leukocytes across the BBB [22, 41]. In a mouse model of mTLE, ICAM-1 levels were locally induced in the hippocampus [22].

Neurosurgical resection of the epileptic focus significantly reduced elevated blood levels of IL-1β, TNF-α, and MIP-1α in mTLE patients [11]. TNF-α levels were highest in the hippocampus, consistent with the implications of prior findings. However, brain levels of IL-1β and MIP-1α were lower in the hippocampus compared to the temporal cortex. Moreover, none of these mediators showed any epilepsy-associated increases, as might have been predicted from that study [11].

MIP-1α, IL-β, and IL-8 levels were highest in the temporal cortex. MIP-1α belongs to the C–C chemokine family (CCL3) and is involved in the recruitment and activation of macrophages, monocytes, and neutrophils. IL-8 (CXCL8) functions in inflammatory cell chemotaxis and phagocytosis, as well as angiogenesis. IL-8 has also been postulated, through NF-kB- and TNF-α-related mechanisms, to contribute to local inflammatory mechanisms in response to oxidative insults [42]. IL-β and IL-α showed graded levels with cortical levels exceeding those in the hippocampus. IL-1β is involved in a plethora of inflammatory activities, including the induction of many other proinflammatory mediators; the induction of cyclooxygenase-2 (PTGS2) by this cytokine in the CNS is just one response to inflammation. IL-1β secreted by hypoxic astrocytes upregulated MCP-1 and ICAM-1 levels that are thought to play a crucial role in leukocyte recruitment [43]. IL-α also mediates numerous inflammation-related activities, including TNF induction. Both are acute-phase cytokines that operate in the picomolar-femtomolar range. MIP-1β, which acts as a chemoattractant for natural killer cells, monocytes, and other immune cells, was also greater in the temporal cortex than in the entorhinal cortex.

Intriguingly, CRP levels were lower in the temporal cortex than in the hippocampus or entorhinal cortex. As a well-documented inflammatory biomarker, its levels follow those of proinflammatory cytokines; this may reflect an increased inflammatory load proximal to the site(s) of epileptogenesis. Paradoxically, IL-10, an anti-inflammatory cytokine, was found at higher levels in the hippocampus than in the entorhinal cortex but not significantly different from temporal cortical levels.

In the entorhinal cortex, IL-α and TNF-β levels were highest, compared to the hippocampus and temporal cortex. TNF-β (aka lymphotoxin alpha) is a highly inducible, cell surface molecule that mediates a variety of inflammatory responses, as well as apoptotic cell death.

Findings of neuroanatomic mediator level differences suggest brain-specific regulation; however, these might be confounded by blood levels, with brain tissue levels reflecting only differences in vascularization. If true, it could be expected that more vascularized brain tissue would regularly demonstrate higher mediator levels, but this was not the case. Moreover, a review of the recent literature on blood and CSF inflammatory mediator levels indicated, at least for many mediators, that individual CSF levels were greater than blood levels [35, 44, 45]. In comparing brain tissue levels in this study with consensus blood levels from multiple studies (Additional file 2: Table S4J, K), median brain levels exceeded median blood levels for IP-10 (~threefold), MCP-1 (~fourfold), MIP-1β (~threefold), IL-8 (~fivefold), IL-17A (~fourfold), VEGF (~threefold), CRP (>tenfold), and ICAM-1 (~sixfold). Thus, the neuroanatomic differences observed were likely due to brain-related regulatory mechanisms rather than contamination from the blood or CSF.

Epilepsy-related differences

Differences in inflammation-related mediators between epileptic and nonepileptic subjects were further hypothesized to suggest some significance for AED-resistant epileptogenicity. Caution must be taken when comparing these epilepsy cases with nonepilepsy cases as the nonepileptic subjects were (i) emergent neurosurgical patients and not healthy controls, (ii) comprised only four cases, and (iii) had an age distribution (64.5 ± 6.3) different from that of the epileptic group (38.5 ± 1.5)(nonetheless, there was no instance where an epilepsy-related difference could be fully explained by the age difference). Moreover, no data were available regarding circulating AED levels (or other medications) at the time of surgery for these cases, so confounding influences on mediator levels due to drug effects cannot be ruled out.

Eotaxin levels were lower in epilepsy specimens overall and particularly in the entorhinal cortex. Interestingly, phase 2 patients appeared to have higher eotaxin levels than cases without prior electrode placement. Higher levels in the hippocampus would suggest eotaxin is involved in both acute (nonepileptic) and chronic (epileptic) neuroinflammation. Although IP-10 levels were also reduced in the entorhinal cortex of epilepsy cases, this finding is suspect due to several high nonoutlier values in the nonepileptic group.

Proinflammatory cytokines IL-1β and IL-6 were higher in the nonepileptic cases. Both are acutely upregulated, so it is likely the emergent conditions warranting neurosurgical intervention contributed to the elevations. It is interesting to note that, for both mediators, the primary region of increase was in the hippocampus, suggesting that local control of these cytokines dominated, perhaps in the early phase of neuroinflammation.

Epileptic brain exhibited higher levels of IL-12 p70 overall; most of the nonepileptic specimens had no measurable levels. IL-12 p70 was also elevated in the cerebral cortex of pediatric epilepsy patients, compared to nonepileptic controls [46]. The ratio of bioactive IL-12 p70 (p40:p35 heterodimer) to its p40 subunit appeared elevated both in the hippocampus and temporal cortex, indicating a more active IL-12 in these regions relative to the entorhinal cortex. IL-12/23 p40 levels were much greater than IL-12 p70 levels (Additional file 2: Table S3B), indicating that the manifestation of IL-12 bioactivity would be more dependent upon p35 subunit availability and/or the rate of heterodimer formation. In the periphery, IL-12 p70 stimulates T cell proliferation and differentiation, as well as natural killer cell activation. It also promotes induction of IFN-γ and TNF-α in T cells, through which it may block the formation of new blood vessels. Elevated brain IL-12 p70 in epileptics may be associated with transient leukocyte changes observed postictally, manifested by increased lymphocytes, neutrophils, NK cells, and NK-like T cells, with decreased T cells and CD4$^+$/CD8$^+$ ratios [19]. These peripheral changes were all resolved by 24 h postictally. Elevated IL-12 p70 may also relate to alterations in specific blood cytokines and leukocyte numbers in adult epileptics that were differentially ameliorated by various AEDs [13].

Vascular mediators CRP, ICAM-1, and VCAM-1 all showed epilepsy-related differences. Epileptic CRP levels were about half those of nonepileptics in the hippocampus and temporal cortex and 63 % in the entorhinal cortex. This was likely due to the emergent medical condition(s) of the nonepileptic cases. Unexpectedly, epileptic ICAM-1 levels in the entorhinal cortex were about half those of nonepileptic cases. Interestingly, blood levels of ICAM-5, a related gene located predominantly on neural cells, were ~fivefold lower in a group of epileptic patients than in age-matched controls [47]. ICAMs are endothelial-, leukocyte-, and tissue-associated proteins important in cell-cell adhesion and leukocyte extravasation [41, 48]. In this study, ICAM-1 levels were highest in the hippocampus, particularly among the epilepsy cases. Conversely, VCAM-1 levels were much lower in the epileptic cases across all three brain regions (11 % in the hippocampus, 23 % in the entorhinal cortex, 24 % in the temporal cortex). Moreover, the regional VCAM-1 differences noted in the nonepileptic cases were not apparent in the larger group of epileptic cases. While nonepileptic cases comprised a very small, nonage-matched sample, this might have implications for epilepsy-related changes in hippocampal VCAM-1. Not much is known about the contribution of human VCAM-1 to neuroinflammation, though its levels increased acutely in the blood and CSF after brain injuries [49, 50]. Again, the emergent nature of the nonepileptic cases might explain these differences.

Though the epilepsy-related differences will require further investigation to corroborate, several other notable findings were derived from these results. Distinct regional levels of inflammation-related mediators likely have significance in neuroinflammatory physiology. For example, correlations of mediator levels within and between individual brain regions reveal the influences of intrinsic and extrinsic controls on neuroinflammatory regulation. These are summarized below.

Mediator-to-mediator correlations

Of the inflammation-related mediators with significant correlation(s), 70 % were with other mediators within a single brain region. Intraregional correlations support the notion of local control of multiple mediators, whereas correlations between different brain regions support more external mechanisms. Half of the observed correlations within a single brain region were in the temporal cortex, suggesting greater local regulatory mechanisms, compared to those of the hippocampus and entorhinal cortex.

Correlations of different mediators in different regions suggested more external control mechanisms (e.g., by diffusible factors or distributed neural cell inputs). Over 90 % of these types of correlations were between the hippocampus and the cortical brain regions (temporal cortex, 57 %; entorhinal cortex, 36 %). Only 7 % of interregional correlations of different mediators were between the entorhinal and temporal cortices. Although it cannot be known from these data in which direction controls may be exerted, the preponderance of hippocampal involvement along with their neuroanatomical relationships suggest a focus of hippocampal control of inflammation-related mediator levels between these regions.

Only IL-1α, IP-10, MCP-1, IL-2, VEGF, ICAM-1, and VCAM-1 levels were correlated between different brain regions. Of these, except for VCAM-1, tissue level differences were observed. IL-1α was greatest in the entorhinal cortex and diminished from the temporal cortex to the hippocampus; IP-10 was also lowest in the hippocampus, whereas MCP-1 was greater in the hippocampus and temporal cortex than in the entorhinal cortex; and IL-2, VEGF, and ICAM-1 were higher in the hippocampus than in both cortical regions. Thus, individual mediators showing tissue level differences *and* interregional correlations suggest the existence of common, external regulatory mechanisms with local gain controls.

Functional implications

Systemic inflammatory cells, as well as activated intrinsic neuroinflammatory cells, likely contribute to neurochemical and neurophysiologic dysfunction in the affected brain regions. Inflammatory mediators produced by both types of cells can uniquely affect the brain, with little or no manifestation in the periphery [23]. It has been proposed that glial cells establish a cytokine/chemokine network in the ischemic brain—"activated microglia produce... various types of cytokines... which activate astrocytes to synthesize chemokines.... Chemokines in turn activate and/or recruit microglial cells in the injured site" [43]. Cytokines IL-1 and TNF-α, as well as chemokines MCP-1, RANTES, and IL-8 were implicated in these networks [43].

Interestingly, the majority (110/141) of mediator-to-mediator associations observed in this study were accounted for by only eight mediators, namely, eotaxin (22), ICAM-1 (17), MCP-1 (16), IL-4 (14), IL-6 (14), IL-8 (11), MIP-1α (9), and VCAM-1 (8). This observation implies a hierarchical dynamic in which mediators with multiple correlations may regulate, directly or indirectly, the levels of other mediators. These could be one basis of neuroinflammatory functional networks.

Conclusions

Both brain region-specific and epilepsy-associated differences in inflammation-related mediator levels were detected. The hippocampus had the majority of regional increases. Correlations in mediator levels within and between brain regions indicated local and global regulation, respectively. The hippocampus showed the majority of interregional associations, suggesting a focus of inflammatory control between these regions. Thus, it would be important to further characterize the range of inflammation-related mediator levels in the normal brain and in neurologic disorders like epilepsy, with recognized inflammatory components. Finally, further characterization of differences between epilepsies and patient responses to medications would clarify whether AED-resistant seizures resulted from underlying differences in the inflammatory status of the affected brain regions.

Abbreviations

AED: Antiepileptic drug; ANOVA: Analysis of variance; BBB: Blood-brain barrier; CHI: Moderate-to-severe closed head injury; CNS: Central nervous system; CRP: C-reactive protein; CSF: Cerebral spinal fluid; EDTA: Ethylenediaminetetraacetic acid; ERCx: Entorhinal cortex; GM-CSF: Granulocyte-macrophage colony-stimulating factor; HC: Hippocampus; ICAM: Intercellular adhesion molecule; IFN: Interferon; IL: Interleukin; IP-10: Interferon gamma-induced protein 10; LLOD: Lower limit of detection; LLOQ: Lower limit of quantification; MANOVA: Multiple analyses of variance; mCHI: Mild closed head injury; MCP: Monocyte chemoattractant protein; MIP: Macrophage inflammatory protein; MSD: Meso Scale Discovery Corp.; mTLE: Mesial temporal lobe epilepsy; n.s.d.: Not significantly different; SEM: Standard error of the mean; TARC: Thymus- and activation-regulated chemokine; TNF: Tumor necrosis factor; Tukey's HSD: Tukey's honest significant difference test, the Tukey-Kramer method; VCAM: Vascular cell adhesion molecule; VEGF: Vascular endothelial growth factor

Acknowledgements

This work was supported through the Seed Grant program of The American Epilepsy Society. The authors wish to express appreciation for excellent technical assistance provided by Adam Driscoll and Erik Olsen, to Dr. Lena Brundin for use of the MSD Sector 6000 plate reader used in these studies and to the MSD support group.

Funding

This work was supported, in part, by the Seed Grant program of The American Epilepsy Society (AES). The AES had no role in the design of the study and collection, analysis, and interpretation of data or in writing the manuscript.

Authors' contributions

KIS designed and performed all the biochemical aspects of the study, analyzed the data, wrote the draft manuscript, and edited the manuscript. KVE originated the concept, designed all the clinical and surgical components of the study, contributed to the manuscript content, and edited the manuscript. Both authors read and approved the final manuscript.

Competing interest

The authors declare that they have no competing interests.

Ethics approval and consent to participate

This study was undertaken through an institutional review board approved process at the Henry Ford Health System (Detroit, MI USA) where the harvest of tissues took place between 2002 and 2008.
Subsequent analyses took place at the Spectrum Health System and Michigan State University (Grand Rapids, MI USA) and were exempted from further IRB approval (see IRB statement below).
"It was determined that the proposed activity is research but is *not* considered to be human subject research because it does not meet the definition of human subjects as defined by DHHS and FDA regulations. Specifically, there will be no intervention or interaction with human subjects or use of their data that is private and identifiable." SH IRB#: 2012-262.

Author details

[1]College of Human Medicine, Michigan State University, 333 Bostwick Ave NE, Grand Rapids, MI, USA. [2]Department of Clinical Neurosciences, Spectrum Health System, Grand Rapids, MI, USA. [3]Division of Neurosurgery, Michigan State University, East Lansing, USA.

References

1. England MJ, Liverman CT, Schultz AM, Strawbridge LM. Summary: a reprint from epilepsy across the spectrum: promoting health and understanding. Epilepsy Curr. 2012;12(6):245–53.
2. Kohrman MH. What is epilepsy? Clinical perspectives in the diagnosis and treatment. J Clin Neurophysiol. 2007;24(2):87–95.
3. Engel Jr J. Surgery for seizures. N Engl J Med. 1996;334(10):647–52.
4. Marchi N, Angelov L, Masaryk T, Fazio V, Granata T, Hernandez N, Hallene K, Diglaw T, Franic L, Najm I, et al. Seizure-promoting effect of blood-brain barrier disruption. Epilepsia. 2007;48(4):732–42.
5. Oby E, Janigro D. The blood-brain barrier and epilepsy. Epilepsia. 2006; 47(11):1761–74.
6. Vezzani A, Granata T. Brain inflammation in epilepsy: experimental and clinical evidence. Epilepsia. 2005;46(11):1724–43.
7. Bazan NG, Birkle DL, Tang W, Reddy TS. The accumulation of free arachidonic acid, diacylglycerols, prostaglandins, and lipoxygenase reaction products in the brain during experimental epilepsy. Adv Neurol. 1986;44:879–902.
8. De Simoni MG, Perego C, Ravizza T, Moneta D, Conti M, Marchesi F, De Luigi A, Garattini S, Vezzani A. Inflammatory cytokines and related genes are induced in the rat hippocampus by limbic status epilepticus. Eur J Neurosci. 2000;12(7):2623–33.
9. Christensen KV, Leffers H, Watson WP, Sanchez C, Kallunki P, Egebjerg J. Levetiracetam attenuates hippocampal expression of synaptic plasticity-related immediate early and late response genes in amygdala-kindled rats. BMC Neurosci. 2010;11:9.
10. Vezzani A. Epilepsy and inflammation in the brain: overview and pathophysiology. Epilepsy Curr. 2014;14(1 Suppl):3–7.
11. Quirico-Santos T, Meira ID, Gomes AC, Pereira VC, Pinto M, Monteiro M, Souza JM, Alves-Leon SV. Resection of the epileptogenic lesion abolishes seizures and reduces inflammatory cytokines of patients with temporal lobe epilepsy. J Neuroimmunol. 2013;254(1-2):125–30.
12. Li G, Bauer S, Nowak M, Norwood B, Tackenberg B, Rosenow F, Knake S, Oertel WH, Hamer HM. Cytokines and epilepsy. Seizure. 2011;20(3):249–56.
13. Nowak M, Bauer S, Haag A, Cepok S, Todorova-Rudolph A, Tackenberg B, Norwood B, Oertel WH, Rosenow F, Hemmer B, et al. Interictal alterations of cytokines and leukocytes in patients with active epilepsy. Brain Behav Immun. 2011;25(3):423–8.

14. Lehtimaki KA, Liimatainen S, Peltola J, Arvio M. The serum level of interleukin-6 in patients with intellectual disability and refractory epilepsy. Epilepsy Res. 2011;95(1-2):184–7.

15. Sinha S, Patil SA, Jayalekshmy V, Satishchandra P. Do cytokines have any role in epilepsy? Epilepsy Res. 2008;82(2-3):171–6.

16. Billiau AD, Witters P, Ceulemans B, Kasran A, Wouters C, Lagae L. Intravenous immunoglobulins in refractory childhood-onset epilepsy: effects on seizure frequency, EEG activity, and cerebrospinal fluid cytokine profile. Epilepsia. 2007;48(9):1739–49.

17. Lehtimaki KA, Keranen T, Palmio J, Makinen R, Hurme M, Honkaniemi J, Peltola J. Increased plasma levels of cytokines after seizures in localization-related epilepsy. Acta Neurol Scand. 2007;116(4):226–30.

18. Fabene PF, Bramanti P, Constantin G. The emerging role for chemokines in epilepsy. J Neuroimmunol. 2010;224(1-2):22–7.

19. Bauer S, Koller M, Cepok S, Todorova-Rudolph A, Nowak M, Nockher WA, Lorenz R, Tackenberg B, Oertel WH, Rosenow F, et al. NK and CD4+ T cell changes in blood after seizures in temporal lobe epilepsy. Exp Neurol. 2008;211(2):370–7.

20. Pacifici R, Paris L, Di Carlo S, Bacosi A, Pichini S, Zuccaro P. Cytokine production in blood mononuclear cells from epileptic patients. Epilepsia. 1995;36(4):384–7.

21. Eeg-Olofsson O, Prchal JF, Andermann F. Abnormalities of T-lymphocyte subsets in epileptic patients. Acta Neurol Scand. 1985;72(2):140–4.

22. Zattoni M, Mura ML, Deprez F, Schwendener RA, Engelhardt B, Frei K, Fritschy JM. Brain infiltration of leukocytes contributes to the pathophysiology of temporal lobe epilepsy. J Neurosci. 2011;31(11):4037–50.

23. Shafer LL, McNulty JA, Young MR. Brain activation of monocyte lineage cells: brain-derived soluble factors differentially regulate BV2 microglia and peripheral macrophage immune functions. Neuroimmunomodulation. 2002;10(5):283–94.

24. Lenzlinger PM, Hans VH, Joller-Jemelka HI, Trentz O, Morganti-Kossmann MC, Kossmann T. Markers for cell-mediated immune response are elevated in cerebrospinal fluid and serum after severe traumatic brain injury in humans. J Neurotrauma. 2001;18(5):479–89.

25. Hirschberg DL, Moalem G, He J, Mor F, Cohen IR, Schwartz M. Accumulation of passively transferred primed T cells independently of their antigen specificity following central nervous system trauma. J Neuroimmunol. 1998;89(1-2):88–96.

26. Holmin S, Soderlund J, Biberfeld P, Mathiesen T. Intracerebral inflammation after human brain contusion. Neurosurgery. 1998;42(2):291–8. discussion 298-299.

27. Vezzani A, Ravizza T, Balosso S, Aronica E. Glia as a source of cytokines: implications for neuronal excitability and survival. Epilepsia. 2008;49 Suppl 2:24–32.

28. Ravizza T, Gagliardi B, Noe F, Boer K, Aronica E, Vezzani A. Innate and adaptive immunity during epileptogenesis and spontaneous seizures: evidence from experimental models and human temporal lobe epilepsy. Neurobiol Dis. 2008;29(1):142–60.

29. Alapirtti T, Rinta S, Hulkkonen J, Makinen R, Keranen T, Peltola J. Interleukin-6, interleukin-1 receptor antagonist and interleukin-1beta production in patients with focal epilepsy: a video-EEG study. J Neurol Sci. 2009;280(1-2):94–7.

30. de Jong EK, Dijkstra IM, Hensens M, Brouwer N, van Amerongen M, Liem RS, Boddeke HW, Biber K. Vesicle-mediated transport and release of CCL21 in endangered neurons: a possible explanation for microglia activation remote from a primary lesion. J Neurosci. 2005;25(33):7548–57.

31. Hartzfeld P, Elisevich K, Pace M, Smith B, Gutierrez JA. Characteristics and surgical outcomes for medial temporal post-traumatic epilepsy. Br J Neurosurg. 2008;22(2):224–30.

32. Gompertz RH. Specific gravity of the brain. J Physiol. 1902;27(6):459–62.

33. Rosner B. Percentage points for a generalized ESD many-outlier procedure. Technometrics. 1983;25:165–72.

34. Is M, Coskun A, Sanus GZ, Tanriverdi T, Kafadar AM, Hanimoglu H, Tanriover N, Gezen F, Uzan M. High-sensitivity C-reactive protein levels in cerebrospinal fluid and serum in severe head injury: relationship to tumor necrosis factor-alpha and interleukin-6. J Clin Neurosci. 2007;14(12):1163–71.

35. Yoshio T, Okamoto H, Kurasawa K, Dei Y, Hirohata S, Minota S. IL-6, IL-8, IP-10, MCP-1 and G-CSF are significantly increased in cerebrospinal fluid but not in sera of patients with central neuropsychiatric lupus erythematosus. Lupus. 2016;25(9):997–1003.

36. Erickson MA, Morofuji Y, Owen JB, Banks WA. Rapid transport of CCL11 across the blood-brain barrier: regional variation and importance of blood cells. J Pharmacol Exp Ther. 2014;349(3):497–507.

37. Villeda SA, Luo J, Mosher KI, Zou B, Britschgi M, Bieri G, Stan TM, Fainberg N, Ding Z, Eggel A, et al. The ageing systemic milieu negatively regulates neurogenesis and cognitive function. Nature. 2011;477(7362):90–4.

38. Sutton C, Brereton C, Keogh B, Mills KH, Lavelle EC. A crucial role for interleukin (IL)-1 in the induction of IL-17-producing T cells that mediate autoimmune encephalomyelitis. J Exp Med. 2006;203(7):1685–91.

39. Yuhas Y, Weizman A, Ashkenazi S. Bidirectional concentration-dependent effects of tumor necrosis factor alpha in Shigella dysenteriae-related seizures. Infect Immun. 2003;71(4):2288–91.

40. Stellwagen D, Malenka RC. Synaptic scaling mediated by glial TNF-alpha. Nature. 2006;440(7087):1054–9.

41. Etienne-Manneville S, Chaverot N, Strosberg AD, Couraud PO. ICAM-1-coupled signaling pathways in astrocytes converge to cyclic AMP response element-binding protein phosphorylation and TNF-alpha secretion. J Immunol. 1999;163(2):668–74.

42. Vlahopoulos S, Boldogh I, Casola A, Brasier AR. Nuclear factor-kappaB-dependent induction of interleukin-8 gene expression by tumor necrosis factor alpha: evidence for an antioxidant sensitive activating pathway distinct from nuclear translocation. Blood. 1999;94(6):1878–89.

43. Minami M, Katayama T, Satoh M. Brain cytokines and chemokines: roles in ischemic injury and pain. J Pharmacol Sci. 2006;100(5):461–70.

44. Ichiyama T, Suenaga N, Kajimoto M, Tohyama J, Isumi H, Kubota M, Mori M, Furukawa S. Serum and CSF levels of cytokines in acute encephalopathy following prolonged febrile seizures. Brain Dev. 2008;30(1):47–52.

45. Kothur K, Wienholt L, Brilot F, Dale RC. CSF cytokines/chemokines as biomarkers in neuroinflammatory CNS disorders: a systematic review. Cytokine. 2016;77:227–37.

46. Choi J, Nordli Jr DR, Alden TD, DiPatri Jr A, Laux L, Kelley K, Rosenow J, Schuele SU, Rajaram V, Koh S. Cellular injury and neuroinflammation in children with chronic intractable epilepsy. J Neuroinflammation. 2009;6:38.

47. Pollard JR, Eidelman O, Mueller GP, Dalgard CL, Crino PB, Anderson CT, Brand EJ, Burakgazi E, Ivaturi SK, Pollard HB. The TARC/sICAM5 ratio in patient plasma is a candidate biomarker for drug resistant epilepsy. Front Neurol. 2012;3:181.

48. Lyck R, Enzmann G. The physiological roles of ICAM-1 and ICAM-2 in neutrophil migration into tissues. Curr Opin Hematol. 2015;22(1):53–9.

49. Rhind SG, Crnko NT, Baker AJ, Morrison LJ, Shek PN, Scarpelini S, Rizoli SB. Prehospital resuscitation with hypertonic saline-dextran modulates inflammatory, coagulation and endothelial activation marker profiles in severe traumatic brain injured patients. J Neuroinflammation. 2010;7:5.

50. Whalen MJ, Carlos TM, Kochanek PM, Wisniewski SR, Bell MJ, Carcillo JA, Clark RS, DeKosky ST, Adelson PD. Soluble adhesion molecules in CSF are increased in children with severe head injury. J Neurotrauma. 1998; 15(10):777–87.

5

Overexpression of zinc-α2-glycoprotein suppressed seizures and seizure-related neuroflammation in pentylenetetrazol-kindled rats

Ying Liu[1†], Teng Wang[1†], Xi Liu[1], Yuetao Wen[2], Tao Xu[1], Xinyuan Yu[1], Xin Wei[1], Xueying Ding[1], Lijuan Mo[1], Maojia Yin[1], Xinjie Tan[1] and Lifen Chen[1*]

Abstract

Background: Zinc-α2-glycoprotein (ZAG) is a 42-kDa protein reported as an anti-inflammatory adipocytokine. Evidences from clinical and experimental studies revealed that brain inflammation plays important roles in epileptogenesis and seizure. Interestingly, closely relationship between ZAG and many important inflammatory mediators has been proven. Our previous study identified ZAG in neurons and found that ZAG is decreased in epilepsy and interacts with TGFβ and ERK. This study aimed to investigate the role of ZAG in seizure and explore its effect on seizure-related neuroinflammation.

Methods: We overexpressed *AZGP1* in the hippocampus of rats via adeno-associated virus vector injection and observed their seizure behavior and EEG after pentylenetetrazol (PTZ) kindling. The level of typical inflammation mediators including TNFα, IL-6, TGFβ, ERK, and ERK phosphorylation were determined.

Results: The overexpression of *AZGP1* reduced the seizure severity, prolonged the latency of kindling, and alleviated epileptiform discharges in EEG changes induced by PTZ. Overexpression of *AZGP1* also suppressed the expression of TNFα, IL-6, TGFβ, and ERK phosphorylaton in PTZ-kindled rats.

Conclusions: ZAG may inhibit TGFβ-mediated ERK phosphorylation and inhibit neuroinflammation mediated by TNFα and IL-6, suggesting ZAG may suppress seizure via inhibiting neuroinflammation. ZAG may be a potential and novel therapeutic target for epilepsy.

Keywords: Zinc-α2-glycoprotein, Epilepsy, Neuroinflammation, TNFα, IL-6, TGFβ

Background

Zinc-α2-glycoprotein (ZAG) is a 42-kDa, soluble, secretory protein encoded by the *AZGP1* gene located on chromosome 7q22.1 [1, 2]. The structure and amino acid sequence of ZAG are highly homologous to proteins in the major histocompatibility complex class I (MHC-I) family, which has important function in immunity [3]. In our previous study, we found that both ZAG protein and *AZGP1* mRNA levels were

* Correspondence: lifen_chen@163.com
[†]Equal contributors
[1]Department of Neurology, The Second Affiliated Hospital of Chongqing Medical University, 74 Linjiang Road, Yuzhong District, Chonqing 400010, China

significantly decreased in brain tissues of refractory TLE patients and pentylenetetrazol (PTZ)-kindled rats [4], but the role of ZAG in epilepsy and seizure is still unclear.

ZAG is known to be involved in many molecular pathways linked to epilepsy and seizure, and it can regulate many epilepsy- or siezure-related molecules, although its role has never been studied in epilepsy and/or seizure. *AZGP1* overexpression can inhibit the mammalian target of rapamycin (mTOR) pathway activity [5], and ZAG can inhibit transforming growth factor-β (TGFβ)-mediated vimentin expression and extracellular regulated protein kinase (ERK) phosphorylation [6]. Meanwhile, mTOR, TGFβ, ERK, and phosphorylated ERK (pERK) were known to play important roles in epilepsy and seizure. The mTOR pathway regulates various cellular processes involved in growth, metabolism, structure, and cell–cell interactions of neurons and glia [7]. Inhibiting mTOR by rapamycin can suppress seizure, delay seizure development, or prevent epileptogenesis [7]. Increase of TGFβ in neurons was proven to be involved in epileptogenesis via regulating dendrite growth and synaptogenesis [8, 9]. The level of pERK in refractory epilepsy patients is significantly higher than that in controls [10], indicating an increased ERK activity in epilepsy. Inhibiting sodium glucose co transporter 2 (SGLT2) has been proven to increase the level of ZAG via activating PPARγ [11], while activating PPARγ was confirmed to increase *AZGP1* mRNA [12]. Interestingly, both SGLT2 and PPARγ are known to participate in epileptogenesis, especially PPARγ was considered as a promising therapeutic target of epilepsy [13–15]. ZAG can also increase the level of mitochondrial uncoupling proteins (UCP) [16], and PPARγ-upregulated mitochondrial UCP2 expression can ameliorate neuronal death in the hippocampus following status epilepticus [17]. Interactions between ZAG and these epilepsy- or seizure-related molecules or pathways suggest a potential role of ZAG in epilepsy and/or seizure.

Evidences from clinical and experimental studies revealed that brain inflammation plays important roles in epileptogenesis [18]. ZAG was reported as one of the anti-inflammatory adipocytokines including adiponectin, omentin, SFRP5, vaspin, and interleukin-10 (IL-10) [19]. ZAG was reported to block transforming growth factor-β (TGFβ)-mediated extracellular regulated protein kinase (ERK) phosphorylation [7]. While TGFβ plays a significant role in inflammation, inhibition of TGFβ receptor 1 or TGFβ1 diminished TGFβ1-induced inflammation [20]. ERK pathway also plays an important role in the inflammatory response [21–24]. We have verified the interaction between ZAG and TGFβ or pERK previously [4]. Therefore, it is possible that ZAG may participate in the pathogenesis and pathophysiology of epilepsy via regulating TGFβ-mediated ERK phosphorylation. In addition, increase of various inflammation-related cytokines has been observed in epilepsy [25–27]. Proinflammatory cytokines, such as tumor-necrosis factor (TNFα) and interleukin-6 (IL-6), were increased in epilepsy patients and epilepsy models [28–32]. Interestingly, TNFα has been identified to reduce ZAG production [33], while the interaction between ZAG and IL-6 has not been found.

The role of ZAG in seizure and seizure-related inflammation has not yet been discussed. In this study, we injected adeno-associated virus (AAV) that overexpress *AZGP1* to the hippocampus of rats and investigated the effect of *AZGP1* overexpression on PTZ kindling-induced seizures in rats by behavior tests and scalp electroencephalogram. To further explore the molecular mechanism by which ZAG affects seizure and seizure-related inflammation, the effect of *AZGP1* overexpression on pERK, total ERK (tERK), TGFβ, TNFα, and IL-6 were also measured in the hippocampus of PTZ-kindled rats and controls.

Methods

Experimental animals

Adult, male, 200–300 g, specific-pathogen-free Sprague–Dawley rats (Experimental Animal Center of Chongqing Medical University) were raised in a temperature and humidity-controlled room (temperature 27 °C, humidity 55–65%) with a 12-h light/12-h dark cycle (lights on 6:00 and off 18:00), and they were allowed free access to food and water. All rats were housed for 1 week before the experiment.

Adeno-associated virus (AAV) vector construction and stereotaxic injections

A DNA sequence that amplifies *AZGP1* expression was incorporated into the adeno-associated virus (AAV) vector (pHBAAV-CMV-ZsGreen) containing green fluorescent protein (GFP) sequence and was named AAV–*AZGP1*. The same AAV vector containing only GFP was used as a control and named as AAV–GFP. Both vectors were manufactured by Hanbio Biotechnology (Shanghai, China). The final titer was 1.35×10^{12} vector genomes/ml for AAV–*AZGP1* and 1.5×10^{12} vector genomes/ml for AAV–GFP.

To verify the successful transfection of AAV, 60 rats were randomly divided into 4 groups and treated as following ($n = 15$ for each group): (1) controls: rats received stereotaxic injection of saline; (2) GFP group: rats received AAV–GFP injection; (3) *AZGP1*-3W group: rats received AAV–*AZGP1* injection and recovered for 3 weeks; (4) *AZGP1*-9W group: rats received AAV–*AZGP1* injection and recovered for 9 weeks. After injection, GFP fluorescence was observed in the hippocampus of rats from GFP group, *AZGP1*-3W group and *AZGP1*-9W group ($n = 5$ for each group) as described below. Quantitative real-time polymerase chain reaction (qrt-PCR) ($n = 5$ for each group) and western blot ($n = 5$ for each group) were also performed in controls, GFP group, *AZGP1*-3W group, and *AZGP1*-9W group as described below.

When performing stereotaxic injection, rats were anesthetized by intraperitoneal injections of pentobarbital (60 mg/kg) and then placed in a stereotaxia frame (RWD Life Science, Shenzhen, China). After disinfection, skin of the dorsal surface of rat skull was cut apart, and two parallel holes were created using dental drill in the skull. The stereotactic coordinates of bilateral hippocampus region were 3.0 mm posterior to bregma, 2.0 mm lateral to median line of the skull, and 2.8 mm deep beneath the skull. 4 μL AAV–*AZGP1* or AAV–GFP was injected into the hippocampus through a glass pipette at a speed of 0.2 μL/min. To prevent backflow of vectors, the pipette was kept in the hippocampus for an additional 5 min and then retracted steadily and slowly. For the controls, an equal volume of saline was injected in the same way. In most cases, the surgical procedure last about 45 min for each rat, and most rats recovered from anesthesia 1 h after surgery ending, subsequent injection of pentobarbital was not necessary in our experiment. Rarely, rats had respiratory failure after surgery was rescued using atropine (1 mg/kg, intraperitoneally).

PTZ kindling

After the AAV transfection and *AZGP1* expression was verified successful, another 45 rats were randomly divided into three groups (*n* = 15 for each group): controls, *AZGP1* + PTZ group and GFP + PTZ group. Rats in *AZGP1* + PTZ group and GFP + PTZ group recovered for 3 weeks after AAV injection and then received intraperitoneal injection of PTZ (35 mg/kg, Sigma-Aldrich, St. Louis, USA) for 28 days daily. After each injection of PTZ, all rats were observed for 30 min in plastic cages to assess and record the seizure severity according to a modified Racine scale as follows [34]: grade 0, no response; grade 1, facial myoclonus; grade 2, head nodding; grade 3, forelimb clonus; grade 4, rearing and severe forelimb clonus; grade 5, rearing, falling, and severe forelimb clonus. Controls (*n* = 15) received equal amount of saline instead of AAV and PTZ. Rats that exhibited stage 4 or 5 seizures on 3 consecutive days were considered to be fully kindled. Latency was defined as the days between the first PTZ injection and fully kindling. PTZ injection was conducted between 13:00 and 16:00 in order to minimize possible complicating effects on the behavior of the animals' circadian rhythms.

Scalp EEG recording

Scalp EEG was performed at the last time of PTZ injection. Two unipole scalp electrodes were placed on bilateral temporal skin of rats. After the place of electrodes, rats were allowed to move freely in plastic cages. EEG baseline was recorded for approximately 5 min before the injection of PTZ or saline, then EEG was recorded for at least 30 min using the nicolet vEGG system (natus, USA) and analyzed using nicoleton bms 5000 (natus, USA). The parameters of EEG are set as follows: filtering 30 Hz, paper speed 30 mm/s, and sensitivity 70 μV/mm. All remaining rats that received PTZ injection for 28 days were sacrificed for further research.

Tissue processing

Rats were deeply anesthetized by intraperitoneal injection of pentobarbital (60 mg/kg). For western blot and quantitative real-time polymerase chain reaction (qrt-PCR), rat brains were removed and stored at −80 °C. For GFP fluorescence observation, the rat brains were removed after perfusion with saline and 4% paraformaldehyde in phosphate-buffered saline (PBS) by cardiac puncture via the left ventricle. For comparing level of ZAG protein and *AZGP1* mRNA 3 and 9 weeks after AAV injection, some rat brain tissues were stored for 6 weeks at −80 °C before western blot and qrt-PCR examination. The rest rat brain tissues were examined in 2 weeks after removal.

qrt-PCR

Total RNA was extracted from the brain tissue using RNAiso plus (Takara, Dalian, China) and was reverse transcribed into complementary deoxyribonucleic acid (cDNA) with the Applied Biosystems Veriti-Well Thermal Cycler (Thermo, Wilmington, USA) using the PrimeScript RT reagent Kit with genome DNA Eraser (Takara, Dalian, China) following the manufacturer's instructions. Briefly, 2 μg total RNA was mixed with 4 μl Reverse Transcriptase and 0.5 μg oligo (dT) primer and incubated at 37 °C for 15 min, and the reaction was then terminated at 85 °C for 5 s. Each qrt-PCR reaction contained 2 μl cDNA, 0.8 μl forward primer, 0.8 μl reverse primer, 6.4 μl DEPC water, and 10 μl SYBR Premix ExTaq II (Takara, Dalian, China). The PCR protocol consisted of an initial denaturation step at 95 °C for 30 s, followed by 40 cycles of amplification at 95 °C for 5 s and at 60 °C for 34 s, and then terminated at 95 °C for 15 s. Melting curve analyses were also performed (65.0 to 95.0 °C, 0.5 °C increments for 5 s). The relative gene expression levels in the hippocampus of PTZ-kindled rats were calculated using the $2^{-\Delta\Delta Ct}$ method [35]. The primer sequences for rat were as follows: *AZGP1*: forward 5′-TTCAAGCCACCGCATTTCTC-3′, reverse 5′-TCCTTCTCCCAGTCCTCCATTC-3′. GAPDH: forward 5′-ACGGTCAGGTCATCACTATCG-3′, reverse 5′-GGCATAGAGGTCTTTACGGATG-3′.

Observation of fluorescence of GFP

The fixed brain tissues were successively immersed in 20 and 30% sucrose solution for 48 h (24 h per solution) and sliced into 10-μm-thick frozen sections. Finally, the sections were mounted using 80% glycerol. Images were collected using laser scanning confocal microscopy (Nikon 1R, Japan).

Western blot

Brain tissue was homogenized in RIPA lysis buffer (Beyotime, Haimen, China) containing proteinase inhibitor mixture and phosphorylase inhibitor mixture and centrifuged at 12000 rpm, 4 °C for 25 min. The protein concentrations in the supernatant were determined using a BCA Protein Assay Kit (Beyotime, Haimen, China). The extracted total proteins were mixed with 5× sodium dodecylsulfate (SDS) loading buffer and boiled for 5 min. Equal amounts of total protein (80 μg/lane) were separated by SDS-polyacrylamide gel electrophoresis (PAGE) and then transferred onto polyvinylidene fluoride (PVDF) membranes (Immobilon, Merck Millipore, Darmstadt, Germany). The membranes were blocked with 5% BSA at room temperature for 2 h and then incubated with the anti-ZAG antibody (1:400, Santa Cruz, USA), anti-TNFα antibody (1:500, Bosterbio, USA), anti-IL6 antibody (1:500, Bosterbio, USA), anti-pERK antibody (1:2000, Cell Signaling Technology, Danvers, USA), anti-tERK antibody (1:2000, Proteintech, Wuhan, China), anti-TGFβ antibody (1:1000, Proteintech, Wuhan, China), or anti-glyceraldehyde 3-phosphate dehydrogenase (GAPDH) antibody (1:3000, Proteintech, Wuhan, China) at 4 °C overnight. After washed with tris-buffered saline with Tween-20 (TBST), the membranes were incubated with the horseradish peroxidase-conjugated rabbit anti-mouse antibody (1:3000, Abcam, Cambridge, UK) or mouse anti-rabbit antibody (1:3000, Abcam, Cambridge, UK) at room temperature for 1 h and washed again. Immunoreactivity was visualized using chemiluminescence substrate kit (Beyotime,

Haimen, China) and quantified by densitometric scanning with the Fusion-FX7 system (Vilber Lourmat, Collégien, France). The mean optic density (OD) was normalized by GAPDH.

Statistical analysis

The results were expressed as mean ± standard deviation (SD). SPSS 20.0 (IBM, Armonk, USA) and GraphPad prism 6.01 (GraphPad software, La Jolla, USA) were used for data analysis and graph drawing. Mann–Whitney U test was used to compare the differences of Racine's scores between AAV–$AZGP1$ group and AAV–GFP group. Student's t test was used to compare the differences of latency between AAV–$AZGP1$ group and AAV–GFP group. One-way ANOVA with Bonferroni or Dunnett's T3 post hoc analysis was used to compare the level of proteins between the three groups. $p < 0.05$ (two tailed) was regarded statistically significant.

Results

The transfection of AAV and the overexpression of $AZGP1$

To confirm the efficiency and stability of AAV-induced $AZGP1$ expression, we detected GFP distribution and measured the level of $AZGP1$ mRNA and ZAG protein in rat hippocampus 3 weeks and 9 weeks after AAV injection. The GFP-positive cells in the CA3 region of hippocampus were visualized (Fig. 1a). The level of

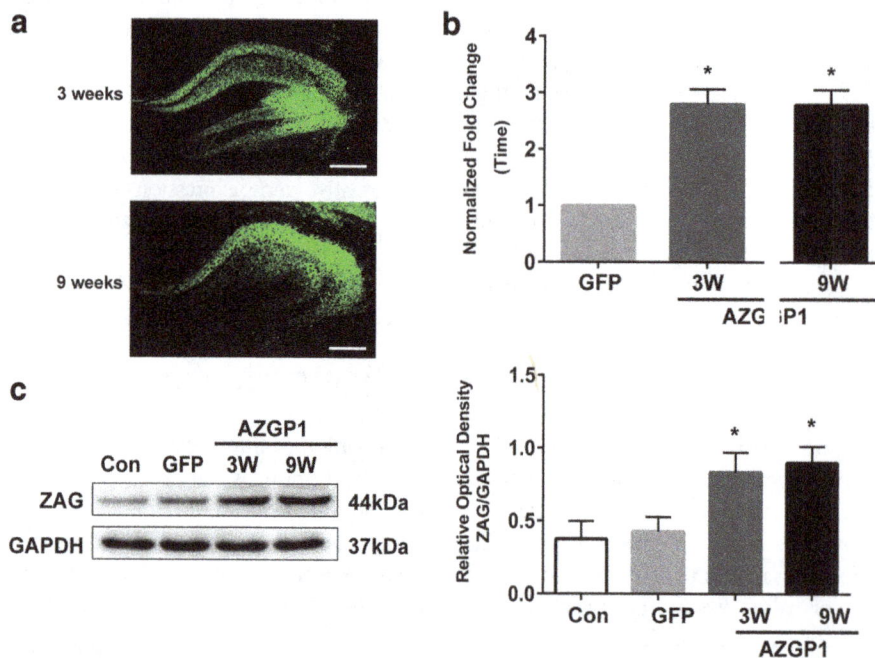

Fig. 1 Expression of GFP and $AZGP1$ after injection of AAV vectors. **a** Fluorescent images showing GFP expression in the hippocampus of rats 3 and 9 weeks after AAV injection. The scale bar = 500 μm. **b** qrt-PCR showed increased $AZGP1$ mRNA level in the hippocampus of rats in AAV–$AZGP1$ group compared to AAV–GFP group 3 and 9 weeks after AAV injection. **c** Western blots showed increased ZAG protein level in the hippocampus of rats in AAV–$AZGP1$ group compared to AAV–GFP group 3 and 9 weeks after AAV injection. Optic density was normalized by GAPDH. $n = 5$ for each group, *$p < 0.05$

AZGP1 mRNA (Fig. 1b) and ZAG protein (Fig. 1c, d) was significantly increased on 3 and 9 weeks in *AZGP1* group compared to GFP group. There was no difference of *AZGP1* mRNA (Fig. 1b) and ZAG protein (Fig. 1c, d) levels between 3 and 9 weeks in *AZGP1* group, suggesting a steady expression of *AZGP1*. In addition, no significant difference of *AZGP1* mRNA (Fig. 1b) and ZAG protein (Fig. 1c, d) level was found between GFP group and controls, suggesting no effect of AAV vectors on *AZGP1* mRNA and ZAG protein expression.

Overexpression of *AZGP1* suppresses seizures in PTZ-treated rats

ZAG protein level in rats of *AZGP1* + PTZ group (OD 1.496 ± 0.086) was significantly higher than in the GFP + PTZ group (OD 0.778 ± 0.080) and controls (OD 1.104 ± 0.074) ($n = 5$, $p = 0.0001$, degrees of freedom (df) = 12, one-way ANOVA) (Fig. 2a). Rats in *AZGP1* + PTZ group had significantly milder seizure severity (Fig. 2b) before being fully kindled and longer latency (Fig. 2c) compared to rats in GFP + PTZ group (latency: *AZGP1* + PTZ 16.07 ± 2.786, $n = 14$ vs. GFP + PTZ 20.00 ± 2.530, $n = 11$, $p = 0.0014$, df = 23, Student's *t* test). In addition, scalp EEG results showed significant decrease in the frequency and amplitude of seizure spike wave in *AZGP1* + PTZ groups compared to GFP + PTZ group (Fig. 3).

Overexpression of *AZGP1* decreased the level of TGFβ and pERK in PTZ-kindled rats without affecting total ERK level

To explore the possibility that ZAG affects seizure via TGFβ-mediated ERK signaling pathway, we measured the level of pERK, total ERK, and TGFβ in the hippocampus of rats in the three groups using western blot. The level of pERK (Fig. 4a, c), pERK/total ERK ratio (Fig. 4c), and TGFβ (Fig. 4d, e) was significantly increased in both *AZGP1* + PTZ and GFP + PTZ groups compared to controls, while rats in *AZGP1* + PTZ group had decreased pERK (Fig. 4a, c), pERK/total ERK ratio (Fig. 4c), and TGFβ (Fig. 4d, e) compared to rats in GFP + PTZ group (pERK: control 0.674 ± 0.045, GFP + PTZ 1.344 ± 0.071, *AZGP1* + PTZ 0.787 ± 0.070, $p = 0.0001$, df = 12, one-way ANOVA); (pERK/total ERK ratio: control 0.410 ± 0.026, GFP + PTZ 0.840 ± 0.073, *AZGP1* + PTZ 0.482 ± 0.040, $p = 0.0001$, df = 12, one-way ANOVA); (TGFβ: control 0.490 ± 0.021, GFP + PTZ 0.862 ± 0.070, *AZGP1* + PTZ 0.660 ± 0.072, $p = 0.001$, df = 12, one-way

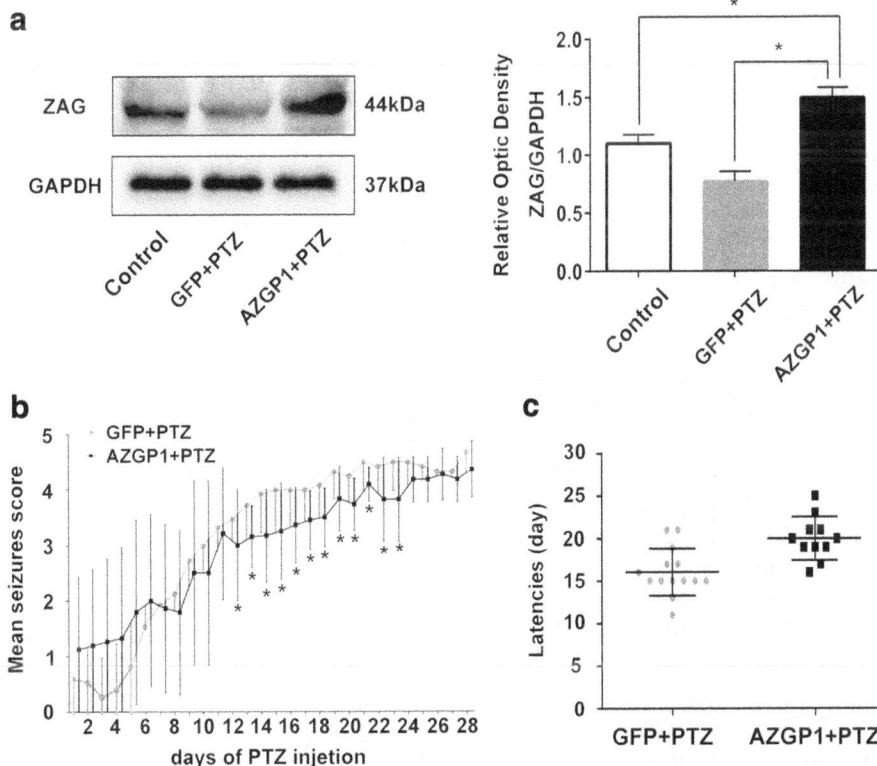

Fig. 2 Overexpression of *AZGP1* suppressed seizure in PTZ-treated rats. **a** ZAG protein level in rats of *AZGP1* + PTZ group was significantly increased compared to GFP + PTZ group and controls. **b** Rats in *AZGP1* + PTZ group had significantly alleviated seizure severity during 12th to 23rd day of PTZ injection compared to GFP + PTZ group, while after 24th day of PTZ injection, there is no difference in seizure severity. **c** Overexpression of *AZGP1* significantly prolonged the latency of PTZ kindling. $n = 15$ for each group, $*p < 0.05$

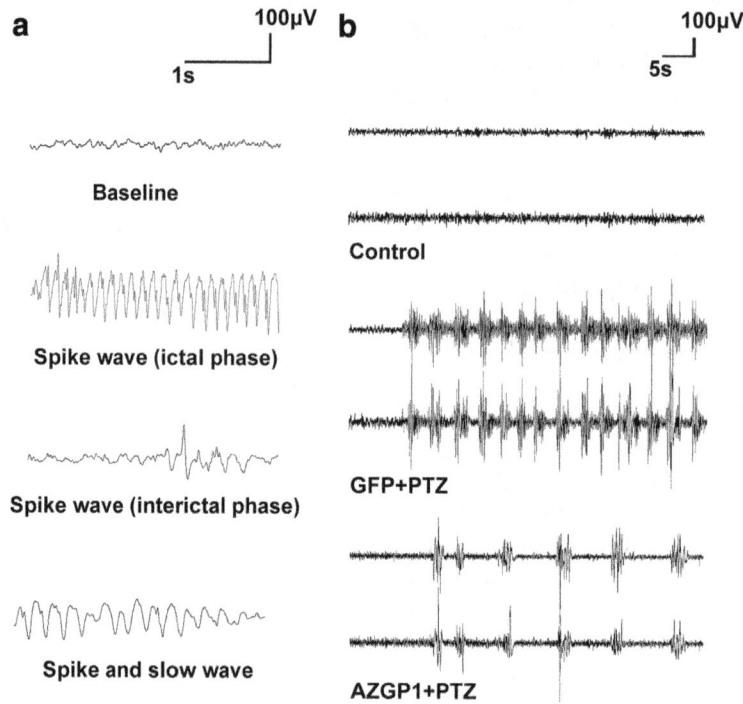

Fig. 3 Scalp electroencephalogram (EEG) changes in *AZGP1* + PTZ group and GFP + PTZ group after PTZ kindling. **a** Typical EEG record of seizure. **b** Representative EEG record among the three groups of rats. Rats in *AZGP1* + PTZ group had significantly decreased frequency and amplitude of epileptiform spike waves in EEG compared to GFP + PTZ group

ANOVA), (*n* = 5 for each group). In addition, there was no significant difference in total ERK level between the three groups (Fig. 4b) (control 1.642 ± 0.123, GFP + PTZ 1.614 ± 0.183, *AZGP1* + PTZ 1.636 ± 0.133, *p* = 1.000, df = 12, one-way ANOVA).

Overexpression of *AZGP1* suppressed the increase of TNFα and IL-6 in PTZ-kindled rats

To assess the inflammatory state of the hippocampus, two typical pro-inflammatory cytokines, TNFα and IL-6, were measured using western blot in the hippocampus of *AZGP1* + PTZ and GFP + PTZ group rats and controls. Hippocampal TNFα (Fig. 5a) level was increased in *AZGP1* + PTZ and GFP + PTZ groups compared to controls, while in *AZGP1* + PTZ group, TNFα (Fig. 5a) was significantly decreased compared to GFP + PTZ group (TNFα: control 0.415 ± 0.055, GFP + PTZ 0.722 ± 0.032, *AZGP1* + PTZ 0.554 ± 0.029, *p* = 0.001, df = 12, one-way ANOVA). Hippocampal IL6 level was significantly decreased in *AZGP1* + PTZ group compared to GFP + PTZ group (IL6: *AZGP1* + PTZ 0.472 ± 0.068, GFP + PTZ 0. 692 ± 0.081, *p* = 0.001, df = 12, one-way ANOVA) while there is no statistical significance between *AZGP1* group and control (IL6: *AZGP1* + PTZ 0.472 ± 0.068, control 0.413 ± 0.058, *p* = 0.609, df = 12, one-way ANOVA) (Fig. 5b).

Discussion

In our previous study, we had found that the level of *AZGP1* mRNA and ZAG protein was significantly decreased in the neocortex of refractory epilepsy patients as well as in the hippocampus and neocortex of PTZ-kindled rats compared to controls [4]. However, the specific role of ZAG in epilepsy and/or seizure remains unclear.

In this study, behavior tests showed that overexpression of *AZGP1* in the hippocampus prolonged the latency of PTZ kindling and alleviated the seizure severity in PTZ-treated rats. Similarly, in scalp EEG recording, decreased frequency and amplitude of spike wave were also identified in AAV–*AZGP1* group. These results indicate a protective role of ZAG against seizure. Interestingly, we found that the seizure severity score of AAV–*AZGP1* group was significantly lower than AAV–GFP group during 12–23 days of PTZ treatment, while after the 24th day of PTZ treatment, the seizure severity was of no difference between the two groups, indicating that overexpression of ZAG can delay but not fully prevent the kindling. Moreover, on the 28th day of PTZ treatment, although the seizure severity of rats in both AAV–*AZGP1* group and AAV–GFP group were similar, the scalp EEG recording demonstrated decreased frequency and amplitude of spike waves in AAV–*AZGP1* group compared to AAV–GFP group. This result indicates that

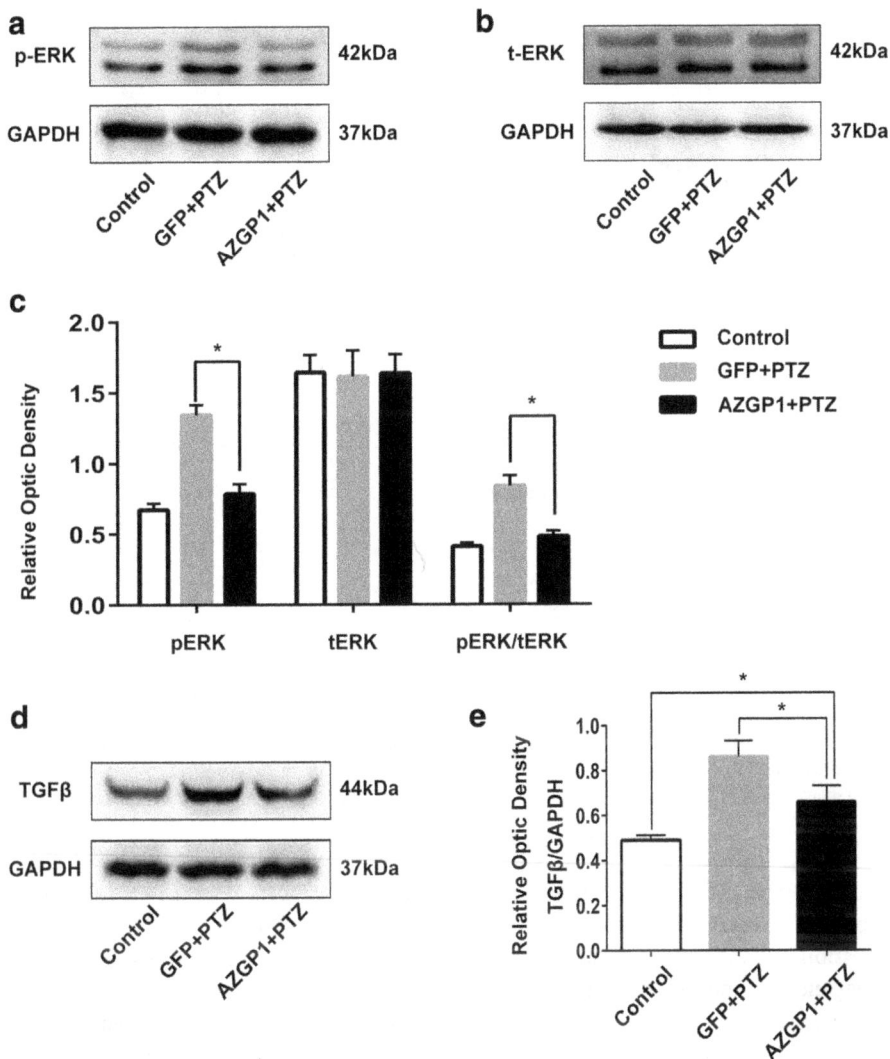

Fig. 4 Overexpression of *AZGP1* decreased the level of TGFβ and pERK in PTZ-kindled rats without affecting total ERK level. **a**, **b** Representative western blot bands of p-ERK and t-ERK in hippocampal tissues of rats. **c** Western blot showed GFP + PTZ group had significantly increased level of p-ERK and p-ERK/t-ERK ratio in hippocampal tissues compared to controls, and rats in *AZGP1* + PTZ group had significantly decreased the level of pERK and pERK/tERK ratio compared to GFP + PTZ group. The level of tERK in hippocampal tissues is of no significant difference among the three groups. **d** Representative western blot bands of TGFβ in hippocampal tissues of rats. **e** Western blot showed increased level of TGFβ in the hippocampal tissues of rats in GFP + PTZ group compared to controls, and rats in *AZGP1* + PTZ group had significantly decreased the level of TGFβ compared to GFP + PTZ group. Optic density was normalized by GAPDH, $n = 5$ for each group, $*p < 0.05$

although rats in the two groups had similar seizure severity in behavior, their epileptiform discharge in brain is different. It is possible that overexpression of ZAG may have protective effect on seizure even if the rats are fully kindled. Although ZAG only delayed PTZ kindling in this study, it also alleviated the epileptiform discharges after the rats were fully kindled. It is possible that ZAG may prevent seizure in the early stage of kindling and has protective effect in the late stage of kindling, indicating a possible role of ZAG in different stage of epileptogenesis or seizure. This is the first study on the role of ZAG in seizure;

further study is needed to explore its effect on seizure and mechanism.

ZAG was reported as an anti-inflammatory adipocytokine [24]. Clinical and experimental evidences have revealed that brain inflammation plays an important role in epileptogenesis [23]. The most extensively studied prototypical inflammatory cytokines in the central nervous system are TNFα and IL-6 [36–38]. The enhanced production of pro-inflammatory cytokines, including TNFα and IL-6, were known to play pro-epileptic roles in the brain [39]. The dynamic modulation of inflammatory processes has potential to be a novel therapeutic

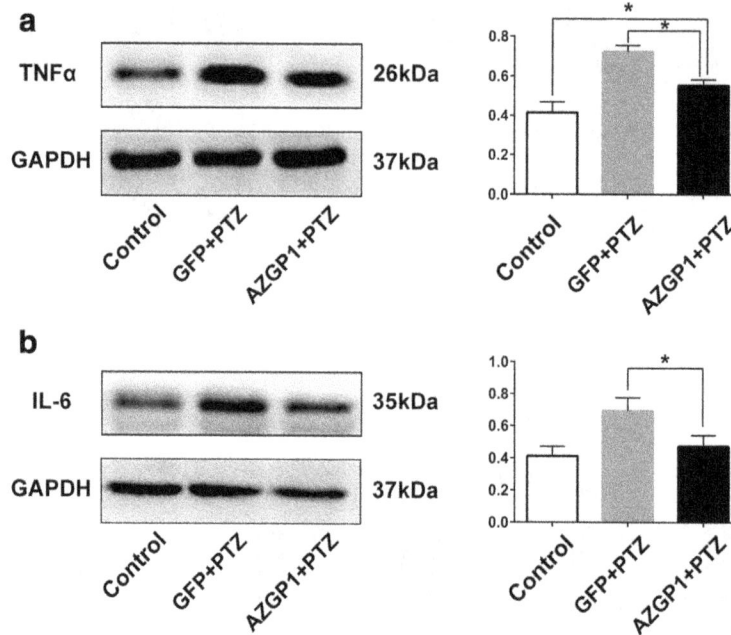

Fig. 5 Overexpression of *AZGP1* suppressed the increase of TNFα and IL-6 in PTZ-kindled rats. **a** Representative western blot bands and expression level of TNFα in the hippocampal tissues of rats. Western blot showed increased level of TNFα in the hippocampal tissues of rats in GFP + PTZ group compared to controls, and rats in *AZGP1* + PTZ group had significantly decreased the level of TNFα compared to GFP + PTZ group. **b** Representative western blot bands and expression level of IL-6 in the hippocampus of rats. Western blot showed increased level of IL-6 in the hippocampal tissues of rats in GFP + PTZ group compared to controls, and rats in *AZGP1* + PTZ group had significantly decreased the level of IL-6 compared to GFP + PTZ group. Optic density normalized by GAPDH, $n = 5$ for each group, $*p < 0.05$

strategy for pharmacologic treatment to control seizures, delay disease progression, or retard epileptogenesis [40]. Moreover, overexpression of cytokines such as TNFα or IL-6 results in age-dependent increase of seizure susceptibility and spontaneous seizures [41, 42]. In our study, overexpression of *AZGP1* attenuated the increase of TNFα and IL6 induced by PTZ kindling. Interestingly, TNFα has been identified to reduce ZAG production [33]. This is suggesting that there may be a circuit or feedback regulation mechanism between ZAG and TNFα. Therefore, ZAG may prevent seizure and protect the brain via alleviating neuroinflammation. This is the first time that the relationship between ZAG and IL-6 was identified.

We had previously verified the interaction between ZAG and TGFβ or p-ERK in the hippocampus of rats [4]. In this study, we found that overexpression of ZAG could decrease the level of TGFβ and ERK phosphorylation. Human recombinant ZAG was found to specifically block TGFβ-mediated ERK phosphorylation [6]. And TGFβ and p-ERK/ERK ratio were upregulated in patients with refractory epilepsy [8, 10]. TGFβ can promote epileptogenesis via upregulating IL-6 [43] and inhibiting TGFβ by losartan can suppress epileptogenesis [44]. ERK activation induced by its phosphorylation is known to cause seizure by activating *N*-methy-D-

aspartate (NMDA) receptors [45, 46]. In addition, TGFβ and ERK are known as inflammatory mediators [20–24]. Thus, it is possible that ZAG may prevent seizure via inhibiting TGFβ-mediated ERK signaling pathway and alleviate inflammation induced by seizure. As the effect of ZAG on TGFβ and ERK has not been investigated in epilepsy and/or seizure before, further study is needed to clarify the existence of ZAG–TGFβ–ERK pathway and its specific role in seizure and epilepsy.

Many studies showed that various inflammatory cytokines are associated with seizure susceptibility [47–50]. Overexpressing IL-6 or TNFα can decrease seizure threshold and exacerbate seizure-induced neuronal loss [51, 52]. Inflammatory signaling is also known to worsen the loss of GABAergic neurons in the hippocampus and thus resulted in an increased susceptibility for seizure [53]. TNFα have also been associated with the regulation of seizure duration in amygdala-kindled rats [54]. In our study, overexpression of *AZGP1* in the hippocampus prolonged the latency of PTZ kindling and attenuated PTZ kindling-induced increase of TNFα and IL-6. This result suggests that overexpression of *AZGP1* may decrease seizure susceptibility in PTZ-treated rats, and this effect of overexpression of *AZGP1* may possibly be attributed to its inhibition of neuroinflammation. This is the first study relating ZAG to neuroinflammation in seizure; further study is needed to explore the relationship between ZAG and neuroinflammation in seizure. This study is a preliminary discuss on the role of ZAG in seizure, but more specific mechanism, such as ZAG–TGFβ–ERK pathway and the effect of ZAG on NMDA/AMPA/GABA receptors, still needs to be further researched. Furthermore, researches on the role of ZAG deficiency in epilepsy and/or seizure are also needed.

Conclusion

Our study found that overexpression of *AZGP1* delayed PTZ kindling, alleviated seizure and epileptiform discharges, inhibited TGFβ-mediated ERK phosphorylation, and decreased TNFα and IL-6 in PTZ-treated rats. Our study indicated that ZAG may suppress seizure via inhibiting neuroinflammation. As an anti-inflammatory cytokine, ZAG may be a novel target for research and clinical treatment of seizure and possibly for epilepsy.

Abbreviations
AAV: Adeno-associated virus; cDNA: Complementary deoxyribonucleic acid; EEG: Electroencephalography; ERK: Extracellular regulated protein kinase; GAPDH: Glyceraldehyde 3-phosphate dehydrogenase; GFP: Green fluorescent protein; IL-10: Interleukin-10; IL-6: Interleukin-6; MHC-I: Major histocompatibility complex class I; mTOR: Mammalian target of rapamycin; NMDA: *N*-methy-D-aspartate; OD: Optic density; PAGE: Polyacrylamide gel electrophoresis; PBS: Paraformaldehyde in phosphate-buffered saline; pERK: Phosphorylated extracellular regulated protein kinase; PPARγ: Peroxisome proliferator-activated receptor gamma; PTZ: Pentylenetetrazol; PVDF: Polyvinylidene fluoride; qrt-PCR: Quantitative real-time polymerase chain reaction; SD: Standard deviation; SDS: Sodium dodecylsulfate; SGLT2: Sodium–glucose cotransporter 2; TBST: Tris-buffered saline with Tween-20; TGFβ: Transforming growth factor-β; TNFα: Tumor-necrosis factor; UCP: Uncoupling proteins; ZAG: Zinc-α2-glycoprotein

Acknowledgements
Not applicable.

Funding
This work is funded by the National Natural Science Foundation of China (81771391) and the Chongqing Municipal Public Health Bureau, Chongqing People's Municipal Government (2015ZDXM011). This study is also supported by the Program for Innovative Research Team of Chongqing Kuanren Hospital.

Authors' contributions
LC, XT, and XL designed the research. YL, TW, YW, TX, XY, XW, XD, LM, and MY performed the research. YL and TW analyzed the data. YL and XL wrote the manuscript. All authors read and approved the final manuscript.

Consent for publication
Not applicable.

Competing interests
The authors declare that they have no competing interests.

Author details
¹Department of Neurology, The Second Affiliated Hospital of Chongqing Medical University, 74 Linjiang Road, Yuzhong District, Chonqing 400010, China. ²Department of Neurosurgery, The University-Town Hospital of Chongqing Medical University, Chongqing 401331, China.

References
1. Burgi W, Schmid K. Preparation and properties of Zn-alpha 2-glycoprotein of normal human plasma. J Biol Chem. 1961;236:1066–74.
2. Tada T, Ohkubo I, Niwa M, Sasaki M, Tateyama H, Eimoto T. Immunohistochemical localization of Zn-alpha 2-glycoprotein in normal human tissues. J Histochem Cytochem. 1991; https://doi.org/10.1177/39.9.1918940.
3. Hassan MI, Waheed A, Yadav S, Singh TP, Ahmad F. Zinc alpha 2-glycoprotein: a multidisciplinary protein. Mol Cancer Res. 2008; https://doi.org/10.1158/1541-7786.MCR-07-2195.
4. Liu Y, Wang T, Liu X, Wei X, Xu T, Yin M, Ding X, Mo L, Chen L. Neuronal zinc-α2-glycoprotein is decreased in temporal lobe epilepsy in patients and rats. Neuroscience. 2017; https://doi.org/10.1016/j.neuroscience.2017.05.043.
5. Chang L, Tian X, Lu Y, Jia M, Wu P, Huang P. Alpha-2-glycoprotein 1(AZGP1) regulates biological behaviors of LoVo cells by down-regulating mTOR signaling pathway and endogenous fatty acid synthesis. PLoS One. 2014; 9(6):e99254.
6. Kong B, Michalski CW, Hong X, Valkovskaya N, Rieder S, Abiatari I, Streit S, Erkan M, Esposito I, Friess H, Kleeff J. AZGP1 is a tumor suppressor in pancreatic cancer inducing mesenchymal-to-epithelial transdifferentiation by inhibiting TGF-β-mediated ERK signaling. Oncogene. 2010; https://doi.org/10.1038/onc.2010.258.
7. Ostendorf AP, Wong M. mTOR inhibition in epilepsy: rationale and clinical perspectives. CNS Drugs. 2015;29(2):91–9.
8. Cacheaux LP, Ivens S, David Y, Lakhter AJ, Bar-Klein G, Shapira M, Heinemann U, Friedman A, Kaufer D. Transcriptome profiling reveals TGF-beta signaling involvement in epileptogenesis. J Neurosci. 2009; https://doi.org/10.1523/JNEUROSCI.0430-09.2009.
9. Yu CY, Gui W, He HY, Wang XS, Zuo J, Huang L, Zhou N, Wang K, Wang Y. Neuronal and astroglial TGFβ-Smad3 signaling pathways differentially regulate dendrite growth and synaptogenesis. NeuroMolecular Med. 2014; 16(2):457–72.
10. Xi ZQ, Wang XF, He RQ, Li MW, Liu XZ, Wang LY, Zhu X, Xiao F, Sun JJ, Li JM, Gong Y, Guan LF. Extracellular signal-regulated protein kinase in human intractable epilepsy. Eur J Neurol. 2007; https://doi.org/10.1111/j.1468-1331.2007.01777.x.
11. Liao X, Wang X, Li H, Li L, Zhang G, Yang M, Yuan L, Liu H, Yang G, Gao L. Sodium-glucose cotransporter 2 (SGLT2) inhibitor increases circulating zinc-α2-glycoprotein levels in patients with type 2 diabetes. Sci Rep. 2016; https://doi.org/10.1038/srep32887.
12. Bao Y, Bing C, Hunter L, Jenkins JR, Wabitsch M, Trayhurn P. Zinc-alpha2-glycoprotein, a lipid mobilizing factor, is expressed and secreted by human (SGBS) adipocytes. FEBS Lett. 2005; https://doi.org/10.1016/j.febslet.2004.11.042.
13. Melo IS, Santos YM, Costa MA, Pacheco AL, Silva NK, Cardoso-Sousa L, Pereira UP, Goulart LR, Garcia-Cairasco N, Duzzioni M, Gitaí DL, Tilelli CQ, Sabino-Silva R, Castro OW. Inhibition of sodium glucose cotransporters following status epilepticus induced by intrahippocampal pilocarpine affects neurodegeneration process in hippocampus. Epilepsy Behav. 2016;61:258–68.
14. Auvin S. Fatty acid oxidation and epilepsy. Epilepsy Res. 2012;100(3):224–8.
15. Taha AY, Burnham WM, Auvin S. Polyunsaturated fatty acids and epilepsy. Epilepsia. 2010;51(8):1348–58.
16. Sanders PM, Tisdale MJ. Effect of zinc-alpha2-glycoprotein (ZAG) on expression of uncoupling proteins in skeletal muscle and adipose tissue. Cancer Lett. 2004;212(1):71–81.
17. Chuang YC, Lin TK, Huang HY, Chang WN, Liou CW, Chen SD, Chang AY, Chan SH. Peroxisome proliferator-activated receptors γ/mitochondrial uncoupling protein 2 signaling protects against seizure-induced neuronal cell death in the hippocampus following experimental status epilepticus. J Neuroinflammation. 2012;9:184.
18. Vezzani A, Friedman A, Dingledine RJ. The role of inflammation in epileptogenesis. Neuropharmacology. 2013; https://doi.org/10.1016/j.neuropharm.2012.04.004.
19. Leal Vde O, Mafra D. Adipokines in obesity. Clin Chim Acta. 2013; https://doi.org/10.1016/j.cca.2013.02.003.
20. Patel RK, Prasad N, Kuwar R, Haldar D, Abdul-Muneer PM. Transforming growthfactor-beta1 signaling regulates neuroinflammation and apoptosis in mild traumatic brain injury. Brain Behav Immun. 2017; https://doi.org/10.1016/j.bbi.2017.04.012.
21. Xu G, Feng L, Song P, Xu F, Li A, Wang Y, Shen Y, Wu X, Luo Q, Wu X, Sun Y, Wu X, Xu Q. Isomeranzin suppresses inflammation by inhibiting M1 macrophage polarization through the NF-κB and ERK pathway. Int Immunopharmacol. 2016; https://doi.org/10.1016/j.intimp.2016.05.027.

22. Huang Y, Zeng J, Chen G, Xie X, Guo W, Tian W. Periodontitis contributes to adipose tissue inflammation through the NF-<kappa>B, JNK and ERK pathways to promote insulin resistance in a rat model. Microbes Infect. 2016; https://doi.org/10.1016/j.micinf.2016.08.002.

23. Li C, Yan Y, Shi Q, Kong Y, Gao L, Bao H, Li Y. Recuperating lung decoction attenuates inflammation and oxidation in cigarette smoke-induced COPD in rats via activation of ERK and Nrf2 pathways. Cell Biochem Funct. 2017; https://doi.org/10.1002/cbf.3273.

24. Zeng KW, Yu Q, Liao LX, Song FJ, Lv HN, Jiang Y, Tu PF. Anti-neuroinflammatory effect of MC13, a novel coumarin compound from condiment Murraya, through inhibiting lipopolysaccharide-induced TRAF6-TAK1-NF-κB, P38/ERK MAPKS and Jak2-Stat1/Stat3 pathways. J Cell Biochem. 2015; https://doi.org/10.1002/jcb.25084.

25. Turrin NP, Rivest S. Innate immune reaction in response to seizures: implications for the neuropathology associated with epilepsy. Neurobiol Dis. 2004;16(2):321–34.

26. Oprica M, Eriksson C, Schultzberg M. Inflammatory mechanisms associated with brain damage induced by kainic acid with special reference to the interleukin-1 system. J Cell Mol Med. 2003;7(2):127–40.

27. Vezzani A, Conti N, De Luigi A, Ravizza T, Moneta D, Marchesi F, et al. Interleukin-l beta immunoreactivity and microglia are enhanced in the rat hippocampus by focal kainate application: functional evidence for enhancement of electrographic seizures. J Neurosci. 1999;19(12):5054–65.

28. Tombini M, Squitti R, Cacciapaglia F, Ventriglia M, Assenza G, Benvenga A, Pellegrino G, Campana C, Assenza F, Siotto M, Pacifici L, Afeltra A, Rossini PM. Inflammation and iron metabolism in adult patients with epilepsy: does a link exist? Epilepsy Res. 2013; https://doi.org/10.1016/j.eplepsyres.2013.09.010.

29. Lehtimäki KA, Keränen T, Palmio J, Mäkinen R, Hurme M, Honkaniemi J, Peltola J. Increased plasma levels of cytokines after seizures in localization-related epilepsy. Acta Neurol Scand. 2007; https://doi.org/10.1111/j.1600-0404.2007.00882.x.

30. Peltola J, Palmio J, Korhonen L, Suhonen J, Miettinen A, Hurme M, et al. Interleukin-6 and interleukin-1 receptor antagonist in cerebrospinal fluid from patients with recent tonic-clonic seizures. Epilepsy Res. 2000;41(3):205–11.

31. Virta M, Hurme M, Helminen M. Increased plasma levels of pro- and anti-inflammatory cytokines in patients with febrile seizures. Epilepsia. 2002;43(8):920–3.

32. Bauer S, Cepok S, Todorova-Rudolph A, Nowak M, Köller M, Lorenz R, Oertel WH, Rosenow F, Hemmer B, Hamer HM. Etiology and site of temporal lobe epilepsy influence postictal cytokine release. Epilepsy Res. 2009; https://doi.org/10.1016/j.eplepsyres.2009.05.009.

33. Mracek T, Gao D, Tzanavari T, Bao Y, Xiao X, Stocker C, Trayhurn P, Bing C. Downregulation of zinc-α2-glycoprotein in adipose tissue and liver of obese ob/ob mice and by tumour necrosis factor-alpha in adipocytes. J Endocrinol. 2010; https://doi.org/10.1677/JOE-09-0299.

34. Racine RJ. Modification of seizure activity by electrical stimulation. II. Motor seizure. Electroencephalogr Clin Neurophysiol. 1972;32(3):281–94.

35. Schmittgen TD, Livak KJ. Analyzing real-time PCR data by the comparative C(T) method. Nat Protoc. 2008;3:1101–8.

36. Bartfai T, Sanchez-Alavez M, Andell-Jonsson S, Schultzberg M, Vezzani A, Danielsson E, Conti B. Interleukin-1 system in CNS stress: seizures, fever, and neurotrauma. Ann N Y Acad Sci. 2007; https://doi.org/10.1196/annals.1391.022.

37. Allan SM, Rothwell NJ. Cytokines and acute neurodegeneration. Nat Rev Neurosci. 2001; https://doi.org/10.1038/35094583.

38. Bartfai T, Schultzberg M. Cytokines in neuronal cell types. Neurochem Int. 1993;22(5):435–44.

39. Ho YH, Lin YT, Wu CW, Chao YM, Chang AY, Chan JY. Peripheral inflammation increases seizure susceptibility via the induction of neuroinflammation and oxidative stress in the hippocampus. J Biomed Sci. 2015; https://doi.org/10.1186/s12929-015-0157-8.

40. Yang T, Zhou D, Stefan H. Why mesial temporal lobe epilepsy with hippocampal sclerosis is progressive: uncontrolled inflammation drives disease progression? J Neurol Sci. 2010; https://doi.org/10.1016/j.jns.2010.06.002.

41. Akassoglou K, Probert L, Kontogeorgos G, Kollias G. Astrocyte-specific but not neuron-specific transmembrane TNF triggers inflammation and degeneration in the central nervous system of transgenic mice. J Immunol. 1997;158(1):438–45.

42. Stalder AK, Carson MJ, Pagenstecher A, Asensio VC, Kincaid C, Benedict M, Powell HC, Masliah E, Campbell IL. Late-onset chronic inflammatory encephalopathy in immune-competent and severe combined immune-deficient (SCID) mice with astrocyte-targeted expression of tumor necrosis factor. Am J Pathol. 1998; https://doi.org/10.1016/S0002-9440(10)65620-9

43. Levy N, Milikovsky DZ, Baranauskas G, Vinogradov E, David Y, Ketzef M, Abutbul S, Weissberg I, Kamintsky L, Fleidervish I, Friedman A, Monsonego A. Differential TGF-β signaling in glial subsets underlies IL-6-mediated epileptogenesis in mice. J Immunol. 2015; https://doi.org/10.4049/jimmunol.1401446.

44. Bar-Klein G, Cacheaux LP, Kamintsky L, Prager O, Weissberg I, Schoknecht K, Cheng P, Kim SY, Wood L, Heinemann U, Kaufer D, Friedman A. Losartan prevents acquired epilepsy via TGF-β signaling suppression. Ann Neurol. 2014; https://doi.org/10.1002/ana.24147.

45. Nateri AS, Raivich G, Gebhardt C, Da Costa C, Naumann H, Vreugdenhil M, Makwana M, Brandner S, Adams RH, Jefferys JG, Kann O, Behrens AERK. Activation causes epilepsy by stimulating NMDA receptor activity. EMBO J. 2007;26(23):4891–901.

46. Itoh T, Kaibuchi K, Masuda T, Yamamoto T, Matsuura Y, Maeda A, Shimizu K, Takai Y. A protein factor for ras p21-dependent activation of mitogen-activated protein (MAP) kinase through MAP kinase kinase. Proc Natl Acad Sci U S A. 1993;90(3):975–9.

47. Vezzani A. Anti-inflammatory drugs in epilepsy: does it impact epileptogenesis? Expert Opin Drug Saf. 2015;14(4):583–92.

48. Vezzani A, Friedman A. Brain inflammation as a biomarker in epilepsy. Biomark Med. 2011;5(5):607–14.

49. Frigerio F, Flynn C, Han Y, Lyman K, Lugo JN, Ravizza T, Ghestem A, Pitsch J, Becker A, Anderson AE, Vezzani A, Chetkovich D, Bernard C. Neuroinflammation alters integrative properties of rat hippocampal pyramidal cells. Mol Neurobiol. https://doi.org/10.1007/s12035-018-0915-1.

50. Rao RS, Prakash A, Medhi B. Role of different cytokines and seizure susceptibility: a new dimension towards epilepsy research. Indian J Exp Biol. 2009;47(8):625–34.

51. Cunningham AJ, Murray CA, O'Neill LA, Lynch MA, O'Connor JJ. Interleukin-1 beta (IL-1 beta) and tumour necrosis factor (TNF) inhibit long-term potentiation in the rat dentate gyrus in vitro. Neurosci Lett. 1996;203(1):17–20.

52. Probert L, Akassoglou K, Pasparakis M, Kontogeorgos G, Kollias G. Spontaneous inflammatory demyelinating disease in transgenic mice showing central nervous system-specific expression of tumor necrosis factor alpha. Proc Natl Acad Sci U S A. 1995;92(24):11294–8.

53. Samland H, Huitron-Resendiz S, Masliah E, Criado J, Henriksen SJ, Campbell IL. Profound increase in sensitivity to glutamatergic—but not cholinergic agonist-induced seizures in transgenic mice with astrocyte production of IL-6. J Neurosci Res. 2003;73(2):176–87.

54. Shandra AA, Godlevsky LS, Vastyanov RS, Oleinik AA, Konovalenko VL, Rapoport EN, et al. The role of TNF-alpha in amygdala kindled rats. Neurosci Res. 2002;42(2):147–53.

6

Increased levels of HMGB1 and pro-inflammatory cytokines in children with febrile seizures

Jieun Choi[1*], Hyun Jin Min[2] and Jeon-Soo Shin[2,3*]

Abstract

Objective: Febrile seizures are the most common form of childhood seizures. Fever is induced by pro-inflammatory cytokines during infection, and pro-inflammatory cytokines may trigger the development of febrile seizures. In order to determine whether active inflammation, including high mobility group box-1 (HMGB1) and pro-inflammatory cytokines, occurs in children with febrile seizures or epilepsy, we analyzed cytokine profiles of patients with febrile seizures or epilepsy.

Methods: Forty-one febrile seizure patients who visited the emergency department of Seoul National University Boramae Hospital from June 2008 to May 2009 were included in this study. Blood was obtained from the febrile seizure child patients within 30 minutes of the time of the seizure; subsequently, serum cytokine assays were performed. Control samples were collected from children with febrile illness without convulsion (N = 41) and similarly analyzed. Serum samples from afebrile status epilepticus attacks in intractable epilepsy children (N = 12), afebrile seizure attacks in generalized epilepsy with febrile seizure plus (GEFSP) children (N = 6), and afebrile non-epileptic controls (N = 7) were also analyzed.

Results: Serum HMGB1 and IL-1β levels were significantly higher in febrile seizure patients than in fever only controls ($p < 0.05$). Serum IL-6 levels were significantly higher in typical febrile seizures than in fever only controls ($p < 0.05$). Serum IL-1β levels were significantly higher in status epilepticus attacks in intractable epilepsy patients than in fever only controls ($p < 0.05$). Serum levels of IL-1β were significantly correlated with levels of HMGB1, IL-6, and TNF-α ($p < 0.05$).

Conclusions: HMGB1 and pro-inflammatory cytokines were significantly higher in febrile seizure children. Although it is not possible to infer causality from descriptive human studies, our data suggest that HMGB1 and the cytokine network may contribute to the generation of febrile seizures in children. There may be a potential role for anti-inflammatory therapy targeting cytokines and HMGB1 in preventing or limiting febrile seizures or subsequent epileptogenesis in the vulnerable, developing nervous system of children.

Background

Febrile seizures are the most common form of childhood seizures, occurring in 2%-5% of children younger than 6 years old [1]. Febrile seizures are defined as seizures that occur during a febrile state and without an obvious central nervous system infection. Fever is induced by pro-inflammatory cytokines such as interleukin (IL)-1β, IL-6, and tumor necrosis factor (TNF)-α during infections. The fever threshold temperature for febrile seizures varies among individuals, as well as by age and maturation [2]. Genetic susceptibility to inflammation may influence the fever threshold temperature for febrile seizures, and 17-30% of febrile seizure patients have a family history of febrile seizures [2]. IL-1β biallelic polymorphism in the promoter region at the -511 position is significantly higher in febrile seizure patients than in fever only children, and this polymorphism results in an increase in IL-1β production [3,4]. However, others have failed to demonstrate a significant association between IL-1β (-511) and febrile seizures [5,6]. The association of IL-1β gene polymorphism and susceptibility to febrile

* Correspondence: jechoi66@snu.ac.kr; jsshin6203@yuhs.ac
[1]Department of Pediatrics, Seoul National University Boramae Hospital, Seoul National University, College of Medicine, Seoul, Korea
[2]Department of Microbiology, Yonsei University College of Medicine, Seoul, Korea

seizures is still controversial. Increased levels of IL-6, and IL-1-receptor antagonist/IL-1β ratio have been reported in the plasma of febrile seizure patients [3]. Viruses as causative agents of febrile seizures have been demonstrated in several reports. Neurotropic viruses, such as herpes and influenza A, are commonly associated with febrile seizures [7,8].

Pro-inflammatory cytokines may trigger febrile seizures. In experimental animals, intraventricular injection of IL-1β reduces the seizure threshold in 14-day old mice subjected to hyperthermia, while IL-1β knock-out mice had an increased seizure threshold [9]. IL-1β increases glutamatergic neurotransmission and lowers the peak magnitude of GABA-mediated currents [10], supporting the role of pro-inflammatory cytokine contribution to the generation of fever-induced seizures [9]. Also, IL-1β prolongs the duration of electroencephalographic seizure [11].

High mobility group box-1 (HMGB1) has been shown to be a key mediator of inflammatory diseases. HMGB1 is a nuclear protein that triggers inflammation, binds to lipopolysaccharides (LPS) and IL-1, and initiates and synergizes with a Toll-like receptor (TLR) 4-mediated pro-inflammatory response [12]. After pro-inflammatory stimulation, such as that by LPS, TNF-α, IL-1, IL-6 and IL-8, HMGB1 is actively released from activated monocytes and macrophages. Regulation of HMGB1 secretion is important for control of HMGB1-mediated inflammation and is dependent on various processes such as phosphorylation by calcium-dependent protein kinase C [13], as well as acetylation and methylation [14]. In a recent study, HMGB1 and TLR4 were involved in the generation and recurrence of seizures in experimental animals [15,16].

Cytokine analyses in our previous study showed that pro-inflammatory cytokine levels, including IL-1β, IL-8, IL-12p70, and macrophage inflammatory protein (MIP)-1β, were significantly high in the epileptogenic cortex of intractable epilepsy children [17]. In addition, levels of IL-6 and MCP-1 were significantly high in patients with a family history of epilepsy. Active neuroinflammation, such as a marked activation of microglia and astrocytes as well as marked cellular injury, were also observed in epileptogenic brain tissue, supporting the suggestion that neuroinflammation may contribute to epileptogenesis in the developing brain.

In order to determine whether active inflammation, including HMGB1 and pro-inflammatory cytokines, occurs in children with febrile seizures and pediatric epilepsy, we analyzed cytokine profiles in the serum of child patients with febrile seizures or epilepsy and assessed the correlation between cytokine levels and febrile seizures.

Materials and methods
Patient information
Forty-one febrile seizure patients who visited to emergency department of Seoul National University Boramae Hospital from June 2008 to May 2009 were included in this study (Table 1). Blood was obtained from patients within 30 minutes of the time of seizure, and serum was immediately separated and frozen for subsequent cytokine assay. Patient inclusion criteria were age between 6 months and 6 years, body temperature ≥38.5°C, C-reactive protein (CRP) ≤2.0, and presented no other identifiable cause of the seizure. Clinical data for familial febrile seizure history, earlier febrile seizure attacks, as well as duration and semiology of febrile seizures were obtained from the patients' parents. Family history was regarded as positive when febrile seizures occurred in first-degree relatives. Laboratory findings, including complete blood counts (CBC), blood chemistry, and CRP, were checked at the time of seizure. CRP levels higher than 2.0 were excluded due to presumptive presence of bacterial infection. Febrile seizure patients were classified into two types: typical type for whom febrile seizures persist for < 15 minutes, are generalized tonic-clonic, and only occur once within 24 hours; and atypical types for whom seizures persist for > 15 minutes, or are partial seizures, or recur within 24 hours of the initial attack. Control samples were collected from children with febrile illness, but without convulsion (N = 41). Control groups were matched for age and temperature criteria and had no convulsions during the febrile illness and no known history of previous febrile seizures. Control blood serum was collected and frozen as above. In addition, blood serum was collected and frozen from afebrile status epilepticus attacks in intractable epilepsy children (N = 12), afebrile seizure attacks in GEFSP children (N = 6), and afebrile non-epileptic controls (N = 7) for cytokine assay in order to subtract fever effects from the cytokine levels. The study was approved by the Institutional Review Board at the Seoul National University Boramae Medical Center (20080918/06-2008-74/76). Informed consent was obtained from each child's parents.

Cytokine measurement
Levels of pro-inflammatory cytokines including HMGB1, IL-1β, IL-6, interferon (IFN)-β, TNF-α, and anti-inflammatory cytokine IL-10 were measured using commercially available, enzyme-linked immunosorbent assay (ELISA) kits according to the manufacturer's instructions (for HMGB1, Shino-Test Corp., Tokyo, Japan [17]; for IL-1β, IFN-β, TNF-α, and IL-10, Panomics Inc., Redwood City, CA, USA; for IL-6, R&D Systems, Minneapolis, MN, USA). Samples were analyzed in duplicate and

Table 1 Clinical findings of febrile seizure, epilepsy, and control children

	Fever only control (N = 41)	Febrile seizure (N = 41)	Afebrile control (N = 7)	Afebrile seizure (N = 6)	Afebrile SE (N = 12)
Age (year)	3.1	2.1	7.9	7.6	6.3
Male/Female	24/17	29/12	3/4	4/2	8/4
BT at admission(°C)	38.4	39.0	36.6	37.0	36.5
WBC count (per mm³)	11,719	12,068	7,540	8,716	9,560
CRP	0.91	0.95	0.4	0.6	0.8

SE, status epilepticus; BT, body temperature

compared with controls. The detection limits were 0.2 ng/mL for HMGB1, 0.27 pg/mL for IL-1β, 0.23 pg/mL for IL-6, 0.21 pg/mL for IFN-γ, 0.49 pg/mL for TNF-α and 0.22 pg/mL for IL-10.

Statistical Analysis

The χ^2 test was used to compare the clinical characteristics between febrile seizure patients and the controls. The Mann-Whitney test was used to compare serum cytokine levels and laboratory findings between controls and febrile seizure patients. The Spearman's rank correlation coefficient was calculated to detect significant correlations between cytokine levels. The Kruskal Wallis test was used to compare cytokine levels among afebrile controls, febrile controls, and four seizure groups (first attack febrile seizure, recurrent attack febrile seizure, afebrile seizure attack in GEFSP, and afebrile status epilepticus attacks in intractable epilepsy patients). GraphPad Prism v. 4.0 (GraphPad Software Inc., San Diego, CA, USA) was used to perform the above tests. Values are expressed as means, and statistical significance of differences was set as $p < 0.05$ for all tests.

Results

Patient characteristics

Table 1 summarizes the patient's clinical data. Forty-one febrile seizure patients and 41 control children with febrile illness without convulsion were included in this study. The mean age of febrile seizure patients was 2.1 years. Boys were more prevalent than girls

Table 2 Subgroups of febrile seizure patients

	Febrile seizure patients (N = 41)	
Family history of FS	Positive	11 (27%)
	Negative	30 (73%)
FS history	First attack	28 (68%)
	Recurrent	13 (32%)
FS type	Typical	27 (66%)
	Atypical	14 (34%)

FS, febrile seizure

were (respectively, 71% vs. 29%). Eleven (27%) patients had a family history of febrile seizures and fourteen (34%) patients exhibited atypical types of febrile seizures (Table 2). Twenty-eight patients (68%) had their first febrile seizure attack and thirteen patients (32%) had experienced previous febrile seizure attacks. Febrile seizure patients and febrile children without seizures did not significantly differ by sex, age, and laboratory data.

Serum cytokine levels in the febrile seizure patients; increased IL-1β, IL-6, IL-10 and HMGB levels

In febrile seizure patients, serum IL-1β levels were at a 4-fold increase and HMGB1 levels were at a 1.3-fold increase higher than the fever only controls (Table 3, both $p < 0.05$). Serum levels of IL-6 were at a 1.8-fold increase and IL-10 were at a 2.8-fold increase in febrile seizure patients higher than the fever only controls, although statistically not significant (Table 3, $p = 07$ and $p = 0.05$). There were no differences in serum IFN-γ and TNF-α levels between febrile seizure patients and fever only controls (Table 3).

In comparisons of the subgroups of febrile seizure patients with the fever only control, typical febrile seizure patients showed a 4.2-fold increase of IL-1β and a 1.9-fold increase of IL-6 levels higher than the fever only controls (Table 3, both $p < 0.05$). Both atypical febrile seizure and first attack febrile seizure patients showed a 1.5- and a 1.4-fold increase of HMGB1 levels higher than the fever only controls (Table 3, both $p < 0.05$). The IL-1β levels were at an 8.1-fold increase in patients with recurrent febrile seizure attacks than those with first febrile seizure attack, although statistically not significant (Table 3, $p = 0.27$). IL-10 levels showed a 6.6-fold increase in children with recurrent febrile seizure attacks higher than the fever only controls (Table 3, $p = 0.06$). Febrile seizure patients without a family history of febrile seizures showed a 3.5-fold increase of IL-10 levels (Table 3, $p < 0.05$) above the fever only controls and a 3.7-fold increase above those with FS without a family history of febrile seizures (Table 3, $p = 0.31$).

Table 3 Comparisons of cytokine levels between fever only control and febrile seizure subgroups

Groups (No.)	IL-1β (pg/mL)	IL-6 (pg/mL)	HMGB1 (ng/mL)	IFN-γ (pg/mL)	TNF-α (pg/mL)	IL-10 (pg/mL)
Fever only control (41)	3.1 ± 0.8†	134.0 ± 22.7	24.8 ± 2.5	84.2 ± 38.6	5.6 ± 2.9	8.3 ± 2.6
Febrile seizures (41)	12.0 ± 5.3*	247.1 ± 43.0	32.6 ± 3.0*	73.5 ± 20.9	5.0 ± 1.8	23.6 ± 13.4
Typical FS (27)	12.9 ± 7.6*	260.1 ± 50.4*	30.5 ± 3.8	66.5 ± 21.6	3.0 ± 0.9	28.5 ± 20.3
Atypical FS (14)	10.4 ± 4.9	228.3 ± 81.2	36.6 ± 5.0*	86.9 ± 45.9	9.0 ± 5.0	14.2 ± 3.8
First FS (28)	3.7 ± 0.7	252.7 ± 53.5	35.0 ± 3.9*	74.6 ± 21.3*	1.9 ± 0.6	9.2 ± 2.2
Recurrent FS (13)	30.1 ± 15.7	241.7 ± 73.0	27.3 ± 4.7	70.9 ± 48.8	11.8 ± 5.3	54.6 ± 41.8
FS without FHx (30)	13.0 ± 6.9	241.6 ± 49.3	31.8 ± 3.6	62.8 ± 22.5	5.2 ± 2.4	29. 4 ± 18.2*
FS with FHx (11)	9.4 ± 5.6	270.1 ± 89.2	34.7 ± 5.9	102.6 ± 48.5	4.7 ± 2.1	7.8 ± 2.7

* indicates a significant ($p < 0.05$) difference compared to fever only control (Mann-Whitney test).

FS, febrile seizure; FHx, family history; SE, status epilepticus

†; mean ± standard error of mean

Serum cytokine levels in the afebrile control, febrile control, and afebrile various seizure groups

1. IL-1β

The mean IL-1β level of the afebrile control children was 2.0 pg/mL, while that for the febrile control was 3.1 pg/mL. The mean IL-1β level in afebrile status epilepticus attacks in intractable epilepsy patients was at a 11.7-fold increase higher than that of the afebrile controls (23.4 vs. 2.0 pg/mL) and a 7.5-fold increase higher than of fever only controls (Table 3, 23.4 vs. 3.1 pg/mL, $p < 0.05$). Comparisons of IL-1β levels among afebrile and febrile controls and the four seizure groups (first and recurrent febrile seizures, afebrile seizures in GEFSP and afebrile status epilepticus in intractable epilepsy patients) showed significantly higher levels in the afebrile status epilepticus in intractable epilepsy and the recurrent febrile seizure groups (Figure 1A, $p < 0.05$).

2. IL-6

The mean IL-6 level of afebrile controls was 34.7 pg/mL, while that of febrile controls was 134.0 pg/mL, and that of afebrile status epilepticus attacks in intractable epilepsy patients was 51.4 pg/mL. Comparisons of IL-6 levels among afebrile and febrile controls, and the four seizure groups showed significantly higher IL-6 levels in first and recurrent attack febrile seizure patients (Figure 1B, p < 0.05).

3. TNF-α

The mean TNF-α level of afebrile controls was 3.4 pg/mL, while that in febrile controls was 5.6 pg/mL, and that in afebrile status epilepticus attacks in intractable epilepsy patients was 14.2 pg/mL. Afebrile seizure patients showed a 57% decrease of TNF-α levels of febrile controls (Table 3, $p < 0.05$). Comparisons of TNF-α levels among afebrile and febrile controls, and the four seizure groups showed higher levels in the afebrile status epilepticus attacks in intractable epilepsy patients and the recurrent attack febrile seizure groups (Figure 1C, p = 0.06).

4. HMGB1

The mean HMGB1 level in the serum of afebrile controls was 9.0 ng/mL, that in febrile control was 24.8 ng/mL, and that in afebrile status epilepticus attacks in intractable epilepsy patients was 30.1 ng/mL. In comparisons of HMGB1 levels between afebrile controls, febrile controls and the four seizure groups, there were trends of higher HMGB1 levels in both febrile seizures and afebrile status epilepticus attacks in intractable epilepsy patients than in the febrile and afebrile controls, but this was not statistically significant (Figure 1D, p = 0.11).

5. IFN-γ

The mean IFN-γ level of afebrile controls was 20.8 pg/mL, that in febrile controls was 84.2 pg/mL, and that in afebrile status epilepticus attacks in intractable epilepsy patients was 21.4 pg/mL. Comparisons of IFN-γ levels among afebrile and febrile controls, and the four seizure groups showed no significant differences (Table 3).

6. IL-10

The mean IL-10 level of afebrile controls was 2.7 pg/mL, that in febrile controls was 8.3 pg/mL, and that in afebrile status epilepticus attacks in intractable epilepsy patients was 0.6 pg/mL. Afebrile seizure patients and afebrile status epilepticus patients with intractable epilepsy showed significantly decreased IL-10 levels than that of febrile and afebrile controls (2.6 pg/mL & 0.6 pg/mL, $p < 0.05$). There were no significant differences of IL-10 levels among afebrile controls, febrile controls and the four seizure groups (Table 3).

The correlations between the various cytokines

IL-1β serum levels were significantly correlated with HMGB1, IL-6, and TNF-α levels (respectively: Figures 2A, B, and 2C; $r = 0.28$, $r = 0.25$, and $r = 0.45$; all $p < 0.05$), but not with IL-10 and IFN-γ. Serum IL-6 levels were significantly correlated with IL-1β and TNF-α levels (respectively: Figures 2B and 2D; $r = 0.25$ and $r = $

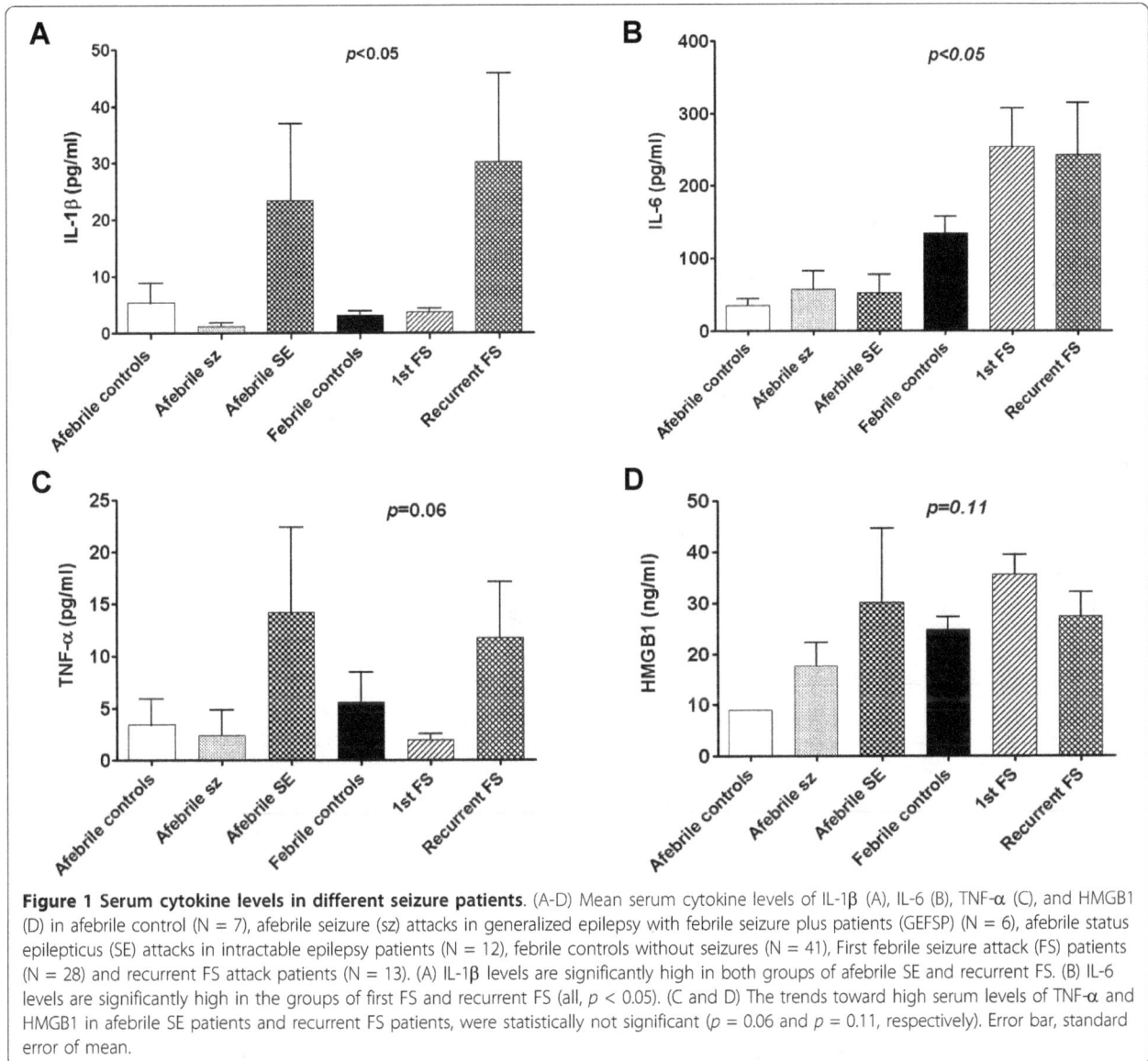

Figure 1 Serum cytokine levels in different seizure patients. (A-D) Mean serum cytokine levels of IL-1β (A), IL-6 (B), TNF-α (C), and HMGB1 (D) in afebrile control (N = 7), afebrile seizure (sz) attacks in generalized epilepsy with febrile seizure plus patients (GEFSP) (N = 6), afebrile status epilepticus (SE) attacks in intractable epilepsy patients (N = 12), febrile controls without seizures (N = 41), First febrile seizure attack (FS) patients (N = 28) and recurrent FS attack patients (N = 13). (A) IL-1β levels are significantly high in both groups of afebrile SE and recurrent FS. (B) IL-6 levels are significantly high in the groups of first FS and recurrent FS (all, *p* < 0.05). (C and D) The trends toward high serum levels of TNF-α and HMGB1 in afebrile SE patients and recurrent FS patients, were statistically not significant (*p* = 0.06 and *p* = 0.11, respectively). Error bar, standard error of mean.

0.28; both $p < 0.05$), but were not correlated with HMGB1, IL-10, and IFN-γ levels.

Discussion

This is the first study demonstrating a significant elevation of HMGB1 in the serum of febrile seizure patients. Moreover, serum levels of other pro-inflammatory cytokines, including IL-1β, IL-6, and the anti-inflammatory cytokine IL-10 were significantly higher among our patients with febrile seizures. IL-1β level increase was related to seizure recurrence and duration, as seen with the higher levels of IL-1β in recurrent febrile seizure or afebrile status epilepticus patients. In addition, IL-1β levels were significantly and positively correlated with HMGB1 levels and with other pro-inflammatory cytokines (IL-6 and TNF-α),

supporting the association of the cytokine network in febrile seizures.

HMGB1 is a highly conserved, ubiquitously expressed protein [18] and is actively secreted from monocytes and macrophages in response to challenges with LPS [19]. HMGB1 binds to and transfers LPS, consequently increasing LPS-induced TNF-α production in human peripheral blood mononuclear cells [13]. HMGB1 is passively released from necrotic cells, but not from apoptotic cells, thereby creating a signal for the organism to distinguish between the two types of cell death [20]. Several clinical studies have reported that serum HMGB1 levels are elevated in patients with infection and/or systemic inflammatory response syndrome, than in healthy control individuals [19,21]. HMGB1 is involved in various diseases without obvious infections;

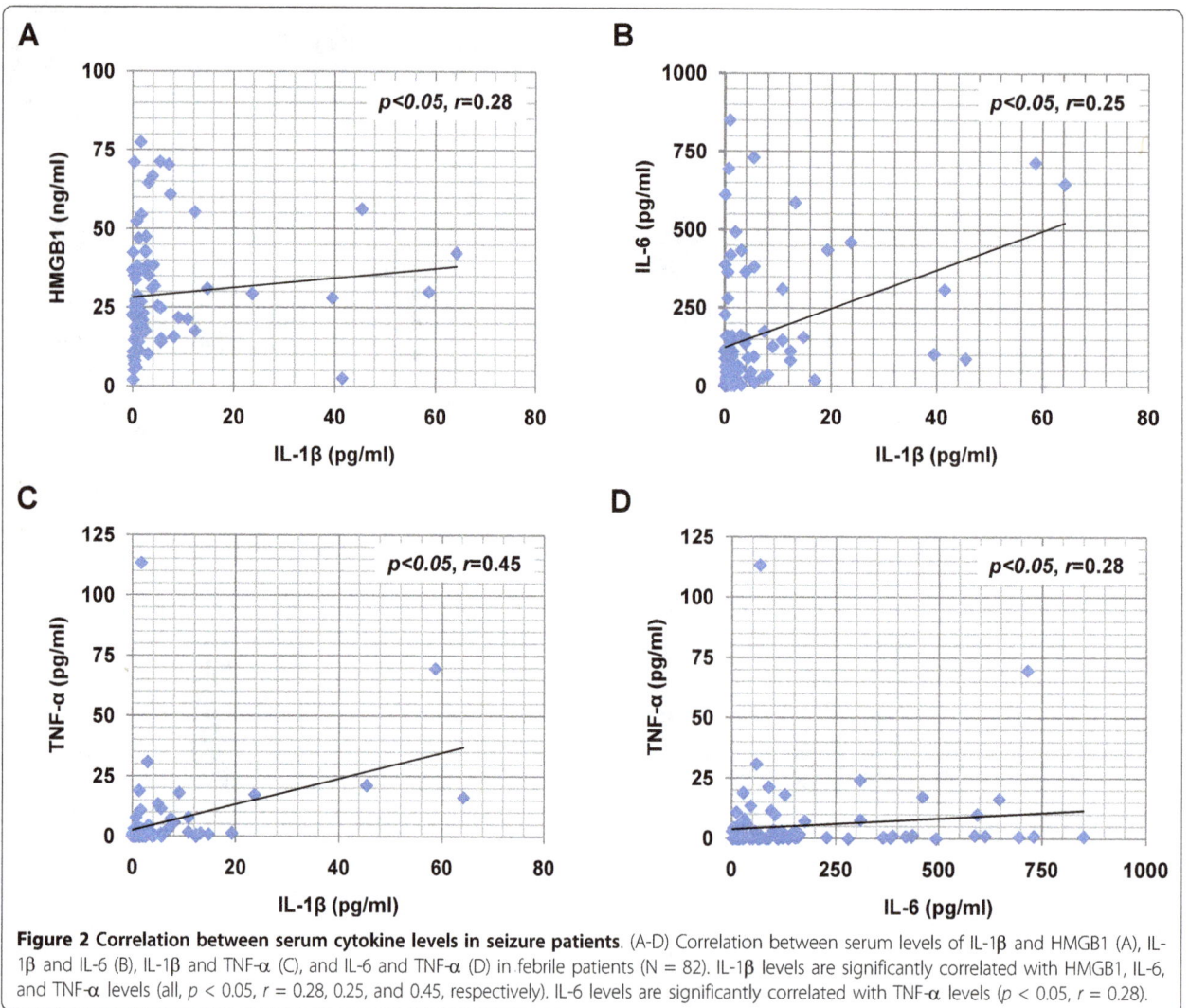

Figure 2 Correlation between serum cytokine levels in seizure patients. (A-D) Correlation between serum levels of IL-1β and HMGB1 (A), IL-1β and IL-6 (B), IL-1β and TNF-α (C), and IL-6 and TNF-α (D) in febrile patients (N = 82). IL-1β levels are significantly correlated with HMGB1, IL-6, and TNF-α levels (all, p < 0.05, r = 0.28, 0.25, and 0.45, respectively). IL-6 levels are significantly correlated with TNF-α levels (p < 0.05, r = 0.28).

for example, rheumatoid arthritis [22], hemorrhagic shock [23], cerebral and myocardial ischemia [24], acute lung injury [25], and acute pancreatitis [26]. HMGB1 is highly expressed in human epileptogenic brain, and antagonists of HMGB1 and TLR4 have been demonstrated to retard seizure precipitation and to decrease acute and chronic seizure recurrence in epilepsy animals [15]. These findings suggest a role for the HMGB1-TLR4 axis in epilepsy. In our study, serum levels of HMGB1 were significantly higher in febrile seizure patients and showed a positive correlation with IL-1β levels. Our results, together with those from other studies, suggest that HMGB1 activation is an important feature associated with epilepsy and febrile seizures.

IL-1β serum levels were significantly higher in our febrile seizures patients than in febrile children without seizures. IL-1β has been shown to have potent pro-convulsant properties in experimental animals [27]. IL-1β acts on astrocytes to increase glutamate release via

TNF-α production [28], resulting in elevated extracellular glutamate levels and hyper-excitability. Also, IL-1β can stimulate IL-6 release [29]. In our patients, IL-1β levels were significantly correlated with IL-6, HMGB1, and TNF-α levels. In our previous work using epileptogenic brain cortices of children with intractable epilepsy, pro-inflammatory cytokines, IL-1β, IL-8, IL-12p70, and MIP-1β were increased significantly above those in non-epileptogenic control brain cortices [30]. Our patients with intractable epilepsy experiencing status epilepticus attacks also showed high IL-1β, IL-6 and HMGB1 levels. These results together suggest that active inflammation does occur in febrile seizures and pediatric epilepsy, and it may play a common pathologic role in febrile seizures and epilepsy.

Since cytokine levels were measured with blood taken 30 min after the seizure, the acute effect of seizures could not be distinguished from a persistent inflammatory tone in febrile seizure patients. Seizures themselves can activate the sympathetic nervous system and induce the release of catecholamines [31,32], resulting in cytokine release from peripheral blood mononuclear cells [33]. However, in our study, patients with recurrent febrile seizure attacks had much higher IL-1β and TNF-α levels than patients with first attack febrile seizures, although interictal cytokine levels were not available after acute seizures. In animal models of prolonged febrile seizures, IL-1β was significantly high in the hippocampus for over 24 hours and was elevated chronically only in rats developing spontaneous limbic seizures after febrile status epilepticus [9,34]. These findings suggest that inflammatory responses in febrile seizures are accentuated by their repetition and increase the likelihood of febrile seizure recurrence.

Interestingly, no increase in serum IL-1β was detected in our children with fever but no seizures (3.1 pg/mL), as compared to controls without fever and with no seizures (2.0 pg/mL). In another study, similarly low IL-1β blood levels of 3.4 pg/mL were reported in the febrile control group [35]. This lack of increase may be the result of excluding patients with presumptive bacterial infections, because LPS is the main inducer for the synthesis of IL-1β [36]. Also, IL-1β is usually difficult to detect because of its binding to large proteins such as α-2 macroglobulin and complement [37]. Furthermore, fever could occur independently of IL-1 or TNF activity during infections, and the cytokine-like property of TLR signal transduction could be one explanation [38].

The sources of the serum cytokine in febrile seizures patients are not clear. The main source of IL-1 is monocytes in the periphery and microglial cells in the nervous system, which upon activation secrete the cytokines. Cytokines are produced by astrocytes and some neurons in the CNS by LPS and other stimuli [39,40]. Under normal conditions, the levels of IL-1 are low, both in the circulation and in the CNS, whereas upon infection or injury, IL-1 levels increase abruptly but transiently, returning to normal within 8 h in healthy, young mouse brain [41]. Therefore, high serum levels of IL-1β may reflect high levels in the CNS. However, conflicting results about IL-1β levels have been reported in peripheral blood and CSF of children with febrile seizures, such as high in plasma but not in CSF [42], or high in CSF but not in serum [43] or increase in neither serum nor CSF [35]. These results potentially reflect difficulties in obtaining clinical samples and measuring free IL-1β. The possible sources of the serum cytokine increases in febrile seizures may be peripheral mononuclear cells, CSF-blood exchange, and leakage from the brain reticuloendothelial system.

A dual role of IL-6 in seizures has been demonstrated in several animal models. IL-6 knockout mice showed an increased seizure susceptibility to glutamate receptor agonists [44]. Transgenic mice over-expressing IL-6 in astrocytes were also reported to have an increased seizure susceptibility to glutamate receptor agonists, probably due to reduced GABA-mediated inhibition [45]. In developing rats, intra-nasal administration of IL-6 prolonged the latency and shortened the duration of hyperthermia-induced seizures, suggesting an anti-convulsant effect to febrile seizures [46]. On the other hand, intranasal administration of IL-6 in adult rats exacerbated the severity of seizures induced by pentylenetetrazole, supporting a pro-convulsant effect [47]. In our patients including only presumptive viral infections, serum IL-6 was higher in febrile seizure children than in fever only controls. Moreover, IL-6 levels in febrile seizure patients were much higher than in afebrile seizure attack patients. Higher IL-6 and IFN-α levels have been reported in patients with influenza-associated febrile seizures compared to those without febrile seizures [3,48]. These findings, with our results, may support the pro-convulsant action of IL-6 in febrile seizures.

IL-10 is a multifunctional anti-inflammatory cytokine produced by monocytes, macrophages, lymphocytes, as well as microglia and inhibits the production of pro-inflammatory cytokines, including IL-1, IL-6, IL-8, and TNF-α [49]. Peripheral blood mononuclear cells from febrile seizure patients have shown increased IL-10 production by LPS [50]. In IL-10 injected animals, the febrile seizure threshold was significantly higher than that in controls, suggesting that IL-10 is associated with a resistance to febrile seizures [51]. Previously, plasma IL-10 levels showed no difference between febrile seizures and controls [3]. However, in our patients, IL-10 levels were higher in recurrent febrile seizure patients than in first attack febrile seizure patients and were also higher in patients without a family history of febrile seizures than in patients with family history. These findings may reflect compensatory activation of anti-inflammatory or anti-convulsive mechanisms, or mechanism defects in the anti-inflammatory role of IL-10 in febrile seizure families; further studies into the role of IL-10 are warranted.

TNF-α causes both detrimental and beneficial effects on brain function depending on its concentration, targeted cells, duration of exposure and the specific receptor subtypes [52,53]. TNF-α is rapidly upregulated in the CNS by seizures, and intrahippocampal injection of TNF-α potently inhibit seizure in a mice model of epilepsy [54]. In our children with acute and brief seizures, either febrile or afebrile, serum TNF-α was decreased, or at least not increased, supporting that TNF-α is not involved in the mechanisms by which seizures are triggered. On the other hand, transgenic mice over-expressing high amounts of TNF-α in astrocytes developed spontaneous seizures, [55] and TNF-α has been shown to increase excitatory postsynaptic currents in hippo-campal neurons [56] and to decrease GABA$_A$-mediated inhibitory synaptic strength, leading to increased seizure susceptibility [57,58]. Our recurrent febrile seizure patients showed higher serum TNF-α levels than first attack febrile seizure patients, and afebrile status epilepticus attacks in intractable epilepsy patients showed higher serum TNF-α level than short-duration seizure attacks in GEFSP patients, supporting that chronic or recurrent expression of TNF-α may change susceptibility to seizures.

The causative role of cytokines in epileptogenesis remains to be elucidated. Cytokines may contribute initially to incite seizures in the developing brain after being induced by seizure or tissue injury, and they may exacerbate tissue injury and promote further seizures. Furthermore, cytokine gene polymorphisms have been linked to epilepsy susceptibility [4]. Thus, it may be worthwhile to explore further a possible link between febrile seizures and genetic susceptibility to inflammation.

In summary, HMGB1 and pro-inflammatory cytokines were significantly higher in febrile seizure patients. Although it is not possible to infer causality from descriptive human studies, our data suggest that HMGB1 and the cytokine network may contribute to the generation of febrile seizures in children. Pro-inflammatory cytokine production may promote seizures, further exacerbate epilepsy, and may cause subsequent intractable epilepsy. If so, there may be a potential role for anti-inflammatory therapy targeting cytokines and HMGB1 as a novel therapeutic strategy to prevent or limit febrile seizures or subsequent epileptogenesis in the vulnerable, developing nervous system of children.

Acknowledgements
This research was supported by the Basic Science Research Program through the National Research Foundation of Korea funded by the Ministry of Education, Science and Technology (800-20110174), the Seoul National University Hospital Research Fund (04-2008-0960), and the Seoul National University Boramae Hospital Research Fund (03-2011-15) to JC, and by the Mid-Career Researcher Program (2009-0081001), NRF (2011-0017611), and the second stage BK21 for Medical Sciences of Yonsei University to JS.

Author details
[1]Department of Pediatrics, Seoul National University Boramae Hospital, Seoul National University, College of Medicine, Seoul, Korea. [2]Department of Microbiology, Yonsei University College of Medicine, Seoul, Korea. [3]Severance Biomedical Science Institute and Institute for Immunology and Immunological Diseases, Yonsei University College of Medicine, Seoul, Korea.

Authors' contributions
JC reviewed and helped in analyzing data, obtained IRB approval and permissions from the patients and their parents, processed serum from the patients, conducted cytokine analyses, and helped draft and prepare the manuscript for publication. HM performed the HMGB1 ELISA analyses. JS reviewed and helped in the data analyses as well as helped with drafting and preparing the manuscript for publication. All authors have read and approved the final version of the manuscript.

Competing interests
The authors declare that they have no competing interests.

References
1. Hauser WA: **The prevalence and incidence of convulsive disorders in children.** *Epilepsia* 1994, **35**(Suppl 2):S1-6.
2. Millichap JG: **Studies in febrile seizures. I. Height of body temperature as a measure of the febrile-seizure threshold.** *Pediatrics* 1959, **23**:76-85.
3. Virta M, Hurme M, Helminen M: **Increased frequency of interleukin-1beta (-511) allele 2 in febrile seizures.** *Pediatr Neurol* 2002, **26**:192-195.
4. Kanemoto K, Kawasaki J, Yuasa S, Kumaki T, Tomohiro O, Kaji R, Nishimura M: **Increased frequency of interleukin-1beta-511T allele in patients with temporal lobe epilepsy, hippocampal sclerosis, and prolonged febrile convulsion.** *Epilepsia* 2003, **44**:796-799.
5. Tilgen N, Pfeiffer H, Cobilanschi J, Rau B, Horvath S, Elger CE, Propping P, Heils A: **Association analysis between the human interleukin 1beta (-511) gene polymorphism and susceptibility to febrile convulsions.** *Neurosci Lett* 2002, **334**:68-70.
6. Chou IC, Lin WD, Wang CH, Tsai CH, Li TC, Tsai FJ: **Interleukin (IL)-1beta, IL-1 receptor antagonist, IL-6, IL-8, IL-10, and tumor necrosis factor alpha gene polymorphisms in patients with febrile seizures.** *Journal of clinical laboratory analysis* 2010, **24**:154-159.
7. Hall CB, Long CE, Schnabel KC, Caserta MT, McIntyre KM, Costanzo MA, Knott A, Dewhurst S, Insel RA, Epstein LG: **Human herpesvirus-6 infection in children. A prospective study of complications and reactivation.** *N Engl J Med* 1994, **331**:432-438.
8. Chiu SS, Tse CY, Lau YL, Peiris M: **Influenza A infection is an important cause of febrile seizures.** *Pediatrics* 2001, **108**:E63.
9. Dube C, Vezzani A, Behrens M, Bartfai T, Baram TZ: **Interleukin-1beta contributes to the generation of experimental febrile seizures.** *Annals of neurology* 2005, **57**:152-155.
10. Wang S, Cheng Q, Malik S, Yang J: **Interleukin-1beta inhibits gamma-aminobutyric acid type A (GABA(A)) receptor current in cultured hippocampal neurons.** *J Pharmacol Exp Ther* 2000, **292**:497-504.
11. Vezzani A, Conti M, De Luigi A, Ravizza T, Moneta D, Marchesi F, De Simoni MG: **Interleukin-1beta immunoreactivity and microglia are enhanced in the rat hippocampus by focal kainate application: functional evidence for enhancement of electrographic seizures.** *J Neurosci* 1999, **19**:5054-5065.
12. Youn JH, Oh YJ, Kim ES, Choi JE, Shin JS: **High Mobility Group Box 1 Protein Binding to Lipopolysaccharide Facilitates Transfer of Lipopolysaccharide to CD14 and Enhances Lipopolysaccharide-Mediated TNF-{alpha} Production in Human Monocytes.** *J Immunol* 2008, **180**:5067-5074.
13. Oh YJ, Youn JH, Ji Y, Lee SE, Lim KJ, Choi JE, Shin JS: **HMGB1 is phosphorylated by classical protein kinase C and is secreted by a calcium-dependent mechanism.** *J Immunol* 2009, **182**:5800-5809.
14. Rauvala H, Rouhiainen A: **Physiological and pathophysiological outcomes of the interactions of HMGB1 with cell surface receptors.** *Biochim Biophys Acta* 2010, **1799**:164-170.
15. Maroso M, Balosso S, Ravizza T, Liu J, Aronica E, Iyer AM, Rossetti C, Molteni M, Casalgrandi M, Manfredi AA, *et al*: **Toll-like receptor 4 and high-mobility group box-1 are involved in ictogenesis and can be targeted to reduce seizures.** *Nat Med* 2010, **16**:413-419.
16. Vezzani A, French J, Bartfai T, Baram TZ: **The role of inflammation in epilepsy.** *Nat Rev Neurol* 2011, **7**:31-40.
17. Yamada S, Inoue K, Yakabe K, Imaizumi H, Maruyama I: **High mobility group protein 1 (HMGB1) quantified by ELISA with a monoclonal antibody that does not cross-react with HMGB2.** *Clin Chem* 2003, **49**:1535-1537.
18. Muller S, Ronfani L, Bianchi ME: **Regulated expression and subcellular localization of HMGB1, a chromatin protein with a cytokine function.** *J Intern Med* 2004, **255**:332-343.
19. Wang H, Bloom O, Zhang M, Vishnubhakat JM, Ombrellino M, Che J, Frazier A, Yang H, Ivanova S, Borovikova L, *et al*: **HMG-1 as a late mediator of endotoxin lethality in mice.** *Science* 1999, **285**:248-251.
20. Scaffidi P, Misteli T, Bianchi ME: **Release of chromatin protein HMGB1 by necrotic cells triggers inflammation.** *Nature* 2002, **418**:191-195.
21. van Zoelen MA, Laterre PF, van Veen SQ, van Till JW, Wittebole X, Bresser P, Tanck MW, Dugernier T, Ishizaka A, Boermeester MA, van der Poll T:

Systemic and local high mobility group box 1 concentrations during severe infection. *Crit Care Med* 2007, 35:2799-2804.

22. Taniguchi N, Kawahara K, Yone K, Hashiguchi T, Yamakuchi M, Goto M, Inoue K, Yamada S, Ijiri K, Matsunaga S, *et al*: High mobility group box chromosomal protein 1 plays a role in the pathogenesis of rheumatoid arthritis as a novel cytokine. *Arthritis Rheum* 2003, 48:971-981.

23. Ombrellino M, Wang H, Ajemian MS, Talhouk A, Scher LA, Friedman SG, Tracey KJ: Increased serum concentrations of high-mobility-group protein 1 in haemorrhagic shock. *Lancet* 1999, 354:1446-1447.

24. Goldstein RS, Gallowitsch-Puerta M, Yang L, Rosas-Ballina M, Huston JM, Czura CJ, Lee DC, Ward MF, Bruchfeld AN, Wang H, *et al*: Elevated high-mobility group box 1 levels in patients with cerebral and myocardial ischemia. *Shock (Augusta, Ga)* 2006, 25:571-574.

25. Ueno H, Matsuda T, Hashimoto S, Amaya F, Kitamura Y, Tanaka M, Kobayashi A, Maruyama I, Yamada S, Hasegawa N, *et al*: Contributions of high mobility group box protein in experimental and clinical acute lung injury. *Am J Respir Crit Care Med* 2004, 170:1310-1316.

26. Yasuda T, Ueda T, Takeyama Y, Shinzeki M, Sawa H, Nakajima T, Ajiki T, Fujino Y, Suzuki Y, Kuroda Y: Significant increase of serum high-mobility group box chromosomal protein 1 levels in patients with severe acute pancreatitis. *Pancreas* 2006, 33:359-363.

27. Balosso S, Maroso M, Sanchez-Alavez M, Ravizza T, Frasca A, Bartfai T, Vezzani A: A novel non-transcriptional pathway mediates the proconvulsive effects of interleukin-1beta. *Brain* 2008, 131:3256-3265.

28. Bezzi P, Volterra A: A neuron-glia signalling network in the active brain. *Current opinion in neurobiology* 2001, 11:387-394.

29. Aronica E, Gorter JA, Redeker S, Ramkema M, Spliet WG, van Rijen PC, Leenstra S, Troost D: Distribution, characterization and clinical significance of microglia in glioneuronal tumours from patients with chronic intractable epilepsy. *Neuropathol Appl Neurobiol* 2005, 31:280-291.

30. Choi J, Nordli DR Jr, Alden TD, DiPatri A Jr, Laux L, Kelley K, Rosenow J, Schuele SU, Rajaram V, Koh S: Cellular injury and neuroinflammation in children with chronic intractable epilepsy. *J Neuroinflammation* 2009, 6:38.

31. Rosenbaum KJ, Sapthavichaikul S, Skovsted P: Sympathetic nervous system response to lidocaine induced seizures in cats. *Acta Anaesthesiol Scand* 1978, 22:548-555.

32. Sakamoto K, Saito T, Orman R, Koizumi K, Lazar J, Salciccioli L, Stewart M: Autonomic consequences of kainic acid-induced limbic cortical seizures in rats: peripheral autonomic nerve activity, acute cardiovascular changes, and death. *Epilepsia* 2008, 49:982-996.

33. Meisel C, Schwab JM, Prass K, Meisel A, Dirnagl U: Central nervous system injury-induced immune deficiency syndrome. *Nat Rev Neurosci* 2005, 6:775-786.

34. Dube CM, Ravizza T, Hamamura M, Zha Q, Keebaugh A, Fok K, Andres AL, Nalcioglu O, Obenaus A, Vezzani A, Baram TZ: Epileptogenesis provoked by prolonged experimental febrile seizures: mechanisms and biomarkers. *J Neurosci* 2010, 30:7484-7494.

35. Lahat E, Livne M, Barr J, Katz Y: Interleukin-1beta levels in serum and cerebrospinal fluid of children with febrile seizures. *Pediatr Neurol* 1997, 17:34-36.

36. Dantzer R, Bluthe RM, Gheusi G, Cremona S, Laye S, Parnet P, Kelley KW: Molecular basis of sickness behavior. *Ann N Y Acad Sci* 1998, 856:132-138.

37. Dinarello CA: Biologic basis for interleukin-1 in disease. *Blood* 1996, 87:2095-2147.

38. Dinarello CA: Infection, fever, and exogenous and endogenous pyrogens: some concepts have changed. *J Endotoxin Res* 2004, 10:201-222.

39. van Dam AM, Poole S, Schultzberg M, Zavala F, Tilders FJ: Effects of peripheral administration of LPS on the expression of immunoreactive interleukin-1 alpha, beta, and receptor antagonist in rat brain. *Ann N Y Acad Sci* 1998, 840:128-138.

40. Eriksson C, Tehranian R, Iverfeldt K, Winblad B, Schultzberg M: Increased expression of mRNA encoding interleukin-1beta and caspase-1, and the secreted isoform of interleukin-1 receptor antagonist in the rat brain following systemic kainic acid administration. *J Neurosci Res* 2000, 60:266-279.

41. Rooker S, Jander S, Van Reempts J, Stoll G, Jorens PG, Borgers M, Verlooy J: Spatiotemporal pattern of neuroinflammation after impact-acceleration closed head injury in the rat. *Mediators Inflamm* 2006, 2006:90123.

42. Tutuncuoglu S, Kutukculer N, Kepe L, Coker C, Berdeli A, Tekgul H: Proinflammatory cytokines, prostaglandins and zinc in febrile convulsions. *Pediatr Int* 2001, 43:235-239.

43. Haspolat S, Mihci E, Coskun M, Gumuslu S, Ozben T, Yegin O: Interleukin-1beta, tumor necrosis factor-alpha, and nitrite levels in febrile seizures. *J Child Neurol* 2002, 17:749-751.

44. De Sarro G, Russo E, Ferreri G, Giuseppe B, Flocco MA, Di Paola ED, De Sarro A: Seizure susceptibility to various convulsant stimuli of knockout interleukin-6 mice. *Pharmacology, biochemistry, and behavior* 2004, 77:761-766.

45. Samland H, Huitron-Resendiz S, Masliah E, Criado J, Henriksen SJ, Campbell IL: Profound increase in sensitivity to glutamatergic- but not cholinergic agonist-induced seizures in transgenic mice with astrocyte production of IL-6. *J Neurosci Res* 2003, 73:176-187.

46. Furukawa K, Mattson MP: The transcription factor NF-kappaB mediates increases in calcium currents and decreases in NMDA- and AMPA/kainate-induced currents induced by tumor necrosis factor-alpha in hippocampal neurons. *J Neurochem* 1998, 70:1876-1886.

47. Kalueff AV, Lehtimaki KA, Ylinen A, Honkaniemi J, Peltola J: Intranasal administration of human IL-6 increases the severity of chemically induced seizures in rats. *Neurosci Lett* 2004, 365:106-110.

48. Masuyama T, Matsuo M, Ichimaru T, Ishii K, Tsuchiya K, Hamasaki Y: Possible contribution of interferon-alpha to febrile seizures in influenza. *Pediatr Neurol* 2002, 27:289-292.

49. Williams K, Dooley N, Ulvestad E, Becher B, Antel JP: IL-10 production by adult human derived microglial cells. *Neurochem Int* 1996, 29:55-64.

50. Straussberg R, Amir J, Harel L, Punsky I, Bessler H: Pro- and anti-inflammatory cytokines in children with febrile convulsions. *Pediatr Neurol* 2001, 24:49-53.

51. Ishizaki Y, Kira R, Fukuda M, Torisu H, Sakai Y, Sanefuji M, Yukaya N, Hara T: Interleukin-10 is associated with resistance to febrile seizures: genetic association and experimental animal studies. *Epilepsia* 2009, 50:761-767.

52. Gary DS, Bruce-Keller AJ, Kindy MS, Mattson MP: Ischemic and excitotoxic brain injury is enhanced in mice lacking the p55 tumor necrosis factor receptor. *J Cereb Blood Flow Metab* 1998, 18:1283-1287.

53. Bruce AJ, Boling W, Kindy MS, Peschon J, Kraemer PJ, Carpenter MK, Holtsberg FW, Mattson MP: Altered neuronal and microglial responses to excitotoxic and ischemic brain injury in mice lacking TNF receptors. *Nat Med* 1996, 2:788-794.

54. Balosso S, Ravizza T, Perego C, Peschon J, Campbell IL, De Simoni MG, Vezzani A: Tumor necrosis factor-alpha inhibits seizures in mice via p75 receptors. *Ann Neurol* 2005, 57:804-812.

55. Akassoglou K, Probert L, Kontogeorgos G, Kollias G: Astrocyte-specific but not neuron-specific transmembrane TNF triggers inflammation and degeneration in the central nervous system of transgenic mice. *J Immunol* 1997, 158:438-445.

56. Wheeler D, Knapp E, Bandaru VV, Wang Y, Knorr D, Poirier C, Mattson MP, Geiger JD, Haughey NJ: Tumor necrosis factor-alpha-induced neutral sphingomyelinase-2 modulates synaptic plasticity by controlling the membrane insertion of NMDA receptors. *J Neurochem* 2009, 109:1237-1249.

57. Beattie EC, Stellwagen D, Morishita W, Bresnahan JC, Ha BK, Von Zastrow M, Beattie MS, Malenka RC: Control of synaptic strength by glial TNFalpha. *Science* 2002, 295:2282-2285.

58. Stellwagen D, Beattie EC, Seo JY, Malenka RC: Differential regulation of AMPA receptor and GABA receptor trafficking by tumor necrosis factor-alpha. *J Neurosci* 2005, 25:3219-3228.

7

The role of inflammation in the development of epilepsy

Amna Rana and Alberto E. Musto[*]

Abstract

Epilepsy, a neurological disease characterized by recurrent seizures, is often associated with a history of previous lesions in the nervous system. Impaired regulation of the activation and resolution of inflammatory cells and molecules in the injured neuronal tissue is a critical factor to the development of epilepsy. However, it is still unclear as to how that unbalanced regulation of inflammation contributes to epilepsy. Therefore, one of the goals in epilepsy research is to identify and elucidate the interconnected inflammatory pathways in systemic and neurological disorders that may further develop epilepsy progression. In this paper, inflammatory molecules, in neurological and systemic disorders (rheumatoid arthritis, Crohn's, Type I Diabetes, etc.) that could contribute to epilepsy development, are reviewed.

Understanding the neurobiology of inflammation in epileptogenesis will contribute to the development of new biomarkers for better screening of patients at risk for epilepsy and new therapeutic targets for both prophylaxis and treatment of epilepsy.

Keywords: Epileptogenesis, Inflammation, Neurological disorders, Systemic inflammatory disorders, Blood–brain barrier (BBB) breakdown

Background

Epilepsy is a multifaceted neurological disease, characterized by recurrent spontaneous seizures. Despite the efficacy of current anti-epileptic drugs, almost 30% of patients with epilepsy are refractory to medical treatment, have progressive cognitive impairment, and may require neurosurgical resection of the epileptic focus to ameliorate seizure recurrence [1].

It has been widely ascertained that the development of epilepsy-epileptogenesis can be owed to a diverse array of factors, including genetic predisposition, developmental dysfunction, and neurological insult, which contribute to morphological synaptic changes and hyper-excitable neuronal transmission [2]. For instance, a history of familial epilepsy, neurodevelopmental abnormality, and generation of complex febrile seizures are associated with the highest risk of epilepsy development in infants [2, 3]. Moreover, neurological insult, such as traumatic brain injury, hyp-

oxia, or febrile seizures, is associated with neuronal death, dysfunctional synaptic modification, and the generation of a hyper-excitable network, which could predispose to spontaneous recurrent seizures [1]. Brain injury induces a highly regulated cascade of biological events, characterized by the release of cytokines, chemokines, lipid mediators, and protectins in the neuronal microenvironment [4, 5]. Physiologically, inflammatory mediators activate their corresponding receptors on different brain cells to stimulate various pathways of molecular signaling and to initiate brain repair [6]. Deregulation of mediator and receptor expression could sustain neuronal damage, which would clinically manifest depending on the region of the brain affected [7]. Although the cellular and molecular mechanisms of epileptogenesis are not clear, it is postulated that focal or systemic unregulated inflammatory processes lead to aberrant neural connectivity and the hyper-excitable neuronal network, which mediate the onset of epilepsy [4, 8].

This review discusses critical inflammatory events, from neuronal tissue (central inflammation), BBB integrity and systemic inflammatory disorders (peripheral inflammation), that could contribute to epilepsy and may

---
* Correspondence: mustoae@evms.edu
Department of Pathology and Anatomy, Department of Neurology, Eastern Virginia Medical School, 700 W. Olney Road, Lewis Hall, Office 2174, Norfolk, VA 23507, USA

hold potential as molecular biomarkers and targets for therapeutic approaches for epilepsy (Fig. 1).

Inflammation in the central nervous system

Epileptogenesis is associated, along with subtle neuronal damage, gliosis, and microgliosis, with an increased, strong, and persistent inflammatory state in the microenvironment of neural tissue [9]. Inflammatory processes may originate in the central nervous system or be acquired from systemic circulation through a breakdown in the blood–brain barrier (BBB) [10]. A wider breadth of research on neuro-inflammation and epilepsy has focused on hippocampal foci as opposed to extra-hippocampal foci of epilepsy due to the well-documented pathology, physiology, and clinical manifestations of hippocampal atrophy and sclerosis. However, evidence has also associated neuro-inflammation with extra-hippocampal neuronal cell death and gliosis [11]. Various clinical trials with TSPO (translocator protein expressed by activated microglia) positron emission tomography (PET) have linked seizures, induced in temporal lobe epilepsy, frontal lobe epilepsy, and focal cortical dysplasia, with ensuing acute neuro-inflammation. The acute bout of neuro-

inflammation is thought to contribute to and worsen a pre-existing state of chronic neuro-inflammation [12]. For instance, patients with multiple sclerosis (MS) have increased risk for epilepsy development when MS is associated with the development of pure intracortical lesions, which cause extensive cortical inflammation [13]. A deeper understanding of the chemical mediators and receptors relevant to neuro-inflammation may elucidate their neurobiological mechanistic contribution to epileptogenesis.

Cytokines

Cytokines, proteins that modulate inflammatory processes, are primarily produced by glial cells and neurons during brain inflammation [9]. Pro-inflammatory cytokines, interleukin-1β (IL-Iβ), IL-2, and IL-6, typically concentrated in low quantities within the brain, increase after seizures [14]. In a clinical study, febrile seizures increased levels of cytokines IL-1β, IL-6, and tumor necrosis factor- α (TNF-α) in cerebrospinal fluid [15]. In addition, mRNA expression of cytokines IL-1β, IL-6, and TNF-α, along with transforming growth factor- beta 1 (TGF-β1) and vascular endothelial growth factor (VEGF) , is upregulated in the hippocampus following seizures

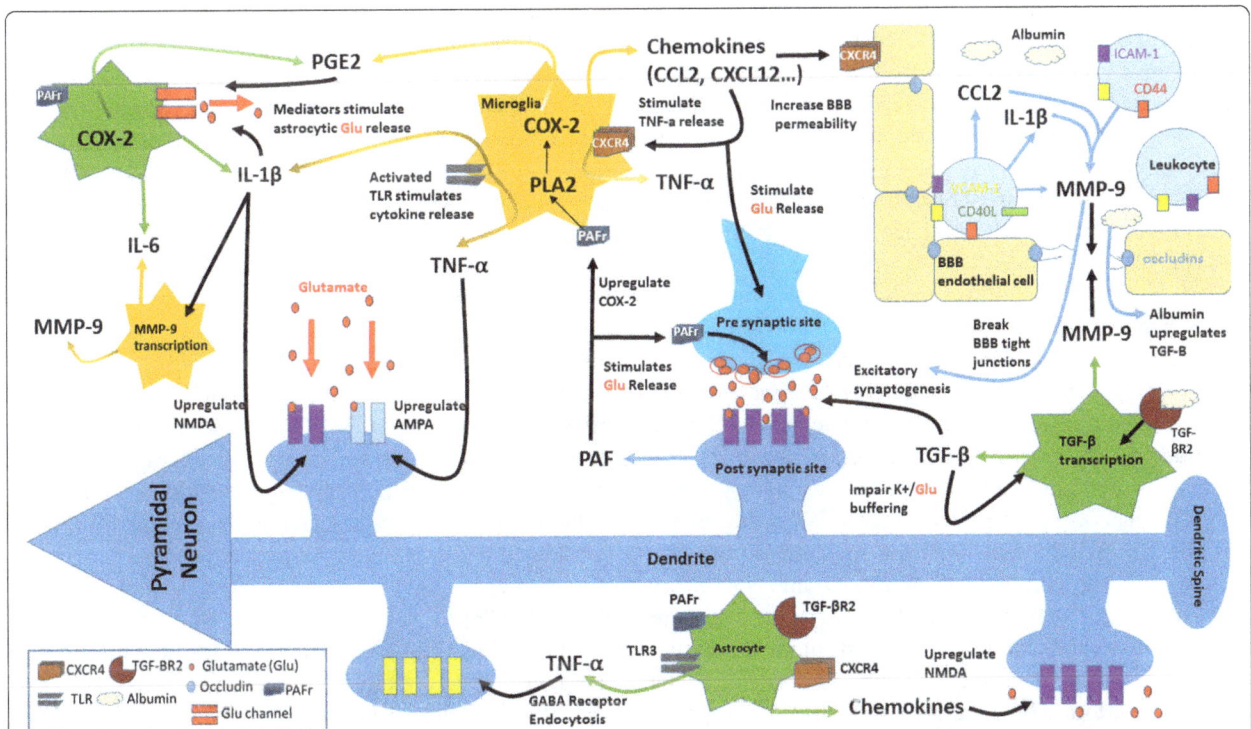

Fig. 1 Sources and targets of unregulated and overlapped components of inflammation in epileptogenesis. Brain injury induces central inflammation and aberrant neuronal connectivity within the hippocampus. Systemic inflammatory disorders generate peripheral inflammation which can further contribute to the buildup of inflammatory mediators. Peripheral and central inflammation allow for the breakdown of the blood–brain barrier due to the upregulation of inflammatory mediators. BBB breakdown permits leukocyte infiltration which generates neuronal hyper-excitability and further upregulates inflammatory mediators. Unregulated peripheral and central inflammation and breakdown of the blood–brain barrier lead to morphological synaptic changes within the hippocampus and ultimately, the development of epilepsy

[14, 16, 17]. Such key cytokines and cytokine receptors implicate various mechanistic inflammatory pathways which cause detrimental synaptic changes and neuronal hyper-excitability.

Interleukin-1β

Pro-inflammatory cytokine IL-Iβ, expressed in activated microglia and astrocytes, enhances the release of glutamate from astrocytes and decreases glutamate re-uptake, thereby increasing glutamate availability in neuronal synapses and promoting neuronal hyper-excitability [9]. It has been suggested that IL-1β induces seizures through the upregulation of NMDA receptors on post-synaptic cells via an activation of the GluN2B subunit of the NMDA receptor [18]. Postnikova et al., using models of epilepsy, found that the production of the GluN2B mRNA increases 24 h after seizures and that changes in NMDA receptors may lead to impaired synaptic plasticity [19]. It has also been reported that induced seizures decreased long-term potentiation (LTP), a physiological marker of synaptic strength via normal plasticity, while IL-1β antagonist anakinra increased LTP. These findings suggest that unregulated levels of IL-1β impair physiologic synaptic plasticity and may cause potential neuronal dysfunction [16]. Another study by Roseti et al. shows that the pathophysiological concentrations of IL-1β in TLE decrease GABA-mediated neurotransmission by up to 30% and lead to seizure generation due to neuronal hyper-excitability [20]. Cytokine IL-1β has also been found to be significantly increased within the cerebrospinal fluid (CSF) in the epileptic pediatric population as opposed to the control group, suggesting the cytokine's important role in epilepsy initiation and progression [21].

Tumor necrosis factor-α

Pro-inflammatory cytokine TNF-α is released from activated microglia and astrocytes. Glial cells sense extracellular glutamate levels and, upon detection of low levels of glutamate, release TNF-α to upregulate synapses and maintain a certain level of neuronal excitatory input [22]. It has been reported that TNF-α regulates N-cadherin, an adhesion molecule involved in the formation and organization of excitatory and inhibitory synapses [23]. Furthermore, TNF-α has been found to increase microglial glutamate release through the upregulation of glutaminase and gap junctions in microglia [24]. In addition, TNF-α upregulates AMPA receptors, augmenting glutamergic transmission. Increased AMPA receptors allow for the over-uptake of calcium, causing neurotoxicity [25]. TNF-α not only amplifies the number of glutamate receptors but also induces GABA receptor endocytosis, reducing the inhibitory drive and causing pertinent changes in excitability [26]. Although TNF-α

may have an important role in epileptogenesis, anti-TNF-α therapy for epilepsy is under debate due to the suspected risks of infection and cancer development. Within the TNF and TNF receptor (TNFR) family, certain ligands have come to light as possible pharmacological targets. In patients with TLE, TNF-related apoptosis-inducing ligand (TRAIL) expression is increased to significant levels and is thought to modulate chemokine (C-X3-C motif) ligand 1 (CX3CL1)-induced cell death [9, 27]. There may be an association with hippocampal sclerosis but the effects of TRAIL and TRAIL receptors must be further analyzed to be fully understood [9].

Interleukin-6

IL-6, a pro-inflammatory cytokine, is typically found in low quantities in the central nervous system, but stimulation of astrocytes and microglia can lead to increased production of IL-6 [28]. IL-6 is also upregulated by increased levels of other cytokines such as TNF-α, IL-Iβ, IFN-gamma, and IL-17 [29]. Studies indicate that IL-6 upregulation decreases LTP and hippocampal neurogenesis while increasing gliosis, creating conditions that may contribute to epileptogenesis [29, 30]. Although in one study IL-6 knockout (KO) mice were found to be more sensitive to pro-convulsant stimuli, in other studies, transgenic IL-6 expression and intranasal IL-6 administration within mice proved to be pro-convulsive [29]. IL-6 has also been found to bi-directionally transfer across human placenta [31, 32]. It is suggested that prenatal exposure to IL-6 results in higher risk of neurodegeneration of the hippocampus, leading to changes in both hippocampal structure and morphology [33]. Polyinosinic–polycytidylic acid (PIC) induces maternal immune activation (MIA) in experimental pregnancy, leading to hippocampal hyper excitability and faster progression of epileptogenesis in the offspring by increasing pro-inflammatory cytokines IL-6 and IL-1β within the offspring hippocampus [34]. These findings further implicate the role of IL-6 in epileptogenesis. However, although it is clear that IL-6 contributes to neural inflammation-induced epilepsy, more research is required for IL-6 to be considered in disease-modifying therapy.

Prostaglandins

Prostaglandins (PG) are formed from arachidonic acid by the constitutively expressed cyclooxygenase-1 (COX-1) and the inducible COX-2 enzymes and are secreted mainly by astrocytes and microglia. Prostaglandin E2 (PGE2) is coupled with its receptors EP1, EP2, EP3, and EP4 [35–37]. PGE2 stimulates EP3 on astrocytes, increasing astrocytic glutamate release and inducing hyper excitability and neuronal cell death; meanwhile, inhibition of EP3 may delay seizure induction [35]. mPGES (membrane-bound PGE2 synthase) increases production of glial fibrillary acidic protein (GFAP)-positive astrocytes following seizure kindling, whereas PGE2 antagonists reduce seizure severity and seizure-induced neurological damage in experimental epilepsy [35, 38]. Although PGE2 synthesis may be an effective therapeutic target, the role of COX-2 as a therapeutic target remains unclear. Studies show that COX-2 deficiency in immature mouse brains leads to greater seizure susceptibility due to decreased production of anticonvulsants PGF-2a and PGD-2 [39, 40]; PGD-2 is reported as essential to seizure suppression [41]. However, in a recent study conducted by Iwasa et al., the blockade of PG production ameliorated delayed neuronal death mediated by PGD-2 [42]. Current evidence is inconclusive on the effectivity of COX-2 therapy, and many have reported that the effects of COX-2 therapy may be highly dependent on the type of inhibitor used and the timing at which the medication is administered in relation to seizure onset. Such conflicting results are drawing attention to other targets within PG synthesis and mechanistic pathways [43]. COX-2 is upregulated by platelet-activating factor (PAF) and NMDA activation [7, 44].

Platelet-activating factor

PAF, a potent pro-inflammatory lipid mediator, has both physiological and pathological implications in the brain. PAF stimulates glutamate release and is a retrograde-messenger for LTP [45]. PAF also activates transcriptional signaling pathways of COX-2 gene expression [45, 46]. The action of PAF is mediated through its interaction with distinct binding sites on presynaptic and intracellular membranes [44]. PAF binding sites have been successfully blocked by PAF receptor antagonists, which are neuroprotective in brain damage and down-regulate cytokine production and COX-2 induction in human neuronal cells [47–49]. Epileptogenesis and aberrant plasticity associated with epilepsy are attenuated by PAF receptor antagonists [7, 50].

CD44

Adhesion molecules such as CD44 are also implicated in epileptogenesis. CD44 is physiologically expressed on glial cells and neurons and acts as a signaling molecule that guides neuron development [51]. In response to stress such as glutamate mediated neuronal hyper excitability, CD44 has been found to induce Src kinase activation, leading to actin remodeling and alterations of dendritic morphology such as hippocampal dendritic shortening [51]. Changes in dendritic morphology, though under debate, have been shown to contribute to epileptogenesis [52]. CD44 is also upregulated in epileptogenesis and is thought to play a role in neuronal

reorganization and mossy fiber sprouting (MFS), a process of hippocampal synaptic rearrangement [53]. In addition, the CD44 ligand, hyaluron, has been found to have a 146% increase in the hippocampus of patients with mesial TLE and the upregulation of hyaluron has been implicated in mossy fiber sprouting [54–56]. CD44 silencing decreased dendritic morphology changes, which suggests CD44 silencing to be a therapeutic mechanism for epileptogenesis [51].

Matrix metalloproteinase-9

Matrix metalloproteinase-9 (MMP-9) is a proteolytic enzyme secreted primarily by astrocytes and microglia in the hippocampus, cerebral cortex, and cerebellum. MMP-9 transcription increases in response to depolarization of neurons and upregulation of other inflammatory factors such as IL-Iβ and chemokines. MMP-9 has various roles within the brain, ranging from structural modifications to facilitation of inflammatory processes. Chronic levels of MMP-9 cause thinning and elongation of dendritic spines, leading to morphological changes in synapses, and are associated with impaired synaptic plasticity [57–59]. Moreover, increased expression of MMP-9 indicates greater susceptibility to epileptogenesis as MMP-9 facilitates cell death through various mechanisms including excitotoxicity, apoptosis, and impairment of extracellular matrix-cell interactions [57, 58]. MMP-9 also loosens the BBB by directly damaging the tight junctions. Furthermore, MMP-9 activity increases in neural and glial cells, within the CA1 and CA2 regions of the hippocampus in patients with mesial TLE (MTLE) with hippocampal sclerosis, and is implicated as an important factor in drug resistant MTLE, suggesting a potential therapeutic target in patients with drug-resistant epilepsy [58].

Toll-like receptors

Toll-like receptors (TLR 1, 2, 3), expressed primarily by microglia and astrocytes, mediate innate and adaptive immunity. TLRs induce secretion of cytokines such as IL-1β and other inflammatory mediators which mediate epileptogenesis [60]. In an experimental model of epilepsy, deletion of TLR3 limits seizures, reduces levels of cytokines TNF-α and IL-1β, decreases levels of microglial activity, and increases survival rates [61]. TLR3 contributes to hippocampal excitability through its upregulation of pro-inflammatory cytokines such as IFN- β [62]. FOX3P, typically found to induce T cell differentiation, is also expressed by microglia to downregulate inflammatory processes through modulation of NFkB, a key inflammatory transcription factor [63]. FOX3P limits TLR4 signaling and inflammation, leading to an inactivation of the NR2B NMDA receptor and attenuation of seizure activity [64]. This research suggests TLRs as possible therapeutic targets due to their intrinsic importance in neuro-inflammation and potential restructuration of neuronal excitability.

Chemokines

Chemokines, expressed in the brain by microglia, astrocytes, and endothelial cells, guide inflammatory mediators towards the source of inflammation and activate leukocytes [65, 66]. Many variants of chemokines can alter neuronal physiology through the modulation of voltage-dependent channels, activation of G-protein-gated potassium influx channels, and increased release of certain neurotransmitters [66]. Chemokines CCL2, CCL3, and CCL4 have been detected in DNA microarray analysis of surgically removed hippocampi of TLE patients [66]. TLE patients also exhibit increased C-X-C chemokine receptor type 4 (CXCR4) expression on microglia and astrocytes, which leads to an increase in CXCL12 binding, stimulating microglia to release TNF-α and then increasing glutamate levels [66]. Chemokine CCL2, which binds to the G-protein-coupled receptor C-C chemokine receptor type 2 (CCR2), is also highly elevated in patients with pharmacoresistant epilepsy and is found on various brain cell types, including neurons, astrocytes, microglia, neural progenitor cells, and microvascular endothelial cells, suggesting that CCL2 and its receptor CCR2 could play an important role in seizure control [65]. Moreover, in patients with intractable epilepsy and in experimental epilepsy models, CXCL13 and CXCR5 are highly upregulated, suggesting a mediation in epileptogenesis [67].

Neurological disorders and epilepsy

Insult to the brain typically induces an acute neuro-inflammatory response, marked by an increase of pro-inflammatory molecules, which mediate onset of recurrent seizure development [4, 8]. Neural inflammation initiated due to other neurological pathologies (see Table 1) may contribute to the development of epilepsy as inflammatory mediators are upregulated. As a result, the treatment and resolution of other neurological conditions may play a key role in the prevention of epilepsy.

Blood–brain barrier breakdown

The CNS is generally protected against many of the conventional reactions present in the immune system due to the BBB, which is impermeable to many molecules, toxins, and cells due to numerous non-infenestrated endothelial cells with inter-endothelial tight junctions. This delicate layer is maintained by the normal function of pericytes, perivascular microglia, astrocytes, and the basal lamina [10]. Physiologic astrocyte production of the sonic hedgehog protein signals endothelial cells to

Table 1 Neural inflammation initiated due to other neurological pathologies

Neurological disorders	Inflammatory contribution to epilepsy development
Traumatic brain injury	Damage associated molecular pattern (DAMP) stimulation of immune system Significant CCL2 increase Neutrophil recruitment —> BBB damage Reactive oxygen species (ROS) release —> activate vascular endothelium —> T cell infiltration of BBB [137]
Status epilepticus	Elevated IL-1β, TNF-α, IL-6 transcript levels Albumin extravasation <—>BBB breakdown EP2-COX2 upregulation TLR pathways stimulated [138]
Multiple sclerosis	Increased oxidative stress and ROS Activation of microglia Recruitment of T-cells, B-cells, and macrophages [139]
GBM	IL-8 up-regulation via EGFRvIII IL-6-mediated STAT3 activation IL-1β-dependent activation of NF-κB, p38 MAPK and JNKs pathways [140]
Stroke	TNF-α, IL-1B, IL-6 upregulation ICAM and VCAM upregulation MMP-9 increase MCP-1,(MIP-1α), fractalkine (CX3CL1) increase [141]
Alzheimer's disease	MCP-1, cytokines (IL-6, TNF-α), CXCL8, CCL5 increase Deposition of Aβ generates ROS Activation of the complement cascade [142]

secrete Netrin 1, a laminin like protein which regulates glial cell migration. Netrin 1 increases endothelial junctional proteins to stabilize the BBB and decreases leukocyte infiltration, suggesting an important role as a BBB protective mediator [68].

Inflammatory mediators overview

Central and peripheral inflammation contributes to the breakdown of the BBB through the upregulation of inflammatory mediators. SE, infections, and traumatic and ischemic injuries have been reported to cause transient changes in the composition and permeability of the BBB. Although the exact mechanism of delayed onset of epilepsy remains unclear, available data suggests that inflammation and breakdown of the BBB are necessary components of epileptogenesis following brain injury [10]. For instance, gram-negative bacterial lipopolysaccharide (LPS) activates macrophages to produce IL-1, IL-6, and TNF alpha, promoting BBB permeability and facilitating entrance of peripherally generated pro-inflammatory cytokines into circumventricular brain regions [69]. TNF-α and IL-6, cytokines that increase the BBB permeability, have been clearly implicated in seizure generation and severity [70–72]. IL-1β is also an etiologic trigger for BBB breakdown and plays a pivotal role in the activation of astrocytes whereas IL-1Ra, an IL-1 antagonist, limits the effects of those cytokines [10]. In addition, the binding of cytokines to receptors located in brain vasculature can cause the production of molecules, such as endothelial cell adhesion molecules, chemokines, nitric oxide, and prostaglandins that may further compromise the integrity of the BBB [69].

Leukocyte adhesion and infiltration

BBB leukocyte-endothelium interactions mediate leakage and infiltration of inflammatory cells into the hippocampus [73]. Epilepsy is typically accompanied by an increase of leukocytes, such as neutrophils, into the hippocampus, and the infiltration is thought to lead to higher levels of neurodegeneration [73, 74]. Spontaneous recurrent seizures lead to the chronic expression of VCAM-1, the ligand for VLA-4 integrin. It has been hypothesized that upregulation of VCAM-1 may contribute to BBB permeability, neuro-inflammation, and subsequent seizure generation [73]. CD44 mediates, in conjunction with the integrin pathway, leukocyte adhesion and rolling on cytokine-activated endothelium [75, 76]. Using induced CD44, VCAM-1, and ICAM-1, leukocytes form endothelial membrane protrusions, called "transmigratory cups", which assist with transendothelial migration of leukocytes across the BBB [76]. Of particular note, one study suggests that CD44 is required for optimal neutrophil recruitment into tissues as CD44 (−/−) mice indicated a 65% decrease in neutrophil adhesion [77]. Certainly, leukocyte-adhesion molecule targets may be looked into for epilepsy treatment [74]. However, genetic and pharmacological interventions to prevent T-cell infiltration or deplete systemic macrophages and cytotoxic inflammatory cells show diverse outcomes, suggesting that the mechanics of neuro-inflammatory signaling in epileptogenesis are incompletely understood [74, 78].

Leukocyte infiltration through dysfunctional BBB leads to the upregulation of inflammatory mediators, such as interleukins, tumor necrosis factors, COX-2, complement, and adhesion molecules which contribute to leakage of the BBB. Specifically, findings show that T cell activation leads to the release of chemokines. CCL2 mediates chemotaxis of neutrophils and enhances local inflammatory responses in the brain [79–82]. Inflowing leukocytes also secrete MMP-9, which then damages the BBB by cleaving the zonula occludens 1 protein, which is integral to the tight junctions of the BBB. By directly damaging the BBB, MMP-9 allows for greater inflow of leukocytes and perpetuates the inflammation. MMP-9 also cleaves dystroglycan, a protein which fixes astrocytic feet to the basement membrane and allows for leukocytic infiltration into the brain's parenchyma [57]. In addition, CD40-L is expressed predominantly on activated CD4+ T lymphocytes and increases after SE [83]. The CD40 Ligand (CD40-L) is a transmembrane glycoprotein belonging to the TNF family, and the soluble trimeric form of CD40-L has the most potent biological activity through oligomerization of cell surface receptor, CD40 [84]. The CD40-CD40L pathways have been implicated in many neurological disorders; however, the research related to epilepsy is sparse. Further research into this pathway may yield important molecular targets.

Astrocyte reactivity

Evidence suggests that the BBB disruption contributes to astrocyte activation and gliosis. Within 24–48 h of the induction of SE, there is activation of glial fibrillary acidic protein-positive astrocytes (GFAP). The reactive gliosis may be detectable for over 3 to 4 months [10]. These reactive astrocytes may have difficulty handling the extracellular glutamate, leading to neuronal hyper excitability and damage. Reactive astrocytes also serve to further release pro-inflammatory cytokines (e.g., IL-1β, IL-6, and TNF-α) and recruit more inflammatory cells by secreting C-C motif chemokine ligands 2, 3, and 5 [57]. As a result, there is increased neuronal excitability, development of seizures, cell death, and subsequent neuro-inflammation [72]. The leakage of serum proteins such as albumin through a disrupted BBB may be a key factor in the initiation of specific signaling cascades within neurovascular cells, specifically astrocytes. Albumin is hypothesized to bind to the astrocytic TGF-βR2, leading to the activation of the TGF-β signaling pathway, production of TGF-β, and astrocyte activation, which causes impaired buffering of potassium and glutamate at the cellular level [85]. ALK5/TGF-β-pathway induces excitatory synaptogenesis whereas SJN2511, a specific ALK5/TGF-β inhibitor, prevents synaptogenesis and epilepsy [86]. Hence, TGF-β pathway inhibition prevents the activation of astrocytes during epileptogenesis, leading to a reduction in spontaneous seizure activity and brain inflammation [85, 87]. The TGF-B pathway may serve as a therapeutic target to prevent seizure development in individuals with brain injury [86].

Systemic inflammation

As discussed, inflammatory molecules are induced in response to brain injury, such as SE, and modulate not only neural connectivity and excitability but contribute to the breakdown of the BBB, allowing for further intrusion of harmful chemicals and mediators. Various experimental models have shown that the systemic administration of LPS leads to the generation of seizures and enhancement of epileptogenesis. LPS-induced peripheral inflammation increases seizure susceptibility through COX-2-dependent microglial activation and upregulation of IL-1β, IL-6, and TNF-α in the hippocampus [88]. Co-administration of LPS and IL-1B receptor antagonist in immature rat brains, however, partially reverses the enhancement of epileptogenesis [89].

Furthermore, the systematic disruption of CCL2 signaling, through intracerebral administration of anti-CCL2 antibodies, results in potent suppression of LPS-induced seizures in chronically epileptic animals [90]. CCL2 is suggested to be a key mediator that bridges peripheral inflammation and epilepsy. These research findings suggest an important association between peripheral inflammatory conditions and epilepsy.

Furthermore, in a population based retrospective cohort study (n = 2,518,034), the relationship between autoimmune diseases, such as SLE, Hashimoto's Thyroiditis, and RA, and epilepsy was examined. It was found that all of the autoimmune disorders examined posed a varying increased risk of epilepsy and, as a whole, autoimmune diseases posed a fivefold increased risk of epilepsy in children and fourfold increased risk of epilepsy in non-elderly adults (age < 65) [91]. An extensive meta-analysis study investigated the relationship between systemic autoimmune disorders (SAD) and epilepsy and found a 2.5-fold increase of epilepsy in SAD, 2.5-fold increase of SAD in epilepsy, and established a stronger association of SAD and epilepsy in individuals younger than 20 [92].

Due to the evident statistical association of epilepsy and systemic inflammatory conditions, combined with the biochemical understanding of peripheral inflammation leading to central inflammation due to the breakdown of the blood–brain barrier, it is imperative to further study the relationship between systemic inflammatory conditions and epilepsy for prevention and treatment. Most mechanistic pathways between these inflammatory conditions and epilepsy remain unelucidated. The following sections present the current understanding of the relationship between epilepsy and inflammatory conditions, as well as note possible contributory inflammatory factors (Table 2).

Systemic inflammatory conditions
Systemic lupus erythematous
Systemic lupus erythematous (SLE) is a chronic autoimmune disease characterized by an increase of antinuclear and anti-glomerular autoantibodies as well as immunological events that affect several organs through the activation of innate and adaptive immunity [93]. The prevalence of epilepsy in SLE is up to eight times higher than that in the general population, and seizures may appear many years before SLE is diagnosed. Some SLE cases are associated with anti-phospholipid and anti-cardiolipin antibodies and are correlated with abnormal MRI findings in the brain [10, 94, 95]. Vasculitis-stroke-like events could trigger seizures in SLE as a consequence of coagulopathy in small brain vessels or circulation of anti-neuronal complexes that invade the brain tissue [96]. In that case, epileptic seizures could indicate repetitive acute immune events that impact a particular neuronal network. SLE may also induce abnormal

Table 2 Inflammatory conditions

Systemic inflammatory condition	Associated inflammatory findings	Odds ratio (compared to control group)	Prevalence of epilepsy	Incidence of epilepsy
Systemic lupus erythematous (SLE)	Antibodies: ANA, dsDNA, SS-A/SS-B.Upregulates anti- MAP-2 and anti NMDR presence in CSF IL-1β, Il-8, IFN gamma activate microglia. IL-10 upregulates spinogenesis	7-fold [91]	2.5% [91] Up to 8 times higher than non-SLE population [92, 93]	2.86-fold greater than non-SLE cohort [96]
Rheumatoid arthritis (RA)	Upregulated TNF-α,IL-1 and IL-6 cytokines	3.5-fold [91]	1.2% [91]	1.27-fold greater than control cohort [130]
Type I diabetes	Autoantibodies GAD 45	5.2-fold [91]	1.8% [91] 2–3.7% [120]	2.2-fold greater than control cohort [143]
Celiac disease	Anti-endomysial antibodies (EMA), anti-tissue transglutaminase antibodies (tTG), and anti-gliadin antibodies (AGA)	4.5-fold [91]	1.5% [91]	–
Sjogrens	Lymphocyte infiltration of CD4+ T cells, B cells, and plasma cells	4.3-fold [91]	1.5% [91]	1.5-fold greater than control [122, 124, 125]
Crohn's Disease	Th1 and Th17 pathways CD44, IL-6, TNF-a upregulated	3.1-fold [91]	1.1% [91] 3.5–5.9% [105]	–
Ulcerative Colitis	IL-5, IL-13, IL-15 with Th2 upregulation	2.5 fold [91]	0.9% [91]	–
Hashimoto's thyroiditis	Circulating immune complexes Anti-thyroid antibodies	2.4-fold [91]	0.8% [91]	–
Behcet's	HLA-B51 Neuronal lymphocytosis	–	2.2–5% [105, 108]	–
Anti-phospholipid syndrome	Antibodies directed against membrane anionic phospholipids	3.2-fold [94, 103, 119]	–	–

plasticity and promote aberrant neuronal connections that are responsible for seizures and eventual development of epilepsy. IL-10 is associated with super antigen polymorphism and SLE [97]. In the presence of BBB damage after SLE vasculitis, IL-10 crosses the BBB and induces spinogenesis, increasing excitatory and inhibitory synaptic contacts [98]. SLE also increases prolactin which modulates neuronal activity [99]. SLE up regulates anti- MAP-2 and anti NMDR presence in CSF and upregulates circulating IL-1β, Il-8, IFN gamma, and antibodies which activate microglia [97, 100–102]. Moreover, increased levels of anti-phospholipid antibodies are associated with increased seizure development [103].

Hashimoto's encephalopathy
Hashimoto's encephalopathy (HE), a rare complication of autoimmune thyroiditis, involves a high anti-thyroid antibody titer, and clinical manifestations include seizures, agitation, and cognitive deterioration [104]. Up to 66% of HE patients present with seizures, and both convulsive and non-convulsive forms of status epilepticus have been reported in patients with HE. Furthermore, in one study, 80% of HE patients presented with elevated protein and lymphocytic pleocytosis. Specifically, the pathophysiology of HE may involve circulating immune complexes or neuronal antibodies [105]. HE patients respond dramatically to corticosteroids, and this response suggests an immune mediated pro-inflammatory reaction as a possible cause of the CNS symptoms [106]. Although thyroid hormones mediate neuronal activity, it is difficult to separate how much involvement of thyroid hormones and neuro-inflammation exists and how their relationship upregulates the neuronal network that could mediate recurrent seizures in epilepsy [104].

Behcet's disease
Behcet's disease (BD), characterized by recurrent oral ulcers, genital ulcers, and inflammation of the middle layer of the eye, is associated with epilepsy [107]. BD is common in individuals of Middle Eastern and Central Asian descent and those with HLA-B51. Amongst these individuals, seizures and epilepsy occur in 2.2–5% of the cases. Most seizures are of the tonic–clonic type, but partial seizures, like epilepsia partialis continua, are also associated with BD [105, 108]. In Caucasian patients with neuro-Behcet's disease, 27% suffered either single or recurrent seizures and 50% of patients had pleocytosis in their CSF [109]. Seizures in BD have shown improvement with immunosuppressant therapy [108].

Type I diabetes
Type I diabetes (T1DM) is a condition associated with an increase of autoantibodies GAD 45 [110, 111]. These antibodies are present in the CSF of T1DM patients [112–115]. Up to 2–3.7% of patients with T1DM have epilepsy, and patients with type I diabetes have up to six times the increased risk for epilepsy [116].

Crohn's disease
Crohn's disease is a chronic inflammatory disorder characterized by the upregulation of pro-inflammatory cytokines and induction of Th1 and Th17 pathways [117]. According to one study, epilepsy occurs in 3.5 to 5.9% of Crohn's patients, while general neurological manifestations occur in 33 to 67% of Crohn's patients [105]. Crohn's disease is specifically associated with the upregulation of the NF-kB transcription factor with high levels of TNF-α and IL-6 [70–72]. CD44 molecules also double on peripheral blood cells and lymph nodes in Crohn's disease [118]. Further clinical and biomedical research is required to better understand the relationship between Crohn's and epilepsy.

Antiphospholipid syndrome
Antiphospholipid syndrome, a recurrent state of venous or arterial thrombosis, is associated with antibodies directed against membrane anionic phospholipids (i.e., anticardiolipin [aCL] antibody, antiphosphatidylserine) or corresponding plasma proteins, predominantly beta-2 glycoprotein I (apolipoprotein H). Patients with this condition have a 3.2-fold increased risk of developing epilepsy [94, 102, 119].

Sjogren's syndrome
Sjogren's syndrome (SS) is a chronic autoimmune disorder characterized by the lymphocyte infiltration of CD4+ T cells, B cells, and plasma cells in exocrine glands, mainly in salivary and ophthalmic glands. The disorder is also associated with involvement in other organs, including the brain. Although its cause remains unknown, the pathophysiology can be explained by interactions of several molecular factors [120]. Furthermore, between 2 and 60% of patients with SS present neurological complications [121]. SS patients with HDL-c particularly show white matter anomalies [122]. Reports show 1.5% incidence of epilepsy in SS patients and that 1/3 of SS patients have EEG abnormalities [123–125]. However, there is a lack of studies that have explored the relation of SS and epilepsy.

Ulcerative colitis
Ulcerative colitis (UC) is a chronic inflammatory bowel disease of unknown etiology characterized by ulceration of the colon. UC is thought to have extra-intestinal neurological manifestations associated with the peripheral nervous system [126].

Rheumatoid arthritis

Rheumatoid arthritis (RA) is an autoimmune inflammatory disorder characterized by the anti-IgG antibody (RF Factor) and anti-CCP antibody. It is associated with an upregulation of TNF-α, IL-1 and IL-6 [127–129]. The development of epilepsy within RA patients is 1.27-fold higher than the control patients without RA. Duration of non-steroidal anti-inflammatory drug (NSAID) therapy in RA patients negatively correlated with epilepsy development while patients with minimal NSAID therapy had a greater risk of epilepsy development [130]. This suggests that limiting the inflammatory process induced by RA reduces risk of epileptogenesis. Offspring of women, who had RA during pregnancy, are at a significantly higher risk of developing childhood-onset epilepsy as compared to the offspring of women who developed RA post-pregnancy. Paternal RA is suggested to have a relatively low association to epilepsy development within offspring. These findings suggest that the inflammatory conditions induced within RA impact the intrauterine environment and increase the risk of epileptogenesis within children [131].

Celiac disease

Celiac disease (CD) is an autoimmune disorder characterized by gluten sensitivity, predisposing factors such as HLA DQ2/8, and different antibodies including anti-endomysial antibodies (EMA), anti-tissue transglutaminase antibodies (tTG), and anti-gliadin antibodies (AGA) [132, 133]. Exposure to gluten induces an immune reaction which leads to villous atrophy, crypt hyperplasia, and increased intraepithelial lymphocytes [133]. Per a meta-analysis on epilepsy and systemic autoimmune disorders, patients with epilepsy have a 2.6-fold increased risk for celiac disease [92]. In an epidemiologic study of nearly 29,000 subjects with CD and 143,000 controls, it was found that CD increased risk of epilepsy by 1.4-fold [103]. Many case studies have reported an association between CD and epilepsy with occipital calcifications and cerebellar degeneration [133–135]. Another study established an association between TLE, hippocampal sclerosis, and celiac disease [135]. Furthermore, the implementation of a gluten-free diet in epileptic patients may contribute to a decrease of antiepileptic medication use. On a clinical level, CD screening may be advisable as a gluten free diet could possibly replace the need for medication and reduce the occurrence of seizures [136].

Clinical importance

Considering the aforementioned neurobiological effects of inflammatory mediators, the presence of one of these systemic inflammatory conditions could mediate development of epilepsy by (a) inducing seizures, which then beget further seizures and lead to onset of recurrent seizures and epileptogenesis; (b) altering neuronal network architecture which promotes spontaneous recurrent seizures; and (c) aggravating the course of epilepsy (secondary epileptogenesis). Therefore, it can be suggested that inflammation can be treated as an important factor in the treatment of patients with epilepsy. Certainly, prophylactic anti-inflammatory measures in patients at risk for epilepsy may serve to ameliorate the neuronal damage. Proper treatment and possible resolution of other systemic inflammatory disorders may also play a key role in suppressing epilepsy progression.

Conclusion

The development of epilepsy is characterized by complex unregulated inflammatory molecules and pathways found in both the nervous system and systemic tissue. Understanding the neurobiology of cytokines, chemokines, MMP-9, and adhesion molecules, overlapping with neuronal network physiology, will allow for greater development of treatment and prophylactic measures against epilepsy. The presence of peripheral inflammation, due to systemic diseases such as SLE or RA, has the potential capacity to damage the BBB and initiate or aggravate epileptogenesis. Therefore, the control of inflammation in such disorders may lessen the risk of developing epilepsy.

Abbreviations

BBB: Blood–brain barrier; BD: Behcet's disease; CCL2: Chemokine (C-C motif) ligand 2; CCR2: C-C chemokine receptor type 2; CD: Celiac Disease; CNS: Central nervous system; COX: Cyclooxygenase; CSF: Cerebrospinal fluid; CX3CL1: Chemokine (C-X3-C motif) ligand 1; CXCR4: C-X-C chemokine receptor type 4; GFAP: Glial fibrillary acidic protein; HS: Hippocampal sclerosis; IL: Interleukin; KO: Knock out; LPS: Lipopolysaccharide; LTP: Long-term potentiation; MFS: Mossy fiber sprouting; MIA: Maternal immune activation; MMP-9: Matrix metalloproteinase-9; MTLE: Mesial temporal lobe epilepsy; NSAID: Non-steroidal anti-inflammatory drug; PAF: Platelet activating factor; PG: Prostaglandin; PIC: Polyinosinic–polycytidylic acid; PTZ: Pentylenetetrazole; RA: Rheumatoid arthritis; SE: Status epilepticus; SLE: Systemic lupus erythematous; SS: Sjogren's syndrome; TGF: Transforming growth factor; T1DM: Type I diabetes; TLE: Temporal lobe epilepsy; TLR: Toll-like receptors; TNF: Tumor necrosis factor; TRAIL: TNF-related apoptosis-inducing ligand

Authors' contributions

AEM conceived the idea and wrote, reviewed, and approved the manuscript; AR wrote, reviewed, and approved the manuscript.

Competing interests

The authors declare that they have no competing interests.

References

1. Laxer K, Trinka E, Hirsch L, et al. The consequences of refractory epilepsy and its treatment. Epilepsy Behav. 2014;37:59–70. https://doi.org/10.1016/j.yebeh.2014.05.031.
2. Rakhade SN, Jensen FE. Epileptogenesis in the immature brain: emerging mechanisms. Nat Rev Neurol. 2009;5(7):380. https://doi.org/10.1038/nrneurol.2009.80.
3. Chung S. Febrile seizures. Korean J Pediatr. 2014;57(9):384–95. https://doi.org/10.3345/kjp.2014.57.9.384.

4. Musto A, Gjorstrup P, Bazan N. The omega-3 fatty acid-derived neuroprotectin D1 limits hippocampal hyperexcitability and seizure susceptibility in kindling epileptogenesis. Epilepsia. 2011;52(9):1601–8.

5. Walker LE, Janigro D, Heinemann U, Riikonen R, Bernard C, Patel M. WONOEP appraisal: molecular and cellular biomarkers for epilepsy. Epilepsia. 2016;57:1354–62.

6. Chiang N, Serhan C. Structural elucidation and physiologic functions of specialized pro-resolving mediators and their receptors. Mol Asp Med. 2017; https://doi.org/10.1016/j.mam.2017.03.005.

7. Vezzani A, Granata T. Brain inflammation in epilepsy: experimental and clinical evidence. Epilepsia. 2005;46:1724–43.

8. Musto A, Rosencrans R, Walker C, et al. Dysfunctional epileptic neuronal circuits and dysmorphic dendritic spines are mitigated by platelet-activating factor receptor antagonism. Sci Rep. 2016;6(1) https://doi.org/10.1038/srep30298.

9. Alyu F, Dikmen M. Inflammatory aspects of epileptogenesis: contribution of molecular inflammatory mechanisms. Acta Neuropsychiatrica. 2016;29(01):1–16.

10. Choi J, Koh S. Role of brain inflammation in epileptogenesis. Yonsei Med J. 2008;49(1):1.

11. Jung K-H, Chu K, Lee S-T, Kim J-H, Kang K-M, Song E-C, Kim S-J, Park H-K, Kim M, Lee SK, Roh J-K. Region-specific plasticity in the epileptic rat brain: a hippocampal and extrahippocampal analysis. Epilepsia. 2009;50:537–49.

12. Butler T, Li Y, Tsui W, et al. Transient and chronic seizure-induced inflammation in human focal epilepsy. Epilepsia. 2016;57(9):e191–4. https://doi.org/10.1111/epi.13457.

13. Calabrese M, De Stefano N, Atzori M, et al. J Neurol. 2008;255:581. https://doi.org/10.1007/s00415-008-0752-7

14. Scorza C, Marques M, Gomes da Silva S, Naffah-Mazzacoratti M, Scorza F, Cavalheiro E. Status epilepticus does not induce acute brain inflammatory response in the Amazon rodent Proechimys, an animal model resistant to epileptogenesis. Neurosci Lett. 2017; https://doi.org/10.1016/j.neulet.2017.02.049.

15. Ichiyama T, Nishikawa M, Yoshitomi T, Hayashi T, Furukawa S. Tumor necrosis factor-a, interleukin-I, and interleukin-6 in cerebrospinal fluid from children with prolonged febrile seizures comparison with acute encephalitis/encephalopathy. Neurology. 1998;50(2):407–11. https://doi.org/10.1212/wnl.50.2.407.

16. Han T, Qin Y, Mou C, Wang M, Jiang M, Liu B. Seizure induced synaptic plasticity alteration in hippocampus is mediated by IL-1β receptor through PI3K/Akt pathway. Am J Transl Res. 2016;8(10):4499–509.

17. Plata-Salaman CR, Ilyin SE, Turrin NP, Gayle D, Flynn MC, Romanovitch AE, et al. Kindling modulates the IL-1βeta system, TNF-alpha, Tgf-βeta1, and neuropeptide mRNAs in specific brain regions. Brain Res Mol Brain Res. 2000;75:248–58.

18. Viviani B, Bartesaghi S, Gardoni F, Vezzani A, Behrens MM, Bartfai T, Binaglia M, Corsini E, Di Luca M, Galli CL, Marinovich M. Interleukin-1beta enhances NMDA receptor-mediated intracellular calcium increase through activation of the Src family of kinases. J Neurosci. 2003;23:8692–700.

19. Postnikova T, Zubareva O, Kovalenko A, Kim K, Magazanik L, Zaitsev A. Status epilepticus impairs synaptic plasticity in rat hippocampus and is followed by changes in expression of NMDA receptors. Biochem Mosc. 2017;82(3):282–90.

20. Roseti C, van Vliet E, Cifelli P, et al. GABAA currents are decreased by IL-1β in epileptogenic tissue of patients with temporal lobe epilepsy: implications for ictogenesis. Neurobiol Dis. 2015;82:311–20.

21. Shi L, Chen R, Zhang H, Jiang C, Gong J. Cerebrospinal fluid neuron specific enolase, interleukin-1β and erythropoietin concentrations in children after seizures. Childs Nerv Syst. 2017;33(5):805–11.

22. Stellwagen D, Malenka RC. Synaptic scaling mediated by glial TNF-alpha. Nature. 2006;440:1054–9.

23. Kubota K, Inoue K, Hashimoto R, et al. Tumor necrosis factor receptor-associated protein 1 regulates cell adhesion and synaptic morphology via modulation of N-cadherin expression. J Neurochem. 2009;110(2):496–508.

24. Takeuchi H, Jin S, Wang J, et al. Tumor necrosis factor- induces neurotoxicity via glutamate release from Hemichannels of activated microglia in an autocrine manner. J Biol Chem. 2006;281(30):21362–8.

25. Galic MA, Riazi K, Pittman QJ. Cytokines and brain excitability. Front Neuroendocrinol. 2012;33(1):116–25. https://doi.org/10.1016/j.yfrne.2011.12.002.

26. Stellwagen D. Differential regulation of AMPA receptor and GABA receptor trafficking by tumor necrosis factor-alpha. J Neurosci. 2005;25(12):3219–28.

27. Xu Y, Zeng Y, Han Y, et al. Altered expression of CX3CL1 in patients with epilepsy and in a rat model. Am J Pathol. 2012;180(5):1950–62.

28. Gruol DL. IL-6 regulation of synaptic function in the CNS. Neuropharmacology. 2015;96(0 0):42–54. https://doi.org/10.1016/j.neuropharm.2014.10.023.

29. Erta M, Quintana A, Hidalgo J. Interleukin-6, a major cytokine in the central nervous system. Int J Biol Sci. 2012;8(9):1254–66.

30. Levin S, Godukhin O. Modulating effect of cytokines on mechanisms of synaptic plasticity in the brain. Biochem Mosc. 2017;82(3):264–74.

31. Zaretsky M, Alexander J, Byrd W, Bawdon R. Transfer of inflammatory cytokines across the placenta. Obstet Gynecol. 2004;103(3):546–50.

32. Dahlgren J, Samuelsson A, Jansson T, Holmäng A. Interleukin-6 in the maternal circulation reaches the rat fetus in mid-gestation. Pediatr Res. 2006;60(2):147–51.

33. Samuelsson A. Prenatal exposure to interleukin-6 results in inflammatory neurodegeneration in hippocampus with NMDA/GABAA dysregulation and impaired spatial learning. AJP. 2005;290(5):R1345–56.

34. Pineda E, Shin D, You SJ, Auvin S, Sankar R, Mazarati A. Maternal immune activation promotes hippocampal kindling epileptogenesis in mice. Ann Neurol. 2013;74(1):11–9. https://doi.org/10.1002/ana.23898.

35. Shimada T, Takemiya T, Sugiura H, Yamagata K. Role of inflammatory mediators in the pathogenesis of epilepsy. Mediat Inflamm. 2014;2014: 901902. https://doi.org/10.1155/2014/901902.

36. Sayyah M, Javad-Pour M, Ghazi-Khansari M. The bacterial endotoxin lipopolysaccharide enhances seizure susceptibility in mice: involvement of proinflammatory factors: nitric oxide and prostaglandins. Neuroscience. 2003;122(4):1073–80.

37. Cimino PJ, Keene CD, Breyer RM, Montine KS, Montine TJ. Therapeutic targets in prostaglandin E2 signaling for neurologic disease. Curr Med Chem. 2008;15(19):1863–9.

38. Jiang J, Ganesh T, Du Y, et al. Small molecule antagonist reveals seizure-induced mediation of neuronal injury by prostaglandin E2 receptor subtype EP2. Proc Natl Acad Sci U S A. 2012;109(8):3149–54.

39. Chung J, Kim A, Lee S, Baik E. Seizure susceptibility in immature brain due to lack of COX-2-induced PGF2α. Exp Neurol. 2013;249:95–103.

40. Holtman L, van Vliet E, Edelbroek P, Aronica E, Gorter J. Cox-2 inhibition can lead to adverse effects in a rat model for temporal lobe epilepsy. Epilepsy Res. 2010;91(1):49–56. https://doi.org/10.1016/j.eplepsyres.2010.06.011.

41. Kaushik M, Aritake K, Kamauchi S, et al. Prostaglandin D2 is crucial for seizure suppression and postictal sleep. Exp Neurol. 2014;253:82–90. https://doi.org/10.1016/j.expneurol.2013.12.002.

42. Iwasa K, Yamamoto S, Yagishita S, Maruyama K, Yoshikawa K. Excitotoxicity-induced prostaglandin D 2 production induces sustained microglial activation and delayed neuronal death. J Lipid Res. 2017;58(4):649–55. https://doi.org/10.1194/jlr.m070532.

43. Barbalho PG, Carvalho BS, Lopes-Cendes I, Maurer-Morelli CV. Cyclooxygenase-1 as a potential therapeutic target for seizure suppression: evidences from Zebrafish Pentylenetetrazole-seizure model. Front Neurol. 2016;7:200. https://doi.org/10.3389/fneur.2016.00200.

44. Marcheselli VL, Rossowska MJ, Domingo MT, Braquet P, Bazan NG. Distinct platelet-activating factor binding sites in synaptic endings and in intracellular membranes of rat cerebral cortex. J Biol Chem. 1990;265:9140–9145 RefID.

45. Bazan N. A signal terminator. Nature. 1995;374(6522):501–2. https://doi.org/10.1038/374501a0.

46. Squinto S, Block A, Braquet P, Bazan N. Platelet-activating factor stimulates a Fos/Jun/AP-1 transcriptional signaling system in human neuroblastoma cells. J Neurosci Res. 1989,24(4).558–66. https://doi.org/10.1002/jnr.490240414.

47. Panetta T, Marcheselli V, Braquet P, Spinnewyn B, Bazan N. Effects of a platelet activating factor antagonist (BN 52021) on free fatty acids, diacylglycerols, polyphosphoinositides and blood flow in the gerbil brain: inhibition of ischemia-reperfusion induced cerebral injury. Biochem Biophys Res Commun. 1987;149(2):580–7. https://doi.org/10.1016/0006-291x(87)90407-4.

48. Belayev L, Khoutorova L, Atkins K, Gordon W, Alvarez-Builla K, Bazan NG. LAU-0901 a novel platelet-activating factor antagonist is highly neuroprotective in cerebral ischemia. Exp Neurol. 2008;214(2):253–8.

49. Boetkjaer A, Boedker M, Cui JG, Zhao Y, Lukiw WJ. Synergism in the repression of COX-2 and TNF-Alpha induction in platelet activating factor stressed human neural cells. Neurosci Lett. 2007;426:59–63 RefID.

50. Musto A, Sammi MS. Platelet-activating factor receptor antagonism targets Neuroinflammation in experimental epilepsy. Epilepsia. 2011;52(3):551–61.

51. Skupien A, Konopka A, Trzaskoma P, et al. CD44 regulates dendrite morphogenesis through Src tyrosine kinase-dependent positioning of the Golgi. J Cell Sci. 2014;127(23):5038–51. https://doi.org/10.1242/jcs.154542.

52. Tejada J, Garcia-Cairasco N, Roque AC. Combined role of seizure-induced dendritic morphology alterations and spine loss in newborn granule cells with mossy fiber sprouting on the hyperexcitability of a computer model of the dentate gyrus. PLoS Comput Biol. 2014;10(5):e1003601. https://doi.org/10.1371/journal.pcbi.1003601.

53. Borges K, McDermott D, Dingledine R. Reciprocal changes of CD44 and GAP-43 expression in the dentate gyrus inner molecular layer after status epilepticus in mice. Exp Neurol. 2004;188(1):1–10.

54. Lee T-S, Mane S, Eid T, et al. Gene expression in temporal lobe epilepsy is consistent with increased release of glutamate by astrocytes. Mol Med. 2007;13(1–2):1–13.

55. Perosa S, Porcionatto M, Cukiert A, et al. Glycosaminoglycan levels and proteoglycan expression are altered in the hippocampus of patients with mesial temporal lobe epilepsy. Brain Res Bull. 2002;58(5):509–16.

56. Bausch S. Potential roles for hyaluronan and CD44 in kainic acid-induced mossy fiber sprouting in organotypic hippocampal slice cultures. Neuroscience. 2006;143(1):339–50.

57. Bronisz E, Kurkowska-Jastrzębska I. Matrix metalloproteinase 9 in epilepsy: the role of neuroinflammation in seizure development. Mediat Inflamm. 2016;2016:7369020.

58. Acar G, Tanriover G, Acar F, Demir R. Increased expression of matrix metalloproteinase-9 in patients with temporal lobe epilepsy. Turkish Neurosurgery. 2015;25(5):749–756.

59. Konopka A, Grajkowska W, Ziemiańska K, et al. Matrix metalloproteinase-9 (MMP-9) in human intractable epilepsy caused by focal cortical dysplasia. Epilepsy Res. 2013;104(1–2):45–58.

60. Hanke ML, Kielian T. Toll-like receptors in health and disease in the brain: mechanisms and therapeutic potential. Clin Sci (London). 2011;121(9):367–87.

61. Gross A, Benninger F, Madar R, et al. Toll-like receptor 3 deficiency decreases epileptogenesis in a pilocarpine model of SE-induced epilepsy in mice. Epilepsia. 2017;58(4):586–96.

62. Costello D, Lynch M. Toll-like receptor 3 activation modulates hippocampal network excitability, via glial production of interferon-β. Hippocampus. 2013;23(8):696–707. https://doi.org/10.1002/hipo.22129.

63. Chung H, Lee J, Kim H, et al. Foxp3 is a novel repressor of microglia activation. Glia. 2010;58(10):1247–56. https://doi.org/10.1002/glia.21006.

64. Wang F, Xiong X, Zhong Q, Meng Z, Yang H, Yang Q. Foxp3 exhibits antiepileptic effects in ictogenesis involved in TLR4 signaling. FASEB J. 2017;31(7):2948–62. https://doi.org/10.1096/fj.201600989r.

65. Bozzi Y, Caleo M. Epilepsy, seizures, and inflammation: role of the C-C motif ligand 2 chemokine. DNA Cell Biol. 2016;35(6):257–60.

66. Fabene P, Bramanti P, Constantin G. The emerging role for chemokines in epilepsy. J Neuroimmunol. 2010;224(1–2):22–7. https://doi.org/10.1016/j.jneuroim.2010.05.016.

67. Li R, Ma L, Huang H, et al. Altered expression of CXCL13 and CXCR5 in intractable temporal lobe epilepsy patients and pilocarpine-induced epileptic rats. Neurochem Res. 2016;42(2):526–40.

68. Podjaski C, Alvarez JI, Bourbonniere L, et al. Netrin 1 regulates blood–brain barrier function and neuroinflammation. Brain. 2015;138(Pt 6):1598–612.

69. Wilson C, Finch C, Cohen H. Cytokines and cognition-the case for a head-to-toe inflammatory paradigm. J Am Geriatr Soc. 2002;50(12):2041–56.

70. Sanchez-Muñoz F, Dominguez-Lopez A, Yamamoto-Furusho JK. Role of cytokines in inflammatory bowel disease. World J Gastroenterol. 2008;14(27):4280–8.

71. Yarlagadda A, Alfson E, Clayton AH. The blood brain barrier and the role of cytokines in neuropsychiatry. Psychiatry (Edgmont). 2009;6(11):18–22.

72. Vezzani A, French J, Bartfai T, Baram T. The role of inflammation in epilepsy. Nat Rev Neurol. 2010;7(1):31–40.

73. Fabene PF, Mora GN, Martinello M, et al. A role for leukocyte-endothelial adhesion mechanisms in epilepsy. Nat Med. 2008;14(12):1377–83.

74. Zattoni M, Mura M, Deprez F, et al. Brain infiltration of leukocytes contributes to the pathophysiology of temporal lobe epilepsy. J Neurosci. 2011;31(11):4037–50.

75. Bonder CS, Clark SR, Norman MU, Johnson P, Kubes P. Use of CD44 by CD4 + Th1 and Th2 lymphocytes to roll and adhere. Blood. 2006;107:4798–806.

76. Weiss N, Miller F, Cazaubon S, Couraud P. The blood-brain barrier in brain homeostasis and neurological diseases. Biochim Biophys Acta Biomembr. 2009;1788(4):842–57.

77. Khan A, Kerfoot S, Heit B, et al. Role of CD44 and Hyaluronan in neutrophil recruitment. J Immunol. 2004;173(12):7594–601.

78. Marchi N, Granata T, Freri E, et al. Efficacy of anti-inflammatory therapy in a model of acute seizures and in a population of pediatric drug resistant epileptics. PLoS ONE. 2011;6(3):e18200. doi:https://doi.org/10.1371/journal.pone.0018200.

79. Feniger-Barish R, Ran M, Zaslaver A, Ben-Baruch A. Differential mo0064es of regulation of cxc chemokine-induced internalization and recycling of human CXCR1 and CXCR2. Cytokine. 1999;11(12):996–1009. https://doi.org/10.1006/cyto.1999.0510.

80. Souza D, Vieira A, Soares A, et al. The essential role of the intestinal microbiota in facilitating acute inflammatory responses. J Immunol. 2004;173(6):4137–46. https://doi.org/10.4049/jimmunol.173.6.4137.

81. Zwijnenburg P, Polfliet M, Florquin S, et al. CXC-chemokines KC and macrophage inflammatory protein-2 (MIP-2) synergistically induce leukocyte recruitment to the central nervous system in rats. Immunol Lett. 2003;85(1):1–4. https://doi.org/10.1016/s0165-2478(02)00200-6.

82. Otto V, Heinzel-Pleines U, Gloor S, Trentz O, Kossmann T, Morganti-Kossmann M. sICAM-1 and TNF-? induce MIP-2 with distinct kinetics in astrocytes and brain microvascular endothelial cells. J Neurosci Res. 2000;60(6):733–42. doi:10.1002/1097-4547(20000615)60:6<733::aid-jnr5>3.0.co;2-x.

83. Zhang B, Chen M, Yang H, Wu T, Song C, Guo R. Evidence for involvement of the CD40/CD40L system in post-stroke epilepsy. Neurosci Lett. 2014;567:6–10. https://doi.org/10.1016/j.neulet.2014.03.003.

84. Jin R, Yu S, Song Z, et al. Soluble CD40 ligand stimulates CD40-dependent activation of the β2 integrin mac-1 and protein kinase C Zeda (PKCζ) in neutrophils: implications for neutrophil-platelet interactions and neutrophil oxidative burst. PLoS One. 2013;8(6):e64631. https://doi.org/10.1371/journal.pone.0064631.

85. Friedman A, Dingledine R. Molecular cascades that mediate the influence of inflammation on epilepsy. Epilepsia. 2011;52(0 3):33–9. https://doi.org/10.1111/j.1528-1167.2011.03034.x.

86. Weissberg I, Wood L, Kamintsky L, et al. Albumin induces excitatory synaptogenesis through astrocytic TGF-β/ALK5 signaling in a model of acquired epilepsy following blood-brain barrier dysfunction. Neurobiol Dis. 2015;78:115–25. https://doi.org/10.1016/j.nbd.2015.02.029.

87. Cacheaux LP, Ivens S, David Y, et al. Transcriptome profiling reveals TGF-β signaling involvement in epileptogenesis. J Neuroscience. 2009;29(28):8927–35. https://doi.org/10.1523/JNEUROSCI.0430-09.2009.

88. Ho Y-H, Lin Y-T, Wu C-WJ, Chao Y-M, Chang AYW, Chan JYH. Peripheral inflammation increases seizure susceptibility via the induction of neuroinflammation and oxidative stress in the hippocampus. J Biomed Sci. 2015;22(1):46.

89. Auvin S, Shin D, Mazarati A, Sankar R. Inflammation induced by LPS enhances epileptogenesis in immature rat and may be partially reversed by IL1RA. Epilepsia. 2010;51(Suppl 3):34–8. https://doi.org/10.1111/j.1528-1167.2010.02606.x.

90. Cerri C, Genovesi S, Allegra M, et al. The chemokine CCL2 mediates the seizure-enhancing effects of systemic inflammation. J Neurosci. 2016;36(13):3777–88.

91. Ong M-S, Kohane I, Cai T, Gorman MP, Mandl K. Population-level evidence for an autoimmune etiology of epilepsy. JAMA Neurol. 2014;71(5):569–74. https://doi.org/10.1001/jamaneurol.2014.188.

92. Lin Z, Si Q, Xiaoyi Z. Association between epilepsy and systemic autoimmune diseases: a meta-analysis. Seizure. 2016;41:160–6.

93. Sang A, Yin Y, Zheng Y, Morel L. Animal models of molecular pathology. Progress in molecular biology and translational science. 2012:321–70. https://doi.org/10.1016/b978-0-12-394596-9.00010-x.

94. Cimaz R, Meroni P, Shoenfeld Y. Epilepsy as part of systemic lupus erythematosus and systemic antiphospholipid syndrome (Hughes syndrome). Lupus. 2006;15(4):191–7. https://doi.org/10.1191/0961203306lu2272rr.

95. Appenzeller S, Cendes F, Costallat L. Epileptic seizures in systemic lupus erythematosus. Neurology. 2004;63(10):1808–12. https://doi.org/10.1212/01.wnl.0000144178.32208.4f.

96. Tsai J-D, Lin C-L, Lin C-C, Sung F-C, Lue K-H. Risk of epilepsy in patients with systemic lupus erythematosus—a retrospective cohort study. Neuropsychiatr Dis Treat. 2014;10:1635–43. https://doi.org/10.2147/NDT.S64323.

97. Dar S, Janahi E, Haque S, et al. Superantigen influence in conjunction with cytokine polymorphism potentiates autoimmunity in systemic lupus erythematosus patients. Immunol Res. 2015;64(4):1001–12.

98. Lim S-H, Park E, You B, et al. Neuronal synapse formation induced by microglia and interleukin 10. PLoS One. 2013;8(11):e81218.

99. Yang J, Li Q, Yang X, Li M. Increased serum level of prolactin is related to autoantibody production in systemic lupus erythematosus. Lupus. 2016; 25(5):513–9.

100. Takei K, Sato M, Nakamura M, Shimizu H. Longitudinally extensive transverse myelitis with anti-NMDA receptor antibodies during a systemic lupus erythematosus flare-up. BMJ Case Reports. 2015;2015:bcr2015212112. doi: https://doi.org/10.1136/bcr-2015-212112.

101. Wang J-B, Li H, Wang L-L, Liang H-D, Zhao L, Dong J. Role of IL-1β, IL-6, IL-8 and IFN-γ in pathogenesis of central nervous system neuropsychiatric systemic lupus erythematous. Int J Clin Exp Med. 2015;8(9):16658–63.

102. Ho R, Thiaghu C, Ong H, et al. A meta-analysis of serum and cerebrospinal fluid autoantibodies in neuropsychiatric systemic lupus erythematosus. Autoimmun Rev. 2016;15(2):124–38.

103. Hawro T, Bogucki A, Krupińska-Kun M, Maurer M, Woźniacka A. Intractable headaches, ischemic stroke, and seizures are linked to the presence of anti-β2GPI antibodies in patients with systemic lupus erythematosus. PLoS One. 2015;10(3):e0119911. https://doi.org/10.1371/journal.pone.0119911.

104. Tamagno G, Celik Y, Simó R, et al. Encephalopathy associated with autoimmune thyroid disease in patients with Graves' disease: clinical manifestations, follow-up, and outcomes. BMC Neurol. 2010;10:27. https://doi.org/10.1186/1471-2377-10-27.

105. Devinsky O, Schein A, Najjar S. Epilepsy associated with systemic autoimmune disorders. Epilepsy Currents. 2013;13(2):62–8.

106. Watemberg N, Greenstein D, Levine A. Topical review: encephalopathy associated with Hashimoto thyroiditis: pediatric perspective. J Child Neurol. 2006;21(1):1–5.

107. Kalra S, Silman A, Akman-Demir G, et al. Diagnosis and management of neuro-Behçet's disease: international consensus recommendations. J Neurol. 2014;261(9):1662–76. https://doi.org/10.1007/s00415-013-7209-3.

108. Saleh Z, Arayssi T. Update on the therapy of Behçet disease. Ther Adv Chronic Dis. 2014;5(3):112–34. https://doi.org/10.1177/2040622314523062.

109. Joseph F, Scolding N. Neuro-Behçet's disease in Caucasians: a study of 22 patients. Eur J Neurol. 2007;14(2):174–80.

110. Keezer M, Novy J, Sander J. Type 1 diabetes mellitus in people with pharmacoresistant epilepsy: prevalence and clinical characteristics. Epilepsy Res. 2015;115:55–7.

111. Falip M, Carreño M, Miró J, et al. Prevalence and immunological spectrum of temporal lobe epilepsy with glutamic acid decarboxylase antibodies. Eur J Neurol. 2012;19(6):827–33.

112. Ganelin-Cohen E, Modan-Moses D, Hemi R, Kanety H, Ben-zeev B, Hampe C. Epilepsy and behavioral changes, type 1 diabetes mellitus and a high titer of glutamic acid decarboxylase antibodies. Pediatr Diabetes. 2015;17(8):617–22.

113. YOSHIMOTO T, DOI M, FUKAI N, et al. Type 1 diabetes mellitus and drug-resistant epilepsy: presence of high titer of anti-glutamic acid decarboxylase autoantibodies in serum and cerebrospinal fluid. Intern Med. 2005;44(11):1174–7.

114. Solimena M, Folli F, Denis-Donini S, et al. Autoantibodies to glutamic acid decarboxylase in a patient with stiff-man syndrome, epilepsy, and type I diabetes mellitus. N Engl J Med. 1988;318(16):1012–20.

115. Vincent A, Crino P. Systemic and neurologic autoimmune disorders associated with seizures or epilepsy. Epilepsia. 2011;52:12–7.

116. Fazeli Farsani S, Souverein P, van der Vorst M, Knibbe C, de Boer A, Mantel-Teeuwisse A. Chronic comorbidities in children with type 1 diabetes: a population-based cohort study. Arch Dis Child. 2015;100(8):763–8.

117. Raza A, Yousaf W, Giannella R, Shata MT. Th17 cells: interactions with predisposing factors in the immunopathogenesis of inflammatory bowel disease. Expert review of clinical immunology. 2012;8(2):161-168. doi:https://doi.org/10.1586/eci.11.96.

118. Damjanovich L, Volkó J, Forgács A, Hohenberger W, Bene L. Crohn's disease alters MHC-rafts in CD4+ T-cells. Cytometry Part A. 2011;81A(2):149–64.

119. Liimatainen S, Peltola M, Fallah M, Kharazmi E, Haapala A, Peltola J. The high prevalence of antiphospholipid antibodies in refractory focal epilepsy is related to recurrent seizures. Eur J Neurol. 2009;16(1):134–41.

120. Voulgarelis M, Tzioufas AG. Current aspects of pathogenesis in Sjögren's syndrome. Ther Adv Musculoskelet Dis. 2010;2(6):325–34. https://doi.org/10.1177/1759720X10381431.

121. Colaci M, Cassone G, Manfredi A, Sebastiani M, Giuggioli D, Ferri C. Neurologic complications associated with Sjögren's disease: case reports and modern pathogenic dilemma. Case Rep Neurol Med. 2014;2014:590292. https://doi.org/10.1155/2014/590292

122. Akasbi M, Berenguer J, Saiz A, et al. White matter abnormalities in primary Sjogren syndrome. QJM. 2011;105(5):433–43.

123. Soliotis F, Mavragani C, Moutsopoulos H. Central nervous system involvement in Sjögren's syndrome. Ann Rheum Dis. 2004;63(6):616–20.

124. Bansal S, Sawhney I, Chopra J. Epilepsia partialis continua in Sjögren's syndrome. Epilepsia. 1987;28(4):362–3.

125. Matsuo K, Saburi M, Ishikawa H, et al. Sjögren syndrome presenting with encephalopathy mimicking Creutzfeldt–Jakob disease. J Neurol Sci. 2013; 326(1–2):100–3.

126. Zois C, Katsanos K, Kosmidou M, Tsianos E. Neurologic manifestations in inflammatory bowel diseases: current knowledge and novel insights. J Crohn's Colitis. 2010;4:115–24.

127. Nishimoto N. Interleukin-6 in rheumatoid arthritis. Curr Opin Rheumatol. 2006;18(3):277–81.

128. Uludag I, Duksal T, Tiftikcioglu B, Zorlu Y, Ozkaya F, Kirkali G. IL-1β, IL-6 and IL1Ra levels in temporal lobe epilepsy. Seizure. 2015;26:22–5.

129. Youn Y, Sung IK, Lee IG. The role of cytokines in seizures: interleukin (IL)-1β, IL-1Ra, IL-8, and IL-10. Korean J Pediatr. 2013;56(7):271–4.

130. Chang K-H, Hsu Y-C, Chang M-Y, et al. A large-scale study indicates increase in the risk of epilepsy in patients with different risk factors, including rheumatoid arthritis. Medicine. 2015;94(36):e1485.

131. Rom A, Wu C, Olsen J, et al. Parental rheumatoid arthritis and childhood epilepsy. Neurology. 2016;87(24):2510–6.

132. Gujral N, Freeman HJ, Thomson AB. Celiac disease: prevalence, diagnosis, pathogenesis and treatment. World J Gastroenterol. 2012;18(42):6036–59. https://doi.org/10.3748/wjg.v18.i42.6036.

133. Jackson JR, Eaton WW, Cascella NG, Fasano A, Kelly DL. Neurologic and psychiatric manifestations of celiac disease and gluten sensitivity. Psychiatric Q. 2012;83(1):91–102.

134. Díaz-Marcaccio R, González-Rabelino G, Delfino A. Epilepsy, cerebral calcifications and coeliac disease. The importance of an early diagnosis. Rev Neurol. 2005;40(07):417–20.

135. Peltola M, Kaukinen K, Dastidar P, et al. Hippocampal sclerosis in refractory temporal lobe epilepsy is associated with gluten sensitivity. J Neurol Neurosurg Psychiatry. 2009;80(6):626–30.

136. Bashiri H, Afshari D, Babaei N, Ghadami M. Celiac disease and epilepsy: the effect of gluten-free diet on seizure control. Adv Clin Exp Med. 2016;25(4):751–4.

137. Corps KN, Roth TL, McGavern DB. Inflammation and neuroprotection in traumatic brain injury. JAMA Neurol. 2015;72(3):355–62. https://doi.org/10.1001/jamaneurol.2014.3558.

138. Vezzani A, Dingledine R, Rossetti AO. Immunity and inflammation in status epilepticus and its sequelae: possibilities for therapeutic application. Expert Rev Neurother. 2015;15(9):1081–92. https://doi.org/10.1586/14737175.2015.1079130.

139. Haider L. Inflammation, iron, energy failure, and oxidative stress in the pathogenesis of multiple sclerosis. Oxidative Med Cell Longev. 2015;2015: 725370. https://doi.org/10.1155/2015/725370.

140. Yeung Y, McDonald K, Grewal T, Munoz L. Interleukins in glioblastoma pathophysiology: implications for therapy. Br J Pharmacol. 2013;168(3):591–606. https://doi.org/10.1111/bph.12008.

141. Jin R, Liu L, Zhang S, Nanda A, Li G. Role of inflammation and its mediators in acute ischemic stroke. J Cardiovasc Transl Res. 2013;6(5):834–51. https://doi.org/10.1007/s12265-013-9508-6.

142. Azizi G, Navabi SS, Al-Shukaili A, Seyedzadeh MH, Yazdani R, Mirshafiey A. The role of inflammatory mediators in the pathogenesis of Alzheimer's disease. Sultan Qaboos Univ Med J. 2015;15(3):e305–16. https://doi.org/10.18295/squmj.2015.15.03.002.

143. Chou I, Wang C, Lin W, Tsai F, Lin C, Kao C. Risk of epilepsy in type 1 diabetes mellitus: a population-based cohort study. Diabetologia. 2016;59(6):1196–203.

8

Pro-epileptogenic effects of viral-like inflammation in both mature and immature brains

Nina Dupuis[1,2], Andrey Mazarati[3], Béatrice Desnous[1,2,4], Vibol Chhor[1,2], Bobbi Fleiss[1,2], Tifenn Le Charpentier[1,2], Sophie Lebon[1,2], Zsolt Csaba[1,2], Pierre Gressens[1,2,4], Pascal Dournaud[1,2†] and Stéphane Auvin[1,2,4*†]

Abstract

Background: Infectious encephalitides are most often associated with acute seizures during the infection period and are risk factors for the development of epilepsy at later times. Mechanisms of viral encephalitis-induced epileptogenesis are poorly understood. Here, we evaluated the contribution of viral encephalitis-associated inflammation to ictogenesis and epileptogenesis using a rapid kindling protocol in rats. In addition, we examined whether minocycline can improve outcomes of viral-like brain inflammation.

Methods: To produce viral-like inflammation, polyinosinic-polycytidylic acid (PIC), a toll-like receptor 3 (TLR3) agonist, was applied to microglial/macrophage cell cultures and to the hippocampus of postnatal day 13 (P13) and postnatal day 74 (P74) rats. Cell cultures permit the examination of the inflammation induced by PIC, while the in vivo setting better suits the analysis of cytokine production and the effects of inflammation on epileptogenesis. Minocycline (50 mg/kg) was injected intraperitoneally for 3 consecutive days prior to the kindling procedure to evaluate its effects on inflammation and epileptogenesis.

Results: PIC injection facilitated kindling epileptogenesis, which was evident as an increase in the number of full limbic seizures at both ages. Furthermore, in P14 rats, we observed a faster seizure onset and prolonged retention of the kindling state. PIC administration also led to an increase in interleukin 1β (IL-1β) levels in the hippocampus in P14 and P75 rats. Treatment with minocycline reversed neither the pro-epileptogenic effects of PIC nor the increase of IL-1β in the hippocampus in both P14 and P75 rats.

Conclusions: Hippocampal injection of PIC facilitates rapid kindling epileptogenesis at both P14 and P75, suggesting that viral–induced inflammation increases epileptogenesis irrespective of brain maturation. Minocycline, however, was unable to reverse the increase of epileptogenesis, which might be linked to its absence of effect on hippocampal IL-1β levels at both ages.

Keywords: Encephalitis, Epileptogenesis, Kindling, Microglia, Minocycline, Toll-like receptor, Virus

Background

Infectious encephalitides are most often associated with seizures during the infection period [1, 2] and are established risk factors for the development of epilepsy at later times [1, 3, 4]. Although many infectious encephalitides are of unknown origin, the majority of clinical studies suggest a viral etiology [5, 6]. Common viruses associated with encephalitis-induced seizures are herpes simplex and cytomegalovirus. Children are three times more prone to viral encephalitis than adults are [6, 7], moreover, infants under 1 year are particularly affected [6]. Mechanisms leading to increased seizure occurrence at the time of infection and those underlying encephalitis-induced epileptogenesis are poorly understood. Virus-induced cell injury, brain inflammation, and initial prolonged seizures appear to be key contributors to epileptogenesis after the acute phase of encephalitis [2, 8–10].

* Correspondence: stephane.auvin@inserm.fr
†Equal contributors
[1]INSERM, U1141, 75019 Paris, France
[2]Université Paris Diderot, Sorbonne Paris Cité, INSERM UMR1141, 75019 Paris, France

There are several models of virus-induced encephalitis. However, most experimental animals die during the acute infection period, rendering the study of epileptogenesis impossible [11]. The use of the Daniel's (DA) strain of Theiler's murine encephalomyelitis virus (TMEV) in C57Bl6 mice leads to behavioral seizures during the acute phase in 75% of the animals [10]. A significant proportion (65%) of the animals with acute symptomatic seizures develops spontaneous recurrent seizures later in life [10]. In this model, macrophages have been shown to be associated with seizures during the acute phase of encephalitis, while neuronal loss and inflammation contribute to epileptogenesis [8, 12].

In the central nervous system (CNS), the innate inflammatory response to viral infection primarily involves the activation of microglia, which are cerebral monocyte-like immune cells [13]. The innate inflammatory response is triggered by pattern-recognition receptors, including toll-like receptors (TLRs), RIG1-like receptors, and nucleotide-binding oligomerization domain-like receptors [14]. TLR3 is a receptor for double-stranded RNA, which is released by viruses and necrotic cells. Upon activation, TLR3 triggers cytokine and interferon production pathways [15, 16].

Clinical and experimental data suggest an important role for neuroinflammation in seizure occurrence and epileptogenesis [17]. A direct role of cytokines, and particularly of interleukin 1β (IL-1β), has been demonstrated in the precipitation of seizures during brain inflammation. Cytokines have also been implicated in epileptogenesis. Therapeutic targeting of IL-1β has been proven effective in inhibiting epileptogenesis [18, 19].

Since encephalitis in humans is more frequent in children than in adults, we decided to evaluate the contribution of brain viral-like inflammation to epileptogenesis in not only mature but also in immature brains. To induce brain viral-like inflammation, we injected a TLR3 agonist, polyinosinic-polycytidylic acid (PIC) [20], into the hippocampus, which produces an inflammatory response in the absence of viral replication. Unlike the TMEV model, this model allows us to explore the role of brain inflammation in the absence of viral replication-induced brain injury. Moreover, our kindling model, which is a model of compressed epileptogenesis, allows us to perform the experiment during a precise window of brain maturation.

We first characterized the response to PIC both in vitro and in vivo. Since macrophages contribute to epileptogenesis in the TMEV model, we decided to study microglial cells and macrophages to evaluate potential differences that might derive from specific contributions of these cell types. The second part of the study consisted of the assessment of the effects of intrahippocampal PIC injection on hippocampal excitability and epileptogenesis using the rapid kindling model. We conducted the study in P14 and P75 animals to evaluate whether brain maturation contributes to a higher susceptibility to inflammatory responses and epileptogenesis. Finally, we evaluated the effects of minocycline, an antibiotic described as a modulator of inflammation [21–23], on the inflammatory response to and the modulation of seizures induced by PIC.

Methods

Animals

Male Wistar rats (Charles River, L'Arbesle, France) were used for the rapid kindling and cytokine-dosage experiments. We used P13 and P74 rats at the time of the PIC intrahippocampal injection. Primary microglial and macrophage cell cultures were prepared from the neocortex of OF1 mice (Charles River, L'Arbesle) and 2-month-old OF1 male mice (Charles River). Animals were housed in standard laboratory conditions with controlled temperature/humidity, a 12:12-hour light/dark cycle, and free access to food and water. Studies were approved by the animal ethical institutional review committee (Bichat-Robert Debré ethical committee, Paris, France, #2015072801547679) and met stipulations of the guide for the care and use of laboratory animals (NIH, Bethesda, Maryland, USA), as well as recommendations of reduction, refinement, and replacement (known as the 3 Rs) [24].

Drugs

PIC and minocycline (Sigma, Lyon, France) were dissolved in saline for the in vivo experiments and in phosphate buffered saline (PBS) for the in vitro experiments. PIC (10 µg/rat) was injected stereotaxically into the ventral hippocampus 24 h before rapid kindling at the following coordinates: P13, 3.0 mm posterior, 3.9 mm left, 4.2 mm ventral; P74, 4.8 mm posterior, 5.3 mm left, 6.5 mm ventral, in relation to bregma. The injection of PIC into the hippocampus aims to mimic encephalitis, which is characterized by brain inflammation, rather than meningitis, which is inflammation in the meninges and the cerebrospinal fluid (CSF). Minocycline (50 mg/kg) was administered as 3 consecutive intraperitoneal (i.p.) injections 48, 24, and 4 h before the start of the kindling protocol. Table 1 summarizes the in vitro and in vivo experiments.

Microglia primary cell cultures

Primary mixed glial cell cultures were prepared from the neocortices of P0-P1 OF1 mice, as described previously [25, 26]. Briefly, the cortices were dissected and the meninges were removed in 0.1 M PBS with 6% glucose and 2% penicillin–streptomycin (PS, Gibco, Cergy Pontoise, France). The tissue was subsequently mechanically

Table 1 Experimental plan summarizing treatments and experiment (exp.) numbers included in the study

Cell culture experiments	In vivo experiments
Microglia	Rapid kindling protocol
RT-PCR: PBS vs. PIC, $n = 5$ (x3 exp.)	P14: saline ($n = 5$) vs. PIC ($n = 6$)
Luminex: PBS vs. PIC, $n = 5$ (x1 exp.)	P75: saline ($n = 6$) vs. PIC ($n = 7$)
RT-PCR: PIC vs. PIC + Mino, $n = 5$ (x3 exp.)	P14: mino ($n = 7$) vs. PIC + Mino ($n = 7$)
Luminex: PIC vs. PIC + Mino, $n = $ (x1 exp.)	P75: mino ($n = 5$) vs. PIC + Mino ($n = 5$)
Macrophages	Cytokines dosage by luminex
RT-PCR: PBS vs. PIC, $n = 5$ (x3 exp.)	P14: saline i.p. + saline i.h. ($n = 5$)
Luminex: PBS vs. PIC, $n = 5$ (x1 exp.)	Saline i.p. + PIC i.h. ($n = 5$)
RT-PCR: PIC vs. PIC + mino, $n = 5$ (x3 exp.)	Mino i.p. + saline i.h. ($n = 5$)
Luminex: PIC vs. PIC + mino, $n = 5$ (x1 exp.)	Mino i.p. + PIC i.h. ($n = 5$)
	P75: Saline i.p. + saline i.h. ($n = 5$)
	Saline i.p. + PIC i.h. ($n = 5$)
	Mino i.p. + saline i.h. ($n = 5$)
	Mino i.p. + PIC i.h. ($n = 5$)

dissociated and spun at 1000 rpm for 5 min at 4 °C. The pellet was resuspended in low-glucose Dulbecco's modified Eagle's minimum essential medium (DMEM, 31885, Gibco) supplemented with 10% fetal bovine serum (FBS, Gibco) and 0.01% PS. The cells were then plated in poly-D-L-ornithine-coated T75 flasks. Microglia were isolated from the primary mixed glial cultures on day in vitro 14 by shaking for 20 min. The supernatant was collated and spun at 1800 rpm for 5 min at 4 °C. Microglia were resuspended in DMEM supplemented with 0% FBS in 6-well culture plates and cultured for 1 day before treatment.

Microglia were exposed for 4 h to PBS or PIC (1 µg/ml). Supernatants were collected and stored at –80 °C until cytokine levels were measured. Cells were harvested and RNA was extracted for gene expression analysis.

Peritoneal macrophage primary cell cultures

Primary peritoneal macrophage cultures were prepared from 2-month-old OF1 male mice, as described previously [27]. Macrophages were isolated by peritoneal lavage with ice-cold PBS. After $400 \times g$ centrifugation, cells were resuspended in DMEM/F12 medium (Gibco, Cergy Pontoise, France) supplemented with 10% FBS (Gibco) and 0.01% PS (Gibco) in 6-well culture plates. After 1 h, non-adherent cells were removed by washing and adherent cells were found to be ~95% pure based on

morphological criteria. Cells were cultured for 1 day before treatment.

Similar to microglia, macrophages were exposed to PBS or PIC (4-hour; 1 µg/ml). Supernatants were collected and stored at –80 °C until cytokine level measurements. Cells were harvested and RNA was extracted for gene expression analysis.

RNA extraction and quantitative PCR

Total RNA from primary microglial cell cultures was extracted using the RNeasy mini kit according to the manufacturer's instructions (Qiagen, Courtaboeuf, France). Total RNA (500 ng) was subjected to reverse transcription based on equal amounts of RNA using the iScript™ cDNA synthesis kit (Bio-Rad, Marnes-la-Coquette, France). Quantitative PCR was then performed in duplicate for each sample using the SYBR Green Supermix (Bio-Rad) for 40 cycles with a two-step program (5 s of denaturation at 96 °C, and 10 s of annealing at 60 °C). The primers used are summarized in Table 2. The relative expression of genes of interest was compared with that of the reference gene, glyceraldehyde-3-phosphate dehydrogenase (Gapdh). Analyses were performed using Biorad CFX Manager 3.0 software.

Multiplex cytokine assay

Freshly excised hippocampi from P14 and P75 rats (24 h after ventral hippocampal injection) were homogenized and total protein was extracted in PBS supplemented with protease inhibitors (Roche Diagnostics, Meylan, France). After a 12500-rpm centrifugation for 30 min, supernatants were collected.

IL-1β, interleukin 6 (IL-6), tumor necrosis factor α (TNFα), and interleukin 10 (IL-10) levels were measured in microglia supernatants and hippocampal protein

Table 2 List of PCR primers used in the study

Gene	Forward primer (5′–3′)	Reverse primer (5′–3′)
Gapdh	GGC CTT CCG TGT TCC TAC	TGT CAT CAT ACT TGG CAG GTT
Il1β	GGG CCT CAA AGG AAA GAA TC	TCT TCT TTG GGT ATT GCT TGG
Il6	CAA AGC CAG AGT CCT TCA GA	GCC ACT CCT TCT GTG ACT CC
Tnfα	GCC TCT TCT CAT TCC TGC TT	AGG GTC TGG GCC ATA GAA CT
Il1rn	TTG TGC CAA GTC TGG AGA TG	TTC TCA GAG CGG ATG AAG GT
NfkB	TTA CAT TCC ATC CCG GAG TC	GCA CAA TCT TTA GGG CCA TT
IkB	CTC ACG GAG GAC GGA GAC T	GTC TCC CTT CAC CTG ACC AA
Ifnβ	TGA ACT CCA CCA GCA GAC AG	GGA CAT CTC CCA CGT CAA TC
Trif	GCT CCA GGC TTC ATT CTC C	AAG GCA CCT AGA ATG CCA AA
Tbk1	ATA AGC TTC CTT CGC CCA GT	CCA CAG GGA CAA AAC TCC AT
Irf3	GAT GGC TGA CTT TGG CAT CT	GAC ACG TCC GGC TTA TCC T
Ptgs2	TCA TTC ACC AGA CAG ATT GCT	AAG CGT TTG CGG TAC TCA TT
Nos2	CCC TTC AAT GGT TGG TAC ATG G	ACA TTG ATC TCC GTG ACA GCC

extracts using a Bio-plex 200 and a 96-well magnetic plate assay according to the manufacturer's instructions (Biorad Laboratories, Marnes la Coquette, France). All samples were run in duplicate, and data were analyzed using Bio-Plex Manager software. For hippocampal measurements, cytokine levels were expressed relative to total protein levels (pg of cytokine/mg of total protein).

Immunohistochemistry

Twenty-four hours after the hippocampal PIC injection, P14 and P75 rats ($n = 5$ for each experimental group) underwent transcardiac perfusion with 4% paraformaldehyde. Coronal 30-μm-thick free-floating sections were immunolabeled overnight with rabbit polyclonal anti-ionized calcium binding adaptor molecule 1 (Iba1) (1:1000, Wako) and mouse monoclonal anti-glial fibrillary acidic protein (GFAP) (1:500, Sigma) antibodies and revealed by Alexa Fluor 488- and Cy3-conjugated anti-rabbit and anti-mouse secondary antibodies (1:500, Invitrogen).

Sections of the ventral hippocampus at the PIC or saline injection sites were imaged using a fluorescence microscope (Zeiss Axio Observer Z1). Immunopositive cells were quantified by a cell count in six different areas distant from the injection site in each animal (square; Fig. 3) using ImageJ software.

Rapid kindling protocol

Animals were anesthetized with isoflurane, stereotaxically injected with 10 μg of PIC (1 μl in the left hippocampus), and implanted with a bipolar stimulating electrode (Plastics One Inc., Roanoke, VA) into the left ventral hippocampus. The coordinates in relation to bregma were as follows: P13, 3.0 mm posterior, 3.9 mm left, 4.2 mm ventral; P74, 4.8 mm posterior, 5.3 mm left, 6.5 mm ventral. A tripolar recording electrode was wrapped around the skull screws above the right hemisphere. Electrodes were fixed to the skull using Integrity composite resin (Densply, York, PA, U.S.A.).

Twenty-four hours after surgery, the animals were connected to a DS8000 electrical stimulator via DLS100 stimulus isolators (World Precision Instruments, Sarasota, FL, U.S.A.). Electroencephalograms (EEGs) were acquired using the MP100/EEG100B acquisition system and AcqKnowledge software (BIOPAC, Santa Barbara, CA, U.S.A.). The electrical stimulus used for the assessment of the ictogenesis parameters and the kindling protocol was a square wave biphasic electrical stimulus with the following characteristics: 10-second train duration, 20 Hz, 1-ms pulse duration, delivered every 5 min. At 24 and 48 h post-injection, afterdischarge threshold (ADT) and afterdischarge duration (ADD) were assessed using 0.1 mA incremental currents delivered every 5 min. An AD was defined as paroxysmal epileptiform activity lasting at least 5 s with peak-to-peak amplitude of at least twice the baseline background EEG observed after the end of the hippocampal electrical stimulation.

The kindling protocol consisted of 60 trains delivered every 5 min with a current of 0.1 mA over the ADT with parameters otherwise similar to those described for afterdischarge detection. Animals were video-recorded during the kindling procedure. Behavioral seizures were scored using Racine's scale: 1, motor arrest and twitching vibrissae; 2, chewing, head bobbing; 3, forelimb clonus; 4, forelimb clonus and rearing; 5, rearing and falling. Epileptogenesis was analyzed by calculating the numbers of kindling trials needed to first reach a stage 4–5 seizure and the total numbers of stage 4–5 seizures during the kindling procedure. Ictogenesis was analyzed by calculating changes in afterdischarge properties 24 h after the kindling procedure compared to baseline afterdischarge properties. We also determined the severities of behavioral seizures in response to the threshold stimulation in the kindled animals [28–30].

Statistical analysis

Data were analyzed using Prism 5 software (Graphpad, San Diego, CA, U.S.A.). Data were expressed as mean ± standard errors of the mean. Statistical analyses were performed using Kruskal-Wallis followed by Dunn's posthoc tests and the Mann-Whitney test to compare two groups.

Results

PIC triggers inflammatory responses in both microglia and macrophages

We produced primary cell cultures of both microglia and macrophages to study inflammatory responses to PIC. In microglial cells, PIC treatment increased mRNA levels of Il-1β, Il-6, Tnfα, interferon β (Infβ), and interleukin 1 receptor antagonist (IL-1rn), as well as of activators of TLR3 transduction pathways (i.e., nuclear factor kappa-light-chain-enhancer of activated B cells (NfκB), nuclear factor of kappa light polypeptide gene enhancer in B-cells inhibitor, alpha (IκB), TIR-domain-containing adapter-inducing interferon-β (Trif), and TANK-binding kinase (Tbk1)). Ptgs2 and Nos2 (coding for cyclooxygenase2 and inducible nitric oxide synthase proteins, respectively) mRNA levels were also increased after PIC exposure (Fig. 1a). The levels of pro-inflammatory cytokines were consistent with the reverse transcriptase-PCR findings and indicated increases in the levels of IL-1β, IL-6, and TNFα after PIC exposure (Fig. 1c). In macrophages, we observed a similar profile of inflammatory activation by studying mRNA expression after PIC exposure (Fig. 1b). We found increases of IL-6 and TNFα not of IL-1β in the supernatant after PIC exposure (Fig. 1c).

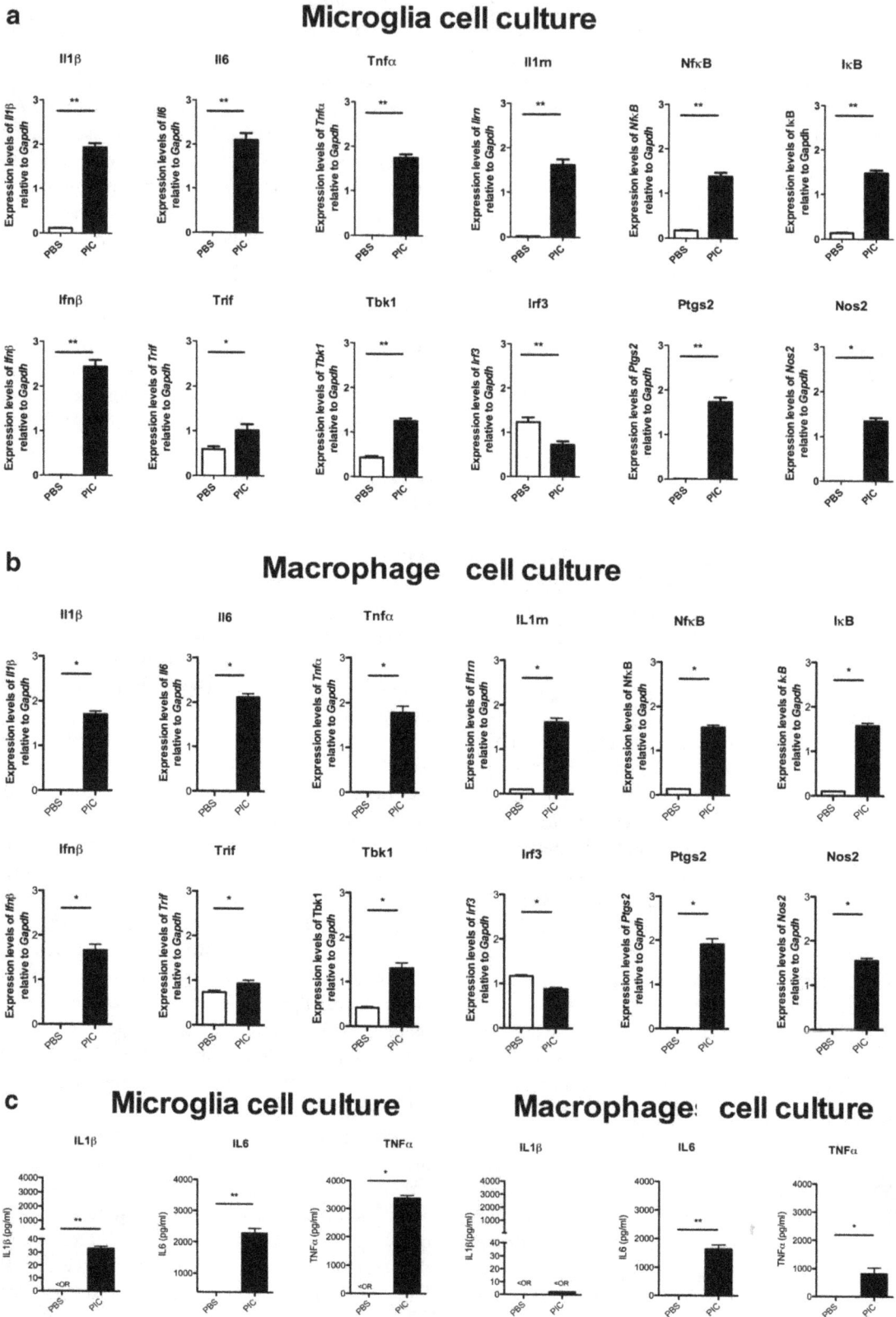

Fig. 1 (See legend on next page.)

(See figure on previous page.)
Fig. 1 Inflammatory response to PIC treatment in microglial and macrophage primary cell cultures. mRNA quantification by RT-qPCR of inflammatory actors in microglial (**a**) and macrophage (**b**) primary cultures 4 h after PBS or PIC exposure (1 µg/ml). Cytokine profile (IL1β, IL6, TNFα) 4 h after PBS or PIC exposure (1 µg/ml) in primary microglial and macrophage cell culture supernatants (**c**). Data are presented as mean ± SEM. *$p < 0.05$, **$p < 0.01$ vs. PBS (Mann-Whitney test)

Hippocampal injection of PIC triggers an inflammatory IL-1β response

Following the injection of PIC into the hippocampus, we observed an increase in IL-1β compared to the controls at both ages (Fig. 2). In contrast, IL-6, TNFα and IL-10 protein levels were unchanged 24 h after PIC injection at both ages (Fig. 2). The intracerebral PIC injection did not result in any change in the blood cytokine levels (Additional file 1).

Hippocampal injection of PIC does not change the numbers of glial cells in vivo

In order to determine whether IL-1β production is associated with glial activation, we analyzed microglia and astrocyte distribution in the hippocampus. Twenty-four hours after the intrahippocampal injection of PIC, the density of Iba1-expressing cells was not different from those found in controls in either age group (Fig. 3). Similarly, in both age groups, the density of GFAP-expressing cells was not different from that of the controls (Fig. 3). Around the injection site, where we observed glial activation (Fig. 3), no difference in the relative intensities of both Iba1- and GFAP immunoreactive

signals was observed in PIC-injected vs. saline control animals (Fig. 3c).

Hippocampal injection of PIC facilitates epileptogenesis in both P14 and P75 rats

We used a rapid kindling model to determine whether intrahippocampal injection of PIC produces pro-ictogenic and/or pro-epileptogenic effects. First, AD parameters were not changed by PIC administration. This suggests that there were no changes in ambient hippocampal excitability at either P14 or P75 (Fig. 4a, b).

Second, kindling epileptogenesis was facilitated by PIC; this was evident as an increase in the numbers of full limbic (i.e., stage 4–5) seizures (P14: 23.3 ± 2.4 vs. 10.2 ± 2.6, $p < 0.01$; P75: 15.6 ± 1.1 vs. 8.8 ± 1.3, $p < 0.01$; comparisons are for PIC vs. saline) and a faster onset of stage 4–5 seizures in P14 animals (number of trials to first stage 4–5 seizure: P14, 11.2 ± 3.5 vs. 27.8 ± 5.0, $p < 0.05$; comparison is for PIC vs. saline) (Fig. 5a, b).

Third, the modification of AD properties after kindling by PIC was more evident in P14 rats. 24 h after the kindling procedure, PIC further increased the scores of seizures induced by threshold stimulation in P14 rats (Fig. 5a). There was no difference in AD threshold

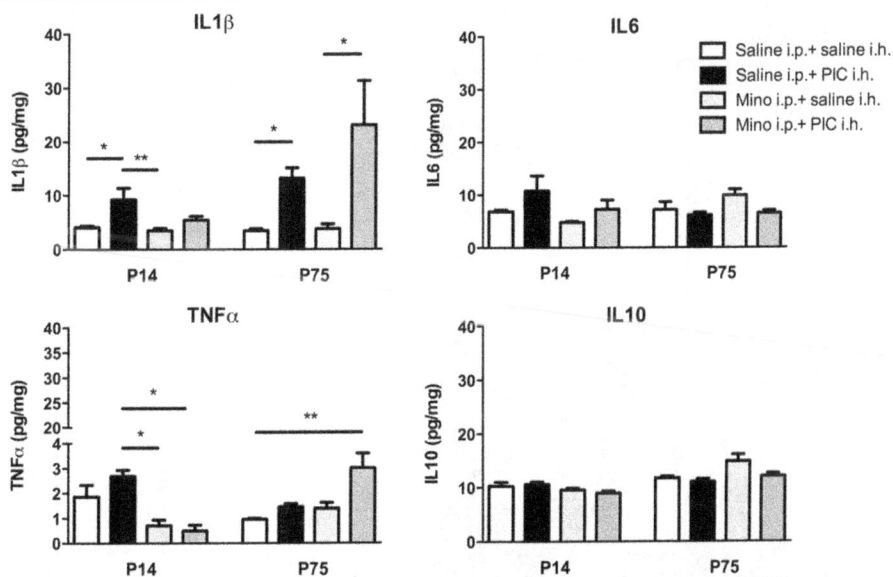

Fig. 2 Hippocampal cytokine levels 24 h after PIC injection. Cytokine profiles (IL1β, IL6, IL10, TNFα) in the hippocampus 24 h after intrahippocampal injection (saline i.p. + saline i.h., saline i.p. + PIC i.h. (10 µg/rat), minocycline i.p. (50 mg/kg) + saline i.h. or minocycline i.p. (50 mg/kg) + PIC i.h. (10 µg/rat)) in P14 and in P75 rats. Data are presented as mean ± SEM. *$p < 0.05$ vs. all other treatment groups according to age group (Kruskal-Wallis test)

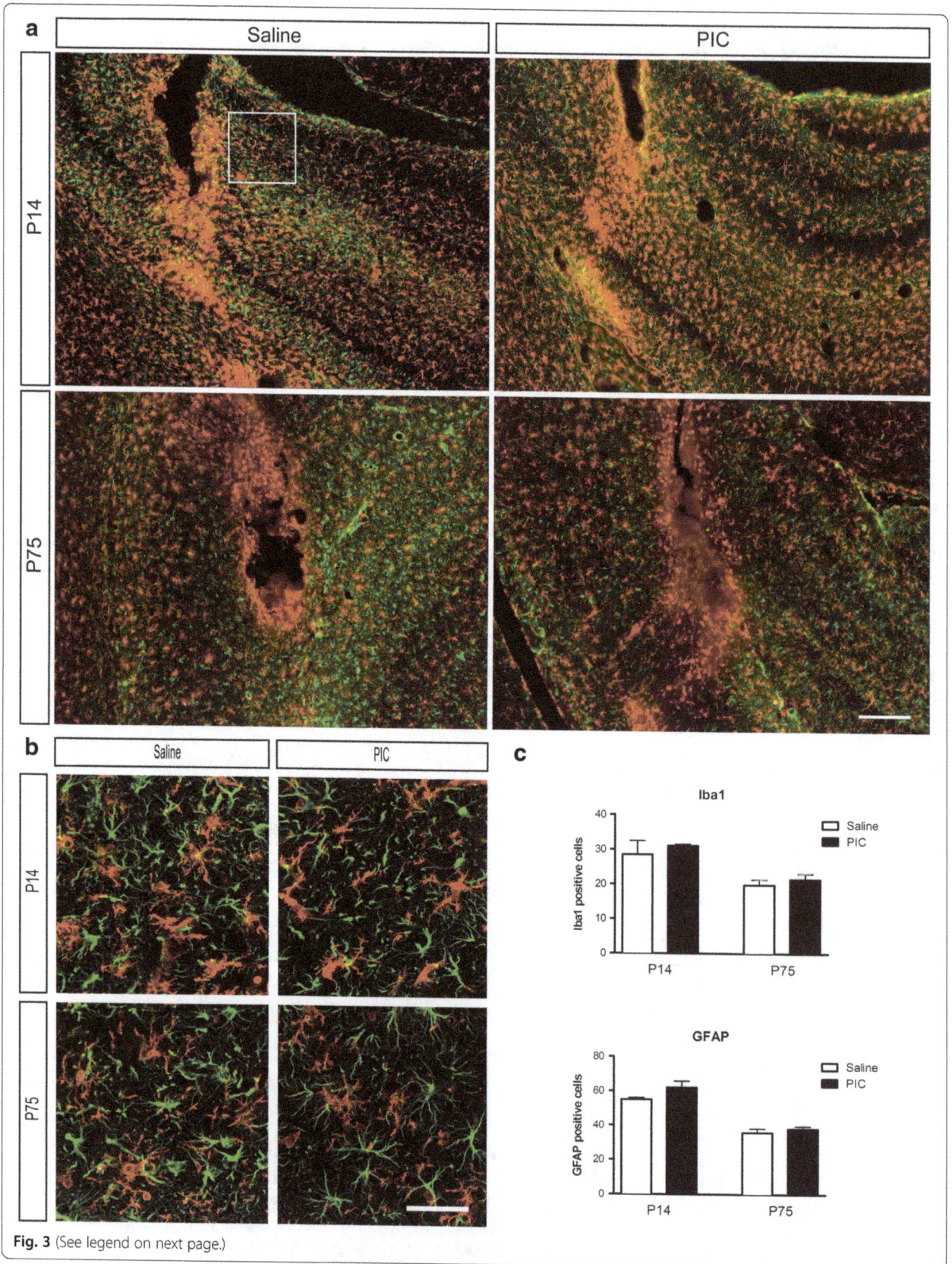

Fig. 3 (See legend on next page.)

between the PIC and control groups at P14 (Fig. 5a). None of these parameters (AD parameters and seizure scores at retest) were changed in P75 rats (Fig. 5b).

Inefficiency of minocycline in the PIC-facilitated epileptogenesis in both P14 and P75 rats

To test possible modulations of the pro-epileptogenic effects of PIC by minocycline, we administered minocycline (50 mg/kg i.p.) over three consecutive days to animals at both ages, with and without intrahippocampal PIC injections (Figs. 4 and 5). First, in AD parameters, we detected a decrease of ADT in minocycline-treated P14 animals as compared to saline controls (Fig. 4a). Second, kindling epileptogenesis facilitated by PIC was not inhibited by minocycline (Fig. 5). Third, after kindling completion, minocycline did not reduce the pro-epileptogenic effects of PIC (Fig. 5). On the contrary, the ADT in minocycline-treated P14 animals was still decreased as compared to saline controls (Fig. 5a).

Minocycline does not modulate IL-1β level in the hippocampus

Hippocampal level of IL-1β increased by PIC was not modified by minocycline treatment at both ages. TNFα was however reduced in the PIC-injected group by minocycline in P14 rats as compared to controls (Fig. 2).

Discussion

In this study, we demonstrated that PIC induced an inflammatory response in both microglial cells and macrophages in vitro. It also led to a pro-inflammatory response in the hippocampi of both P14 and P75 rats

but was limited to an increase of IL-1β. Furthermore, PIC accelerated epileptogenesis at both ages without changing baseline hippocampal excitability. Using minocycline as an anti-inflammatory agent, we were not able to reverse the pro-epileptogenic effects of PIC. This might be attributed to its inability to change the IL-1β hippocampal levels in our experimental settings.

PIC mimics viral infection via binding to TLR3 [15, 16, 20] and results in an inflammatory response [31]. However, there are limited data regarding the exact role of microglial cells in the viral-like inflammatory response induced by PIC [20]. In our primary microglial cultures, PIC resulted in the activation of TLR3 downstream pathways (i.e., increased mRNA expression levels of Trif, NfκB/IκB, and Tbk1) and in the release of IL-1β, IL-6, and TNFα proteins. This is consistent with previous work using higher doses of PIC (50 μg/ml) [20]. We found a similar inflammatory response in both microglia and macrophages, the only difference being that IL-1β was significantly increased by PIC only in microglial cell cultures. This might be a characteristic of our model, as IL-6 release by both infiltrating macrophages and resident microglia has been observed in previous virus-induced encephalitis models, and has been shown to contribute to the precipitation of seizures [8, 9, 32].

The injection of PIC into the hippocampus indeed resulted in an increase in IL-1β levels in both age groups. This was not associated with any extensive cell injury or changes in microglial or astrocytic densities within the hippocampus. In addition, we did not find any difference in blood cytokine levels after PIC injection which excludes the contribution of peripheral inflammation in

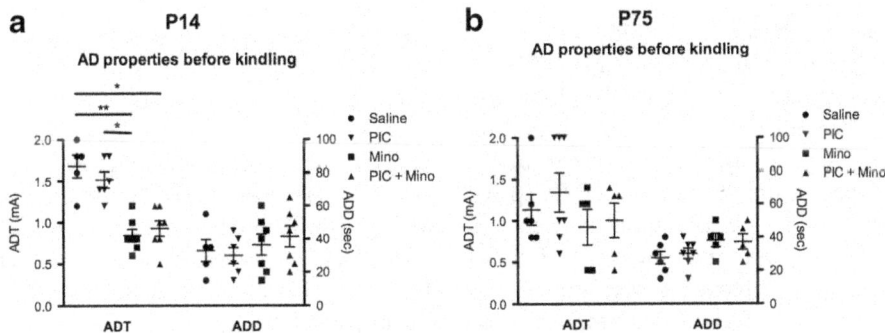

Fig. 4 Effect of PIC and minocycline treatments on hippocampal excitability in P14 and P75 rats. Afterdischarge threshold (ADT) and afterdischarge duration (ADD) 24 h after intrahippocampal injection (saline vs. PIC 10 μg/rat) and the last minocycline intraperitoneal injection (Saline + minocycline vs. PIC 10 μg/rat + minocycline) in P14 (**a**) and in P75 rats (**b**). Data are presented as mean ± SEM. **$p < 0.01$ vs. saline (Mann-Whitney test)

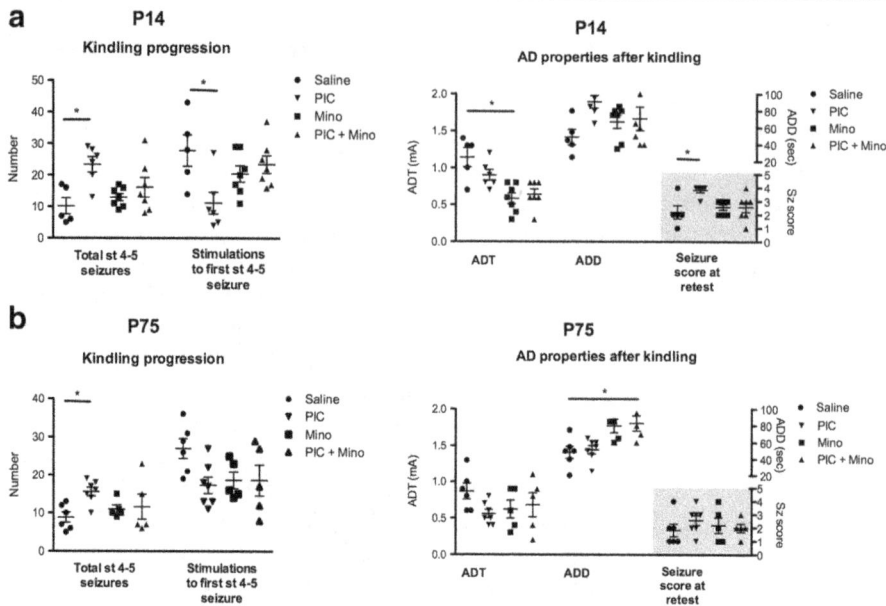

Fig. 5 Effects of PIC and minocycline treatments on epileptogenesis. Kindling progression parameters 24 h after intrahippocampal injection (saline vs. PIC 10 μg/rat) and the last minocycline intraperitoneal injection (Saline + minocycline vs. PIC 10 μg/rat + minocycline) and afterdischarge (AD) properties at retest, 24 h after kindling onset in P14 (**a**) and in P75 rats (**b**). Total number of stages 4-5 seizures and number of stimulations to achieve stage 4–5 seizure in P14 (**a**) and P75 rats (**b**). Afterdischarge threshold (ADT), afterdischarge duration (ADD), and seizure score at retest in P14 (**a**) and P75 rats (**b**) 24 h after kindling onset. Data are presented as mean ± SEM. *$p < 0.05$ vs. saline (Mann-Whitney test)

our model. Together with our in vitro results, one might hypothesize, that even in the absence of cell proliferation, microglial activity is increased by PIC and could be the main source of IL-1β. However, our current data can not exclude the presence of macrophages in the brain tissue. Our results in P14 rats are in line with those of a previous study showing increases in IL-1β in P14 rats after intracerebroventricular (i.c.v.) injection of PIC [33]. TNFα levels were also not changed in this latter study. Further studies are mandatory to determine the exact contribution of the different inflammatory cell types to the production of cytokines in the viral-like inflammation induced by PIC. Moreover, we can not exclude that glial cell activation might occur at later time points.

Intrahippocampal injection of PIC did not change baseline hippocampal excitability in P14 and P75 rats despite leading to increase in IL-1β levels. IL-1β has been consistently described as a factor promoting seizures in both the mature and the immature brain. In adult rats, intrahippocampal injection of IL-1β increases the durations of kainate-induced seizures [34]. In the developing brain, i.c.v. injection of IL-1β leads to pro-convulsant effects in various seizure models [35, 36]. In these former studies, however, IL-1β was directly injected within the brain. By contrast in our model, IL-1β is intrinsically produced thus suggesting that the concentration reached is not sufficient to facilitate ictogenesis.

Interestingly, intrahippocampal injection of PIC facilitated epileptogenesis at both ages. Our results are consistent with the implication that IL-1β has a role in epileptogenesis [37]. This was first suggested by the upregulation of IL-1β in the hippocampi of chronically epileptic mice and in resected hippocampal tissue from patients with temporal lobe epilepsy [38, 39]. The importance of IL-1β in epileptogenesis was further supported by the finding that VX-765, a selective inhibitor of caspase 1, counteracted kindling in adult rats when administered concomitantly with a blockade of IL-1β increase in astrocytes [19]. In agreement with our results, the i.c.v. injection of PIC in P14 rats resulted in an immediate increase in the hippocampal levels of IL-1β without causing any changes in TNFα levels, and was followed by a long-term modification of seizure susceptibility [33], further supporting that IL-1β is a key factor in the facilitation of epileptogenesis by viral-like inflammation.

Minocycline, a semi-synthetic tetracycline antibiotic [40], exerts a variety of biological effects, including proteolysis inhibition, antioxidant effects, and anti-apoptotic and anti-inflammatory activities [23, 41–44]. Minocycline is also well-known to inhibit microglial activation [21, 22, 45]. We first hypothesized that minocycline might modulate the PIC-induced increase in the epileptogenesis through the modulation of inflammation. This assumption was based on previous reports, which have shown that minocycline is able to counteract the long-term increase in brain excitability produced in neonatal rats subjected to an i.c.v. injection of PIC [33]. By decreasing microglial cell activation/proliferation under conditions of status epilepticus induced in juvenile mice by kainate, minocycline limits the kainate-mediated lowering of the seizure threshold [46]. Moreover, the anticonvulsant effects of minocycline have been reported in the amygdala-kindling and the 6-Hz models of adult animals [47, 48]. However, in our model, we did not observe any effect of minocycline on the rapid kindling epileptogenesis and on the pro-epileptic effect of PIC both in P14 and P75 rats. This might be, in part, due to the inability of minocycline to inhibit intrinsic PIC-mediated IL-1β production. Paradoxically, we found a decrease in ADT before and after kindling in P14 rats. This pro-ictogenic effect of minocycline might be associated with some of the paradoxical effects of minocycline described in the developing brain [49] and remains to be studied in details.

Conclusion

The PIC model allowed us to evaluate the involvement of TLR3 agonists in epileptogenesis. Intrahippocampal injection of PIC induced brain inflammation and in particular increased IL-1β levels as well as facilitated kindling epileptogenesis. PIC produced similar effects in P14 and P75 rats, suggesting that mature and immature brains share common mechanisms in our model. Further research is clearly needed to evaluate the key factors involved in the facilitation of epileptogenesis by viral encephalitis, and more specifically to establish the role of IL-1β.

Abbreviations

AD: Afterdischarge; ADD: Afterdischarge duration; ADT: Afterdischarge threshold; CNS: Central nervous system; DA: Daniel's; DMEM: Dulbecco's modified Eagle's minimum essential medium; EEGs: Electroencephalograms; FBS: Fetal bovine serum; i.p.: Intraperitoneal; IL-10: Interleukin 10; IL-1β: Interleukin 1β; IL-6: Interleukin 6; P13: Postnatal day 13; P74: Postnatal day 74; PIC: Polyinosinic-polycytidylic acid; TLR3: Toll-like receptor 3; TLRs: Toll-like receptors; TMEV: Theiler's murine encephalomyelitis virus; TNFα: Tumor necrosis factor α

Acknowledgements

Not applicable

Funding

Stéphane Auvin is partially supported by INSERM Grant (Contrat Interface INSERM 2010). Andrey Mazarati is supported by Research grant R01 NS065783 from the National Institutes of Health (NIH). This work was supported by INSERM, Université Paris-Diderot, Association INJENO, Association Kemil et ses Amis, Fondation Française de Recherche sur l'Epilepsie, Fondation de Spoelberch, Fondation Grace de Monaco, Fondation Leducq.

Authors' contributions

ND, VC, TL, and BF conducted the cell culture experiments. ND, BD, and SL conducted the RT-PCR. ND, BD, and VC conducted the in vivo immuno-assay. ND, BD, ZC, and PD conducted the immunochemistry experiments. AM and SA conducted the kindling experiments. ND and SA coordinated the study. ND, BD, AM, and SA were responsible of the design of the study and the interpretation of the results. ND, AM, and PG, PD, and SA conducted the statistical analysis and the draft of the manuscript. All authors read and approved the final manuscript.

Competing interests

The authors declare that they have no competing interests.

Consent for publication

Not applicable

Author details

[1]INSERM, U1141, 75019 Paris, France. [2]Université Paris Diderot, Sorbonne Paris Cité, INSERM UMR1141, 75019 Paris, France. [3]Department of Pediatrics, Neurology division and Children's Discovery and Innovation Institute, David Geffen School of Medicine at UCLA, Los Angeles, CA 90095, USA. [4]AP-HP, Hôpital Robert Debré, Service de Neurologie Pédiatrique, 75019 Paris, France.

References

1. Getts DR, Balcar VJ, Matsumoto I, Muller M, King NJ. Viruses and the immune system: their roles in seizure cascade development. J Neurochem. 2008;104:1167–76.
2. Misra UK, Tan CT, Kalita J. Viral encephalitis and epilepsy. Epilepsia. 2008;49 Suppl 6:13–8.
3. Annegers JF, Hauser WA, Beghi E, Nicolosi A, Kurland LT. The risk of unprovoked seizures after encephalitis and meningitis. Neurology. 1988;38: 1407–10.
4. Rocca WA, Sharbrough FW, Hauser WA, Annegers JF, Schoenberg BS. Risk factors for complex partial seizures: a population-based case-control study. Ann Neurol. 1987;21:22–31.
5. Whitley RJ. Viral encephalitis. N Engl J Med. 1990;323:242–50.
6. Davison KL, Crowcroft NS, Ramsay ME, Brown DW, Andrews NJ. Viral encephalitis in England, 1989-1998: what did we miss? Emerg Infect Dis. 2003;9:234–40.
7. Nicolosi A, Hauser WA, Beghi E, Kurland LT. Epidemiology of central nervous system infections in Olmsted County, Minnesota, 1950-1981. J Infect Dis. 1986;154:399–408.
8. Cusick MF, Libbey JE, Patel DC, Doty DJ, Fujinami RS. Infiltrating macrophages are key to the development of seizures following virus infection. J Virol. 2013;87:1849–60.
9. Kirkman NJ, Libbey JE, Wilcox KS, White HS, Fujinami RS. Innate but not adaptive immune responses contribute to behavioral seizures following viral infection. Epilepsia. 2010;51:454–64.
10. Stewart KA, Wilcox KS, Fujinami RS, White HS. Development of postinfection epilepsy after Theiler's virus infection of C57BL/6 mice. J Neuropathol Exp Neurol. 2010;69:1210–9.
11. Stringer J. Models available for infection-induced seizures. In: Pitkänen AS PA, Moshé SL, editors. Models of Seizures and Epilepsy. Burlington: Elsevier Academic Press; 2006. p. 521–6.
12. Libbey JE, Fujinami RS. Neurotropic viral infections leading to epilepsy: focus on Theiler's murine encephalomyelitis virus. Futur Virol. 2011;6:1339–50.
13. Kaushik DK, Gupta M, Basu A. Microglial response to viral challenges: every silver lining comes with a cloud. Front Biosci (Landmark Ed). 2011;16:2187–205.
14. Jensen S, Thomsen AR. Sensing of RNA viruses: a review of innate immune receptors involved in recognizing RNA virus invasion. J Virol. 2012;86:2900–10.
15. Alexopoulou L, Holt AC, Medzhitov R, Flavell RA. Recognition of double-stranded RNA and activation of NF-kappaB by Toll-like receptor 3. Nature. 2001;413:732–8.
16. Doyle S, Vaidya S, O'Connell R, Dadgostar H, Dempsey P, Wu T, Rao G, Sun R, Haberland M, Modlin R, Cheng G. IRF3 mediates a TLR3/TLR4-specific antiviral gene program. Immunity. 2002;17:251–63.
17. Vezzani A, Balosso S, Ravizza T. Inflammation and epilepsy. Handb Clin Neurol. 2012;107:163–75.
18. Kwon YS, Pineda E, Auvin S, Shin D, Mazarati A, Sankar R. Neuroprotective and antiepileptogenic effects of combination of anti-inflammatory drugs in the immature brain. J Neuroinflammation. 2013;10:30.

19. Ravizza T, Noe F, Zardoni D, Vaghi V, Sifringer M, Vezzani A. Interleukin converting enzyme inhibition impairs kindling epileptogenesis in rats by blocking astrocytic IL-1beta production. Neurobiol Dis. 2008;31:327–33.

20. Town T, Jeng D, Alexopoulou L, Tan J, Flavell RA. Microglia recognize double-stranded RNA via TLR3. J Immunol. 2006;176:3804–12.

21. Tikka T, Fiebich BL, Goldsteins G, Keinanen R, Koistinaho J. Minocycline, a tetracycline derivative, is neuroprotective against excitotoxicity by inhibiting activation and proliferation of microglia. J Neurosci. 2001;21:2580–8.

22. Tikka TM, Koistinaho JE. Minocycline provides neuroprotection against N-methyl-D-aspartate neurotoxicity by inhibiting microglia. J Immunol. 2001;166:7527–33.

23. Yrjanheikki J, Tikka T, Keinanen R, Goldsteins G, Chan PH, Koistinaho J. A tetracycline derivative, minocycline, reduces inflammation and protects against focal cerebral ischemia with a wide therapeutic window. Proc Natl Acad Sci U S A. 1999;96:13496–500.

24. Scholz S, Sela E, Blaha L, Braunbeck T, Galay-Burgos M, Garcia-Franco M, Guinea J, Kluver N, Schirmer K, Tanneberger K, et al. A European perspective on alternatives to animal testing for environmental hazard identification and risk assessment. Regul Toxicol Pharmacol. 2013;67:506–30.

25. Chhor V, Le Charpentier T, Lebon S, Ore MV, Celador IL, Josserand J, Degos V, Jacotot E, Hagberg H, Savman K, et al. Characterization of phenotype markers and neuronotoxic potential of polarised primary microglia in vitro. Brain Behav Immun. 2013;32:70–85.

26. Thery C, Chamak B, Mallat M. Cytotoxic effect of brain macrophages on developing. Eur J Neurosc. 1991;3:1155–64.

27. Zhang X, Goncalves R, Mosser DM. The isolation and characterization of murine macrophages. In: Coligan JE et al., editors. Current protocols in immunology, Chapter 14:Unit 14 11. 2008.

28. Mazarati A, Shin D, Auvin S, Sankar R. Age-dependent effects of topiramate on the acquisition and the retention of rapid kindling. Epilepsia. 2007;48:765–73.

29. Mazarati A, Wu J, Shin D, Kwon YS, Sankar R. Antiepileptogenic and antiictogenic effects of retigabine under conditions of rapid kindling: an ontogenic study. Epilepsia. 2008;49:1777–86.

30. Sankar R, Auvin S, Kwon YS, Pineda E, Shin D, Mazarati A. Evaluation of development-specific targets for antiepileptogenic therapy using rapid kindling. Epilepsia. 2010;51:39–42.

31. Olson JK, Miller SD. Microglia initiate central nervous system innate and adaptive immune responses through multiple TLRs. J Immunol. 2004;173:3916–24.

32. Libbey JE, Kennett NJ, Wilcox KS, White HS, Fujinami RS. Interleukin-6, produced by resident cells of the central nervous system and infiltrating cells, contributes to the development of seizures following viral infection. J Virol. 2011;85:6913–22.

33. Galic MA, Riazi K, Henderson AK, Tsutsui S, Pittman QJ. Viral-like brain inflammation during development causes increased seizure susceptibility in adult rats. Neurobiol Dis. 2009;36:343–51.

34. Vezzani A, Conti M, De Luigi A, Ravizza T, Moneta D, Marchesi F, De Simoni MG. Interleukin-1beta immunoreactivity and microglia are enhanced in the rat hippocampus by focal kainate application: functional evidence for enhancement of electrographic seizures. J Neurosci. 1999;19:5054–65.

35. Dube C, Vezzani A, Behrens M, Bartfai T, Baram TZ. Interleukin-1beta contributes to the generation of experimental febrile seizures. Ann Neurol. 2005;57:152–5.

36. Heida JG, Pittman QJ. Causal links between brain cytokines and experimental febrile convulsions in the rat. Epilepsia. 2005;46:1906–13.

37. Vezzani A, Friedman A, Dingledine RJ. The role of inflammation in epileptogenesis. Neuropharmacology. 2013;69:16–24.

38. Maroso M, Balosso S, Ravizza T, Iori V, Wright CI, French J, Vezzani A. Interleukin-1beta biosynthesis inhibition reduces acute seizures and drug resistant chronic epileptic activity in mice. Neurotherapeutics. 2011;8:304–15.

39. Ravizza T, Gagliardi B, Noe F, Boer K, Aronica E, Vezzani A. Innate and adaptive immunity during epileptogenesis and spontaneous seizures: evidence from experimental models and human temporal lobe epilepsy. Neurobiol Dis. 2008;29:142–60.

40. Garrido-Mesa N, Zarzuelo A, Galvez J. What is behind the non-antibiotic properties of minocycline? Pharmacol Res. 2013;67:18–30.

41. Jiang X, Wang X. Cytochrome c promotes caspase-9 activation by inducing nucleotide binding to Apaf-1. J Biol Chem. 2000;275:31199–203.

42. Kraus RL, Pasieczny R, Lariosa-Willingham K, Turner MS, Jiang A, Trauger JW. Antioxidant properties of minocycline: neuroprotection in an oxidative stress assay and direct radical-scavenging activity. J Neurochem. 2005;94:819–27.

43. Teng YD, Choi H, Onario RC, Zhu S, Desilets FC, Lan S, Woodard EJ, Snyder EY, Eichler ME, Friedlander RM. Minocycline inhibits contusion-triggered mitochondrial cytochrome c release and mitigates functional deficits after spinal cord injury. Proc Natl Acad Sci U S A. 2004;101:3071–6.

44. Yenari MA, Xu L, Tang XN, Qiao Y, Giffard RG. Microglia potentiate damage to blood-brain barrier constituents: improvement by minocycline in vivo and in vitro. Stroke. 2006;37:1087–93.

45. Henry CJ, Huang Y, Wynne A, Hanke M, Himler J, Bailey MT, Sheridan JF, Godbout JP. Minocycline attenuates lipopolysaccharide (LPS)-induced neuroinflammation, sickness behavior, and anhedonia. J Neuroinflammation. 2008;5:15.

46. Abraham J, Fox PD, Condello C, Bartolini A, Koh S. Minocycline attenuates microglia activation and blocks the long-term epileptogenic effects of early-life seizures. Neurobiol Dis. 2012;46:425–30.

47. Beheshti Nasr SM, Moghimi A, Mohammad-Zadeh M, Shamsizadeh A, Noorbakhsh SM. The effect of minocycline on seizures induced by amygdala kindling in rats. Seizure. 2013;22:670–4.

48. Wang DD, Englot DJ, Garcia PA, Lawton MT, Young WL. Minocycline- and tetracycline-class antibiotics are protective against partial seizures in vivo. Epilepsy Behav. 2012;24:314–8.

49. Arnoux I, Hoshiko M, Diez AS, Audinat E. Paradoxical effects of minocycline in the developing mouse somatosensory Cortex. Glia. 2014;62:399–410.

9

Ex vivo model of epilepsy in organotypic slices— a new tool for drug screening

Daniela M. Magalhães[1,2†], Noémia Pereira[1,2†], Diogo M. Rombo[1,2], Cláudia Beltrão-Cavacas[1,2], Ana M. Sebastião[1,2] and Cláudia A. Valente[1,2*]

Abstract

Background: Epilepsy is a prevalent neurological disorder worldwide. It is characterized by an enduring predisposition to generate seizures and its development is accompanied by alterations in many cellular processes. Organotypic slice cultures represent a multicellular environment with the potential to assess biological mechanisms, and they are used as a starting point for refining molecules for in vivo studies. Here, we investigated organotypic slice cultures as a model of epilepsy.

Methods: We assessed, by electrophysiological recordings, the spontaneous activity of organotypic slices maintained under different culture protocols. Moreover, we evaluated, through molecular-based approaches, neurogenesis, neuronal death, gliosis, expression of proinflammatory cytokines, and activation of NLRP3 inflammasome (nucleotide-binding, leucine-rich repeat, pyrin domain) as biomarkers of neuroinflammation.

Results: We demonstrated that organotypic slices, maintained under a serum deprivation culture protocol, develop epileptic-like activity. Furthermore, throughout a comparative study with slices that do not depict any epileptiform activity, slices with epileptiform activity were found to display significant differences in terms of inflammation-related features, such as (1) increased neuronal death, with higher incidence in CA1 pyramidal neurons of the hippocampus; (2) activation of astrocytes and microglia, assessed through western blot and immunohistochemistry; (3) upregulation of proinflammatory cytokines, specifically interleukin-1β (IL-1β), interleukin-6, and tumor necrosis factor α, revealed by qPCR; and (4) enhanced expression of NLRP3, assessed by western blot, together with increased NLRP3 activation, showed by IL-1β quantification.

Conclusions: Thus, organotypic slice cultures gradually deprived of serum mimic the epileptic-like activity, as well as the inflammatory events associated with in vivo epilepsy. This system can be considered a new tool to explore the interplay between neuroinflammation and epilepsy and to screen potential drug candidates, within the inflammatory cascades, to reduce/halt epileptogenesis.

Keywords: Epilepsy, Organotypic slice cultures, Neuroinflammation, Gliosis, Proinflammatory cytokines, Interleukin-1β, NLRP3 inflammasome

Background

Epilepsy is among the most prevalent neurological disorders worldwide. According to World Health Organization, epilepsy accounts for 1% of global burden of disease [1].

Clinically, epilepsy is characterized by recurrent spontaneous seizures and is defined, by the International

* Correspondence: cvalentecastro@medicina.ulisboa.pt
†Daniela M. Magalhães and Noémia Pereira contributed equally to this work.
[1]Instituto de Farmacologia e Neurociências, Faculdade de Medicina, Universidade de Lisboa, Lisboa, Portugal
[2]Instituto de Medicina Molecular, Faculdade de Medicina, Universidade de Lisboa, Lisboa, Portugal

League Against Epilepsy (ILAE), as "a chronic condition of the brain characterized by an enduring propensity to generate epileptic seizures, and by the neurobiological, cognitive, psychological, and social consequences" [2]. Despite the numerous antiepileptic drugs (AEDs) available, 30% of patients are still refractory to therapy, continue to experience seizures, and a subset suffer progression of the disease, with increasing seizure frequency and cognitive decline. It is therefore imperative to better understand the mechanisms of epileptogenesis, the process by which a normal brain transforms into one capable of producing recurrent spontaneous seizures, and to find novel and specific therapies to prevent/delay the onset of this disorder, as well as to ameliorate its symptoms, and ultimately to cease its progression.

Epileptogenesis is accompanied by several cellular and molecular processes, such as neuronal death, neurogenesis, reactive astrogliosis and microglia activation, and upregulation of inflammatory mediators [3].

The effect of seizures on neuronal death and the role of seizure-induced neuronal death in epileptogenesis have been intensely discussed [4]. αII-Spectrin, a structural protein of the cell cytoskeleton with a molecular weight of 250 kDa, is a major substrate of cytosolic cysteine proteases, such as calpains and caspases [5]. Calpains are the main proteases involved in necrosis, while the effector caspase-3 is considered essential for efficient execution of apoptosis [6, 7]. Neuronal death leads to activation of these cysteine proteases, αII-spectrin cleavage, and formation of spectrin breakdown products (SBDP). Since αII-spectrin occurrence in glial cells is minimal, SBDPs are considered highly specific for neuronal damaged, as well as biomarkers of cell death in brain disorders [8, 9].

Prolonged seizure activity leads to a dramatic increase in cell proliferation in the dentate gyrus (DG) [10, 11] and rostral subventricular zone [12]. In the DG, the accelerated neural stem cell proliferation is reflected by an increased number of cells expressing doublecortin (DCX) [11], a validated marker for newborn neurons [13]. However, the role of new neurons, and their migration, in the epileptic process is still under debate [14].

Non-neuronal cells, especially astrocytes and microglia, play a prominent role in the pathophysiology of epilepsy [15]. Astrocytes are the third element of the tripartite synapse [16–18] and active players in neuroinflammation [19]. They respond to CNS insults by a process commonly referred to as reactive astrogliosis, a graded continuum of progressive alterations [20, 21]. Microglia cells are the main sensors for pathological events in the CNS, and evidence indicates that the unregulated activation of microglia in response to noxious stimulus results in the production of toxic factors that propagate neuronal injury [22, 23]. Moreover, as happens with astrocytes, microglia activation occurs as a graded response with microglia adopting different morphologies, ranging from a highly ramified to an amoeboid-like phenotype [24–26].

Experimental and clinical evidences have also demonstrated that seizures induce high levels of inflammatory mediators in brain regions involved in the generation and propagation of epileptic activity and proinflammatory cytokines, such as interleukin-1β (IL-1β), tumor necrosis factor-α (TNF-α), and interleukin-6 (IL-6), which were found to be upregulated in activated microglia and astrocytes [27]. Recently, NOD-like receptor protein 3 (NLRP3) inflammasome has been associated to central nervous system (CNS)-related disorders [28–30]. NLRP3 is a cytosolic multiprotein complex that assembles in response to invading pathogens (PAMPs, pathogen-associated molecular patterns) and danger signals (DAMPs, damaged-associated molecular patterns), which results in the processing of inactive pro-caspase-1 into the active cysteine-protease enzyme caspase-1, that subsequently processes the pro-IL-1β and pro-IL-18, prompting the production of mature IL-1β and IL-18 and inducing pyroptosis, a highly pyrogenic inflammatory form of cell death. Research suggests that NLRP3-targeted therapies may represent a novel antiepileptogenic strategy [31]. Indeed, NLRP3 inhibition was already reported to provide neuroprotection in a kindling model of epilepsy [32].

Epileptogenesis is difficult to study in humans, due to the heterogeneity of epileptogenic injuries, long latent periods lasting months to decades, and the potentially confusing effects of anticonvulsant treatment after the first spontaneous seizure. Animal models of epilepsy have been crucial in the understanding of the physiological and behavioral changes associated with human epilepsy and they have led to the discovery of many AEDs [33, 34], but they require a large number of animals and data collection is quite slow due to the long latent period until seizures onset [35].

Organotypic hippocampal slice cultures (OHSC), which are prepared from slices of explanted tissue, represent a complex multicellular ex vivo environment and constitute a powerful instrument to elucidate biological mechanisms [36, 37]. These cultures preserve the three-dimensional architecture and local environment of brain cells, including neurons, astrocytes, and microglia, as well as the neuronal connectivity and the complex glial-neuronal interactions. Furthermore, cells in organotypic brain slices develop and mature similarly to their in vivo counterparts [38]. Nowadays, these systems are considered excellent models to study neuroprotection and they are used as a starting point for drug discovery [39, 40]. Ex vivo models of epilepsy in hippocampal slices allow a detailed and well-controlled research of the mechanisms of epileptogenesis, while still preserving the network phenotypic features of epilepsy, particularly the development of spontaneous seizures [41]. Indeed, spontaneous field potential activity was recorded from organotypic slices [42, 43]. It was reported that slices develop epileptiform activity which resembles in vivo epilepsy, including sensitivity to anticonvulsants and increasing seizure incidence over time. Detailed characterization of this system in terms of spontaneous interictal and ictal-like events allowed to present it as a useful model system for investigating the mechanisms of epileptogenesis, as well as to screen potential antiepileptic drugs [42, 44].

In this study, we aimed to further explore organotypic slices as a model of epilepsy. We confirmed the occurrence of spontaneous epileptiform activity in slices maintained in Neurobasal/B27 serum-free medium, and showed the strong incidence of neuroinflammation biomarkers in these slices, as the enhanced expression and activation of NLRP3 inflammasome.

We thus demonstrate that organotypic slice cultures gradually deprived of serum mimic the epileptic-like activity, as well as many inflammatory events associated with in vivo epilepsy. Studies within this system can contribute to a deeper knowledge about the interplay between epilepsy and inflammation. Furthermore, this model can be used as a tool to screen potential therapeutic candidates for epilepsy.

Methods

Animals

Pregnant female Sprague-Dawley rats were acquired from Charles River (Barcelona, Spain). The Portuguese law and European Union guidelines (2010/63/EU) were respected in all procedures regarding the protection of animals for scientific purposes. All efforts were made to minimize animal suffering and to use the minimum number of animals. This study was approved by the "iMM's Institutional Animal Welfare Body–ORBEA-iMM and the National competent authority–DGAV (Direção Geral de Alimentação e Veterinária)."

Organotypic slice cultures

Organotypic slice cultures were prepared from 6- to 7-day-old Sprague-Dawley rats, according to the interface culture method [45]. After decapitation, brains were removed and placed in cold Gey's balanced salt solution (GBSS, Biological Industries, Kibbutz Beit Haemek, Israel) with 25 mM D-glucose (Sigma, St. Louis, MO, USA), under sterile conditions. The hippocampus, together with the entorhinal cortex (EC) and perirhinal cortex (PC), (Fig. 1a), was dissected out and sliced transversely at 350 µm using a McIlwain tissue chopper. Five slices were placed onto porous (0.4 µm) insert membranes (PICM 03050, Millipore, Bedford, MA), which were transferred to six-well culture trays (Corning Costar, Corning, NY). Each well contained 1 ml of culture medium composed of 50% Opti-MEM, 25% Hanks' balanced salt solution (HBSS), 25% heat-inactivated horse serum (HS) (all from Invitrogen, Paisley, UK), 25 mM D-glucose, penicillin (100 units/ml), and streptomycin (100 µg/ml) (Sigma). Slices were maintained at 37 °C with 5% CO_2 and 95% atmospheric air for the following 2 weeks.

Slices were randomly divided in two groups, which undertook different culture conditions (Fig. 1). Those designated control slices (CTL, Fig. 1b) were kept in a serum-based (25% HS) Opti-MEM medium, with medium renewal twice a week, and did not develop epileptiform activity. Those slices which spontaneously develop epileptiform activity (EL, Fig. 1c) were changed at 3 days in vitro (DIV) to a chemically defined serum-free based medium, Neurobasal A (Invitrogen), supplemented with 2% B27 (Invitrogen), L-glutamine (1 mM) (Invitrogen), penicillin (100 units/ml), and streptomycin (100 µg/ml), and decreasing HS concentrations (15%, 10% and 5%), until a serum-free condition was reached at 9 DIV. In EL slices, medium was renewed every second day. Our protocol is different from other reports in the sense that slices are gradually deprived of serum.

Field potential recordings

Field potential recordings were performed in an interface-type chamber as previously described by others [20]. At 14 DIV, slices were transferred to the interface recording chamber, with a humidified (5% CO_2/95% O_2) atmosphere at 36 °C, and with their growth medium continuously superfused and recirculating at a rate of 2 ml/min. Each slice was visually inspected, ensuring slice integrity and organization. After an equilibration period of 20 min, spontaneous field potential recordings were performed with an extracellular microelectrode (4 M NaCl, 2–4 MΩ resistance) positioned in the CA3 pyramidal cell layer over 30–40 min. Recordings were obtained with Axoclamp 2B amplifier, digitized (Axon Instruments, Foster City, CA), and analyzed by the Clampex software version 10.2 (Molecular Devices, Sunnyvale, CA, USA). All recordings were band-pass filtered (eight-pole Bessel filter at 60 Hz and Gaussian filter at 600 Hz).

Patch-clamp recordings

Slices were transferred to an Axioskop 2FS upright microscope (Zeiss, Jena, Germany) equipped with a differential interference contrast-infrared (DIC-IR) CCD video camera (VX44, Till Photonics, Gräfelfing, Germany) and fixed with a grid in a recording chamber continuously superfused by a gravitational superfusion system at 2–3 ml/min with artificial cerebrospinal fluid (aCSF) containing (in mM) NaCl 124, KCl 3, NaH_2PO_4 1.25, $NaHCO_3$ 26, $MgCl_2$ 1, $CaCl_2$ 2, Glucose 10, pH 7.4 (gassed with 95% O_2, 5% CO_2), at room temperature. Patch pipettes (4–9 MΩ) were pulled from borosilicate glass capillaries (1.5 mm outer diameter, 0.86 mm inner diameter, Harvard Apparatus, Holliston, MA, USA) with PC-10 Puller (Narishige Group, London, UK) and were filled with an internal solution containing (in mM) K-gluconate 125, KCl

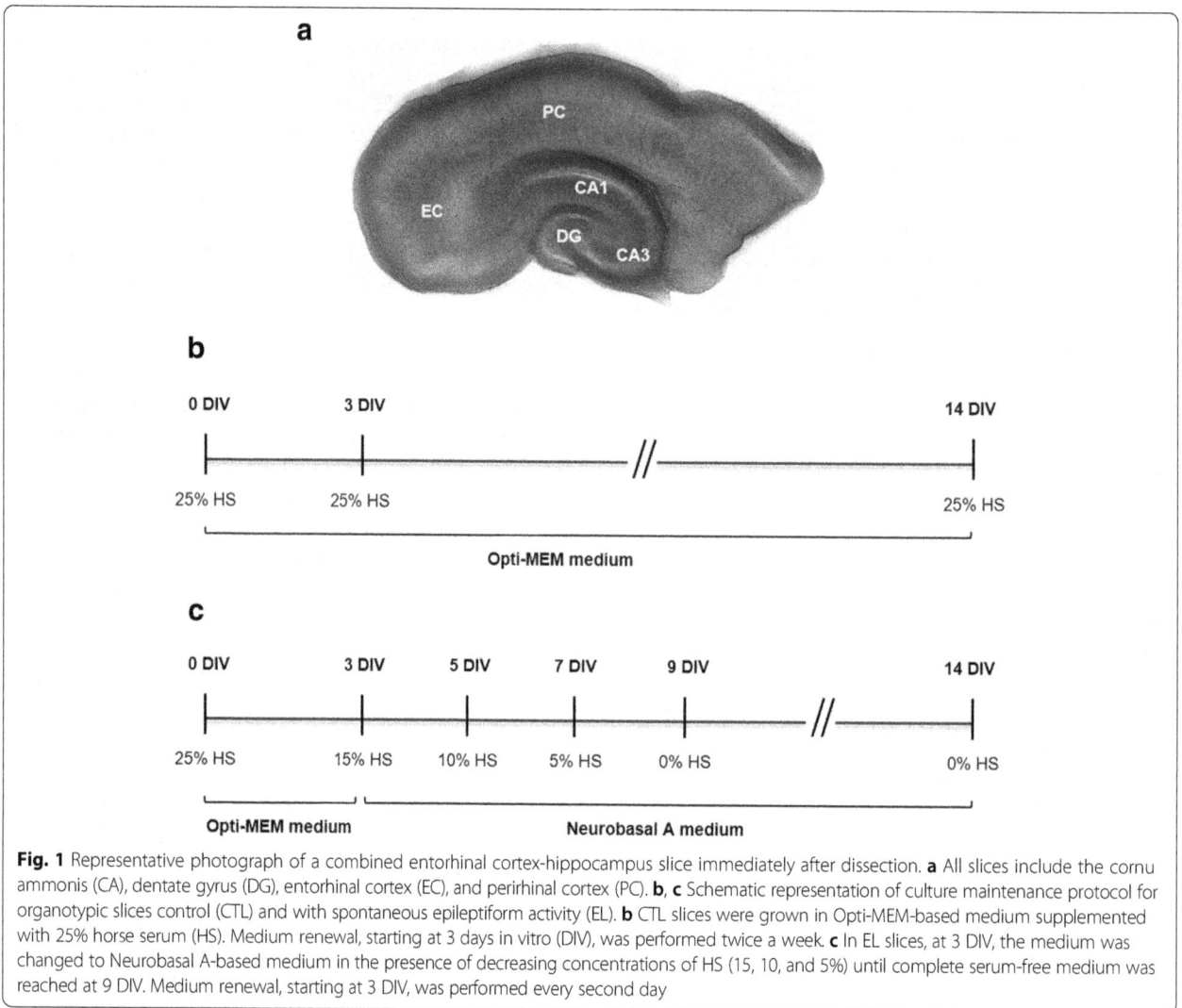

Fig. 1 Representative photograph of a combined entorhinal cortex-hippocampus slice immediately after dissection. **a** All slices include the cornu ammonis (CA), dentate gyrus (DG), entorhinal cortex (EC), and perirhinal cortex (PC). **b, c** Schematic representation of culture maintenance protocol for organotypic slices control (CTL) and with spontaneous epileptiform activity (EL). **b** CTL slices were grown in Opti-MEM-based medium supplemented with 25% horse serum (HS). Medium renewal, starting at 3 days in vitro (DIV), was performed twice a week. **c** In EL slices, at 3 DIV, the medium was changed to Neurobasal A-based medium in the presence of decreasing concentrations of HS (15, 10, and 5%) until complete serum-free medium was reached at 9 DIV. Medium renewal, starting at 3 DIV, was performed every second day

11, CaCl$_2$ 0.1, MgCl$_2$ 2, EGTA 1, HEPES 10, MgATP 2, NaGTP 0.3 and phosphocreatine 10, pH 7.3 adjusted with KOH (1 M), 280–290 mOsm. Recordings were performed in current-clamp mode using an EPC-7 electrical amplifier (List Biologic). Signals were low-pass filtered using a 3- and 10-kHz three-pole Bessel filter of an EPC-7 amplifier, digitized at 10 kHz using a Digidata 1322A board, and registered by the Clampex software version 10.2 (Molecular Devices). Resting membrane potential (RMP) was measured immediately after establishing whole-cell configuration, and action potential firing was systematically evoked in current-clamp mode by injecting current pulses of – 50 to + 300 pA, in 10 or 50 pA increments for 1000 ms from an initial holding potential of – 70 mV. The threshold for action potential (AP) generation was determined as the difference between the resting membrane potential and the membrane potential at which phase plot slope reached 10 mV/ms [46].

Western blot analysis

Hippocampi were dissected from five slices and dissociated by passing 20 times through a 25G needle (Terumo Europe, Leuven, Belgium) in 150 μL of ristocetin-induced platelet agglutination buffer (RIPA, 50 mM Tris pH 8.0, 1 mM EDTA (ethykenediamine tetraacetic acid), 150 mM NaCl, 1% NP40 substitute (Nonyl phenoxlpoylethanol, Fluka Biochemika, Switzerland), and 10% glycerol), containing a mixture of protease inhibitors (Sigma). Dissociated tissue was shaken for 15 min at 4 °C. Tissue lysates were then centrifuged at 13000×g for 10 min to remove cell debris. The supernatant was collected, and total protein was quantified using the Bio-Rad DC Protein Assay Kit (Bio-Rad, Hercules, CA, USA).

Samples (35 μg total protein/well) and protein molecular weight marker (NZYColour Protein Marker II, NZY-Tech, Lisbon, Portugal) were boiled at 95 °C for 10 min, electrophoresed on a 12% SDS-PAGE, and electrotransferred to PVDF membranes (Merck-Millipore, Feltham,

UK). Following blocking, membranes were probed with the primary antibodies and with the appropriate horseradish peroxidase (HRP)-conjugated secondary antibodies (1:10000, Santa Cruz Biotechnology, Heidelberg, Germany) as previously described [47]. Immunoreactions were visualized with ECL Western Blotting Detection System (GE Healthcare, Buckinghamshire, UK). The integrated intensity of each band was calculated using computer-assisted densitometry analysis with ImageJ software 1.44b. Glyceraldehyde-3-phosphate dehydrogenase (GAPDH) was used as the loading control.

Images were prepared for printing in Image Lab software 5.2.1 (software available in ChemiDoc XRS+ system, Bio-Rad). For each protein evaluated, the chemiluminescence image was merged with the colorimetric image of the molecular weight marker.

The primary antibodies used were mouse monoclonal antibody anti-αII-spectrin (1:500) and rabbit polyclonal antibody anti-Caspase-3 (1:1000) from Santa Cruz Biotechnology; rabbit polyclonal antibody anti-GFAP (1:5000) from Sigma; and goat polyclonal antibody anti-Iba1 (1:1000), rabbit polyclonal antibody anti-NLRP3 (1:300), and mouse monoclonal antibody anti-GAPDH (1:5000), all from Abcam, Cambridge, UK.

Quantitative real-time PCR

Hippocampi were isolated from ten slices, and RNA was extracted according to QIAGEN RNeasy Mini Kit (QIAGEN, Hilden, Germany). The collected tissue was dissociated with a 25G needle in the presence of QIAzol lysis reagent. RNA concentration was determined using Nanodrop 1000 (ND-1000 Spectrophotometer, Thermo Fisher Scientific, Waltham, MA, USA).

In vitro reverse transcription was performed from 2 μg of total RNA (in 20 μl) and carried out with SuperScript II Reverse Transcriptase (EC 2.7.7.49, Invitrogen, Carlsband, CA, USA) in a thermoclycler (MyCycle, Bio-Rad), according to the manufacturer's recommendations (SuperScript First Strand Synthesis Systems for RT-PCR, Invitrogen). cDNA amplification was carried out in a Rotor-Gene 6000 real-time rotary analyzer thermocycler (Corbett Life Science, Hilden, Germany) as former described [47]. Briefly, the reactions took place in the presence of SYBR Green Master Mix (Applied Biosystems, Foster City, CA, USA) and 0.2 μM of each gene-specific primers. RT-qPCR parameters included an initial denaturation step for 2 min at 94 °C and 50 cycles with 30 s at 94 °C, 90 s at 60 °C, and 60 s at 72 °C. Reaction specificity was evaluated in all assays by a melting curve (Additional file 1: Figure S1).

The threshold cycle (Ct) and the melting curves required for the relative quantification [48] were acquired with Rotor-Gene 6000 Software 1.7 (Corbett Life Science). GAPDH was used as the reference internal standard.

The primers used for the proinflammatory cytokines (see Table 1) were designed using the OligoAnalyzer 3.1, provided by Integrated DNA Technologies (Coralville, IA, USA) and acquired to Invitrogen. All mRNA sequences from *Rattus norvegicus* were obtained from the GenBank sequence database of the National Centre for Biotechnology Information (http://www.ncbi.nlm.nih.gov/nucleotide/). Accession numbers are indicated in Table 1.

Quantification of cell death by propidium iodide uptake

Cell death was assessed by monitoring the cellular uptake of the fluorescent dye propidium iodide (PI, 3,8-diamino-5-(3-(diethylmethylamino)propyl)-6-phenyl phenanthridinium diiodide, Sigma). PI is a polar compound, which only enters cells with damaged cell membranes and interacts with DNA emitting red fluorescence (630 nm; absorbance 493 nm). It is not toxic to cells and was proven to be a feasible marker of neuronal cell death in organotypic slice cultures [49].

PI imaging was carried out at 14 DIV. CTL and EL slices were incubated with 2 μM sterile PI, diluted in culture medium for 4 h before imaging. Cellular uptake of PI was recorded by fluorescence microscopy on a wide field fluorescence microscope (Axiovert 200, Zeiss, Germany) using a rhodamine filter. Fluorescence photomicrographs were acquired, under identical lighting, with an EC Plan-NeoFluar 5x objective (Zeiss) with a numerical aperture of 0.16. For assessment of PI uptake, the regions of interest (DG, CA1 and CA3) were delineated and the fluorescence intensity was quantified using the software ImageJ 1.44b (NIH). The intensity value of each analyzed region was obtained by correction with a fluorescence background image. PI uptake by each hippocampal region was expressed in arbitrary units of fluorescence intensity.

Immunohistochemical analysis

Slices were fixed, at 14 DIV, for 1 h with 4% paraformaldehyde (PFA, Sigma) diluted in PBS at room temperature (RT), followed by an incubation in increasing concentrations of a sucrose (Sigma) solution (10 and 20% in PBS) at RT. Slices were kept in a 30% sucrose solution at 4 °C until further use.

Slices were cut out of the insert and put in slides. Each slice was surrounded with DAKO pen (Dako, Glostrup, Denmark) to protect staining areas from drying out and from mixing with each other. Following PBS washes, slices were incubated for 3 h at RT in blocking solution containing 10% HS, 10% bovine serum albumin (BSA, Sigma), and 1% Triton X-100 (Sigma) in PBS, which ensure simultaneous permeabilization and blocking of the tissue. Subsequently, slices were incubated with the primary antibodies for 24 h at 4 °C. Slices were rinsed

Table 1 Primers used for the analysis of proinflammatory cytokines by RT-PCR. All primers were designed using the OligoAnalyzer 3.1, provided by Integrated DNA Technologies

Gene	Acession number	Primer sequence (5'–3')	PCR fragment size (bp)
Proinflammatory cytokines			
IL-1β	NM_031512.2	Forward: TCCTCTGTGACTCGTGGGAT	309
		Reverse: GTTTGGGATCCACACTCTCCA	
TNF-α	NM_012675.3	Forward: ATGGGCTCCCTCTCATCAGT	106
		Reverse: GCTTGGTGGTTTGCTACGAC	
IL-6	NM_012589.2	Forward: GCAAGAGACTTCCAGCCAGT	203
		Reverse: TTGCCATTGCACAACTCTTTTCT	
Housekeeping gene			
GAPDH	NM_017008	Forward: GTTTGTGATGGGTGTGAACC	170
		Reverse: TCTTCTGAGTGGCAGTGATG	

The table indicates the gene, the gene accession number, the primer sequence, and the PCR fragment size

with PBST (PBS containing 0.1% Tween-20), and the fluorophores coupled-secondary antibodies were applied to the slices for 4 h at RT. The nuclei were stained with Hoechst 33342 (20 µg/ml, Invitrogen) for 40 min at RT. The slices were mounted in Mowiol (Sigma).

For each marker, images were acquired under identical lighting between conditions, with a frame size of 1024×1024 pixels on an inverted confocal laser scanning microscope (Zeiss LSM 710, Zeiss) equipped with a Plan-Apochromat 20x objective (Zeiss) with a numerical aperture of 0.80. Hoechst 33342 fluorescence was detected with a 405-nm diode laser (30 mW nominal output). Alexa Fluor 488 fluorescence was detected using the 488-nm line of an Argon laser (25 mW nominal output), and Alexa Fluor 568 was detected using a 561-nm DPSS laser (15 mW nominal output). Images were prepared for printing using Illustrator software from Adobe Systems (San Jose, CA, USA).

Doublecortin (DCX) fluorescence intensity was quantified in the DG of CTL and EL slices, using the software ImageJ 1.44b. The final intensity value was obtained by correction with a fluorescence background image. Fluorescence intensity values are presented as a percentage of CTL slices.

The microglia cell body diameter in CTL and EL slices stained with Iba1 was measured, using the software ImageJ 1.44b, in 50–70 microglia cells per each hippocampal area. Whenever the cell body was oval, the cell body diameter was considered the largest distance passing through the center of the ellipse.

The primary antibodies used were mouse monoclonal antibody anti-GFAP (1:1000, Sigma), goat polyclonal antibody anti-Iba1 (1:1000, Abcam), and mouse anti-doublecortin (1:500, Santa Cruz Biotechnology). The secondary antibodies were donkey anti-mouse-Alexa Fluor 488, donkey anti-goat-Alexa Fluor 488, and donkey anti-mouse-Alexa Fluor 568 (1:500, Invitrogen).

ELISA

Hippocampi were dissected from five slices and homogenized, as for western blot, in ice-cold RIPA buffer containing a mixture of protease inhibitors (Sigma). The lysates were centrifuged, and the supernatants, containing the cytosolic and membrane fraction, were collected to measure IL-1β, TNF-α, and IL-6 in the tissue. Total protein was quantified using the Bio-Rad DC Protein Assay Kit (Bio-Rad). IL-1β, TNF-α, and IL-6 protein levels were quantified by ELISA, according to the manufacturers' suggested protocol (R&D Systems, Abingdon, UK), using selective antibodies. Absorbance was read at 405 nm. The detection limit was < 3 pg/ml.

Statistical analysis

All statistical analysis was performed using GraphPad Prism software (San Diego, CA, USA). Most comparisons between CTL and EL slices were made using an unpaired t test. Regarding PI uptake experiments and microglia cell body diameter measurements, statistical analysis was performed with one-way ANOVA, followed by Bonferroni's comparison test. The number of independent cultures or cells (n) used in each assay is indicated in the legend of each figure. In all figures, data are presented as mean ± SEM. Values of $p < 0.05$ were considered to account for statistically significant differences.

Results

Slices maintained in Neurobasal A-serum-free medium exhibit interictal-like activity

As depicted in Fig. 1a, the organotypic slices used throughout this work contain the hippocampal complex, namely the dentate gyrus (DG) and the cornu ammonis areas (CA1 and CA3) of the hippocampus, as well as the entorhinal (EC) and perirhinal (PC) cortex. Indeed, clinical research and animal models of epilepsy have suggested that these cortical areas play an important role in seizure generation [50].

Spontaneous activity of the slices was assessed at 14 DIV. CTL and EL slices were transferred to the interface chamber, and field potentials were recorded (40 min) under a constant superfusion with growth medium. Figure 2 shows representative field potential recordings of spontaneous activity obtained in CA3 area of CTL (Fig. 2a–CTL) and EL (Fig. 2a–EL) organotypic slices at 14 DIV. CTL slices depict a spontaneous typical physiological activity, while EL slices exhibit spontaneous interictal-like discharges, which resemble in vivo epilepsy, in accordance with what was previously described by others [42].

CTL and EL slices have identical resting membrane potential and firing threshold

To evaluate the resting membrane potential of neurons, CTL and EL slices were transferred to the chamber of an upright microscope and RMP values of CA3 pyramidal cells were measured immediately upon establishing whole-cell configuration. We found no statistically significant differences between RMP measured in neurons from CTL slices when compared with neurons from EL slices (CTL – 62.57 ± 1.59 mV and EL – 59.25 ± 1.89 mV, $p > 0.05$, t test) (Fig. 2b).

Action potentials were then evoked under current-clamp mode by injecting current pulses (– 50 to + 300 pA, in 10 or 50 pA increments for 1000 ms) from an initial holding potential of – 70 mV. The threshold for AP generation was measured as the beginning of the upward rise of the AP when dV/dT exceeded 10 mV/ms. The delta between the RMP of each neuron and the threshold potential (Vt), dRMP-Vt, at which they first fired an AP was not significantly different ($p > 0.05$, t test) between CTL (dRMP-Vt 21.63 ± 1.63 mV) and EL (dRMP-Vt 21.40 ± 1.81 mV) slices (Fig. 2c, d).

EL slices have increased doublecortin immunoreactivity

Over the last decade, changes in hippocampal neurogenesis have emerged as a hallmark of temporal lobe epilepsy (TLE) [14].

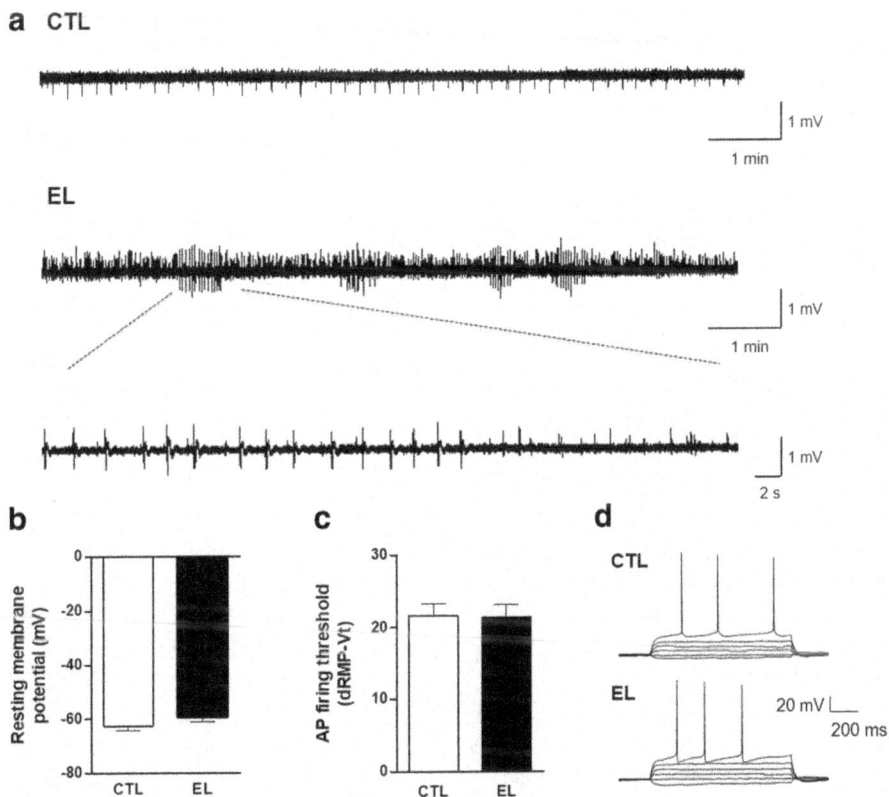

Fig. 2 Electrophysiological properties of organotypic slices control (CTL) and with spontaneous epileptiform activity (EL). **a** Representative field potential recordings of spontaneous activity from CA3 area of CTL and EL organotypic slices. CTL slices depict a regular physiological activity, while EL slices exhibit epileptiform activity at 14 DIV. All vertical bars, 1 mV. **b** Resting membrane potential (RMP) of CA3 pyramidal neurons were measured immediately upon establishing whole-cell configuration and did not significantly differ between CTL and EL slices. **c** There were also no statistically significant changes between the action potential (AP) threshold measured from neurons in CTL and EL slices. **d** Representative tracings for each condition are shown. Data represent the mean ± SEM. $n = 7$–9 cells per condition, from 3 to 4 independent cultures, unpaired t test

Doublecortin (DCX) is a microtubule-associated phosphoprotein, which is widely used as a marker for immature neurons derived from newly generated neural precursor cells and has been validated to assess changes in the level of neurogenesis [11].

Thus, an immunofluorescence protocol was performed to evaluate the DCX staining in the DG of CTL and EL slices at 14 DIV.

As can be observed in Additional file 2: Figure S2, DCX staining was increased in slices that display epileptiform activity. Indeed, DCX fluorescence intensity was found to be significantly higher ($^*p < 0.05$, t test) in the DG of EL slices, thus suggesting increased neurogenesis.

EL slices show higher αII-spectrin cleavage

Neuronal death is considered an important feature of epilepsy. To evaluate if neuronal death was increased in EL slices, we quantified αII-spectrin cleavage and caspase-3 activation by a western blot assay, carried out with protein extracts obtained from the hippocampal region of the slices. Calpain-mediated degradation of αII-spectrin results in the formation of two unique and highly stable SBDPs with a molecular weight of 145 and 150 kDa (SBDP145 and SBDP150), which can be further cleaved by caspase-3 yielding shorter fragments. The presence of the calpain-cleaved fragments is usually indicative of necrotic and excitotoxic neuronal death. On the other hand, caspase-3-mediated αII-spectrin cleavage leads to the formation of a fragment with 150 kDa (SBDP150), which is further degraded by caspase-3, producing the apoptotic-specific SBDP120, with 120 kDa [51].

Thus, an antibody which recognizes the full length αII-spectrin, as well as the calpain- and caspase-3-signature SBDPs, was used. As can be observed in Fig. 3a, this antibody identified two bands: a high molecular weight band, which corresponds to full length αII-spectrin (250 kDa), and a lower one for SBDPs. The expression of SBDP145 and SBDP150 was not possible to visualize separately (Fig. 3a). However, the apoptotic-specific SBDP120, which results from the caspase-3 cleavage of αII-spectrin, was absent from both conditions, indicating that the lower band recognized by αII-spectrin antibody corresponds exclusively to the calpain-signature SBDPs.

CTL and EL slices have a similar expression of full length αII-spectrin (Fig. 3c, $p > 0.05$, t test). The results also indicate that the ratio SBDP145/150 to αII-spectrin was significantly increased (Fig. 3d, $^*p < 0.05$, t test) in EL slices, pointing to a higher αII-spectrin cleavage by calpain in these slices. Furthermore, the band for active caspase-3 (17 kDa) is absent from the immunoblot (Fig. 3b) and no differences are found in pro-caspase 3 expression (Fig. 3e, $p > 0.05$, t test). These results corroborate the sole detection of SBDP145/150 originated by

calpain-mediated cleavage of αII-spectrin and point to an increased necrosis in EL slices.

EL slices show increased PI uptake

To evaluate neuronal death across the different regions of the hippocampus, the PI uptake assay was carried out in CTL and EL slices at 14 DIV.

The representative fluorescence photomicrographs of both groups of slices (Fig. 4a) suggested that PI incorporation was increased in EL slices. This observation was corroborated by the quantification of PI uptake in each hippocampal region, expressed in arbitrary units of fluorescence intensity (Fig. 4b). PI uptake in granular and pyramidal neurons of EL slices was significantly higher ($^*p < 0.05$, one-way ANOVA) than that detected in the same regions of CTL slices. Also, in both groups of slices, CA1 pyramidal neurons show a significantly higher PI uptake than granular neurons ($^\#p < 0.05$, one-way ANOVA). Specifically, for DG, CTL 86.71 ± 8.016 vs EL 121.3 ± 10.51; for CA3, CTL 105.4 ± 6.920 vs EL 135.5 ± 9.846; and for CA1, CTL 130.1 ± 10.67 vs EL 169.8 ± 11.83.

EL slices depict increased gliosis

Activation of astrocytes and microglia are considered a molecular hallmark of epilepsy, and recent findings point to a role of glial cells in the pathogenesis of this disorder [52, 53].

To investigate if gliosis was associated with epileptiform activity, two experimental approaches were used: a western blot assay to evaluate the overall expression of GFAP and Iba1 and an immunohistochemistry assay to evaluate morphological changes in astrocytes and microglia.

The western blot was carried out with 14 DIV hippocampal lysates obtained from CTL and EL slices. The immunoblots (Fig. 5a, c) showed an increased expression of GFAP and Iba1 in EL slices. Indeed, the densitometry analysis (Fig. 5b) attested a significant increase in GFAP expression in EL slices ($^*p < 0.05$, t test). Likewise, the increased Iba1 expression in EL slices, evident in the immunoblot (Fig. 5c), was supported by the densitometry analysis (Fig. 5d), which indicated that Iba1 expression was significantly higher ($^{***}p < 0.001$, t test) in EL slices, when compared to CTL ones.

An immunofluorescence analysis was also performed in CTL and EL slices to assess the morphological features of astrocytes (Fig. 6) and microglia (Fig. 7) in the main hippocampal areas. At 14 DIV, slices were fixed with PFA and handled as described before.

In the DG and CA regions of CTL slices (Fig. 6a–A1, A2, A3), most GFAP-positive astrocytes have thin processes and display preservation of individual domains, which can be observed in the magnified panels, Fig. 6a–A1a, A2a, and

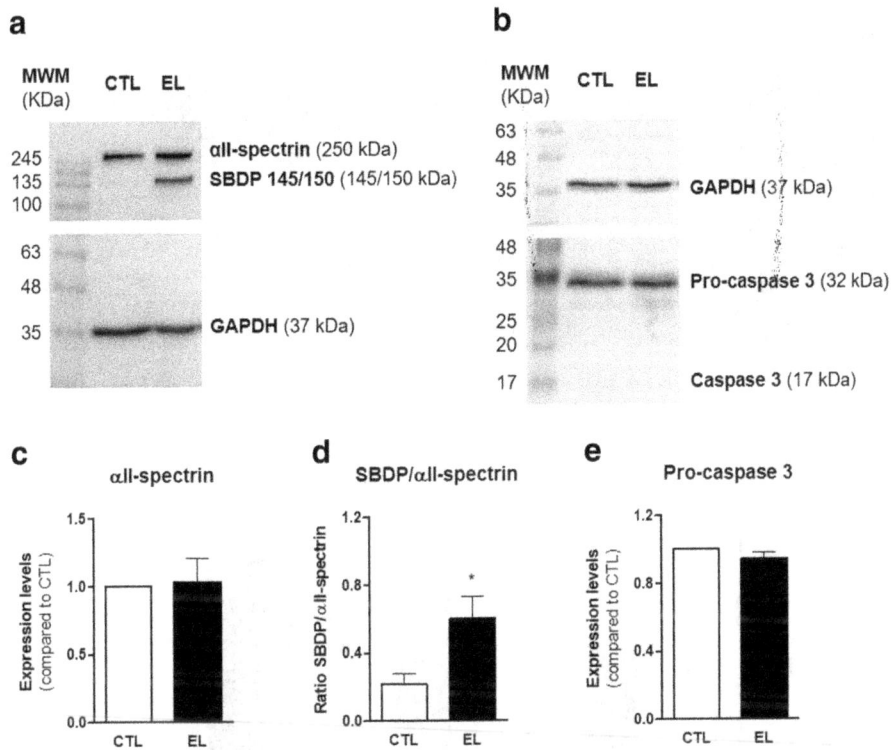

Fig. 3 Western blot analysis of αII-spectrin cleavage and Pro-caspase 3 of organotypic slices control (CTL) and with spontaneous epileptiform activity (EL). **a**, **b** Representative immunoblots of αII-spectrin (250 kDa), SBDP 145/150 (145/150 kDa), Pro-caspase 3 (32 kDa), and GAPDH (37 kDa). **c**–**e** Densitometry analysis was performed with ImageJ software using GAPDH as internal control. **c** Full length αII-spectrin expression was similar between CTL and EL slices, while **d** the ratio SBDP 145/150 to αII-Spectrin was significantly upregulated in EL slices. **e** No differences were found in Pro-caspase 3 expression between CTL and EL slices. All values are mean ± SEM. $n = 4$, $*p < 0.05$, unpaired t test

A3a. However, some hypertrophic cell bodies can also be observed suggestive of a mildly activated state. This basal astrogliosis in organotypic slices has long been reported by others [54]. However, in EL slices (Fig. 6b), a moderate/reactive astrogliosis can be noticed in all regions of the hippocampus, which include the presence of tick and highly superimposed astrocytic processes, resulting in the disruption of individual domains. These features are visible in the magnified panels, Fig. 6b–B1a, B2a, and B3a.

Figure 7 shows the occurrence of microglia cells, identified by Iba1 expression, in all hippocampal regions of CTL and EL slices. In CTL slices (Fig. 7a), most microglia have a ramified morphology, characteristic of a resting state, as can be noticed in Fig. 7a–A1a, A2a, and A3a. In EL slices (Fig. 7b), microglia are more abundant in all regions of the hippocampus, which agrees with the western blot results described above. Furthermore, most microglia have larger cell bodies and have changed their morphology from ramified to bushy-like cells with fewer processes, as observable in Fig. 7b–B1a, B2a, and B3a. In comparison with CTL slices, microglia in EL slices have a significantly increased cell body diameter in all regions

of the hippocampus ($***p < 0.001$, one-way ANOVA), as attested by the quantification depicted in Fig. 7c. Within each condition, no statistical difference was found between hippocampal areas ($p > 0.05$, one-way ANOVA). The mean microglia cell body diameter for CTL slices (DG 11.6 μm ± 0.32; CA3 11.9 μm ± 0.30; CA1 11.5 μm ± 0.31) is higher than 7.5 μm reported by others [55] in resting microglia. This points to a mixed population of resting and reactive microglia in CTL slices, which is in accordance with some basal microglia activation known to occur in organotypic slices [54]. However, in EL slices, the mean microglia cell body diameter increases approximately twofold in relation to CTL ones (DG 18.9 μm ± 0.82; CA3 17.6 μm ± 0.64; CA1 19.8 μm ± 0.63), supporting the qualitative morphological analysis.

Thus, the described morphological alterations depicted by astrocytes and microglia corroborate an increased astrogliosis and microgliosis in EL slices.

Expression of proinflammatory cytokines is increased in EL slices

Recently, inflammatory-related events have been intensely discussed in the context of epilepsy and were

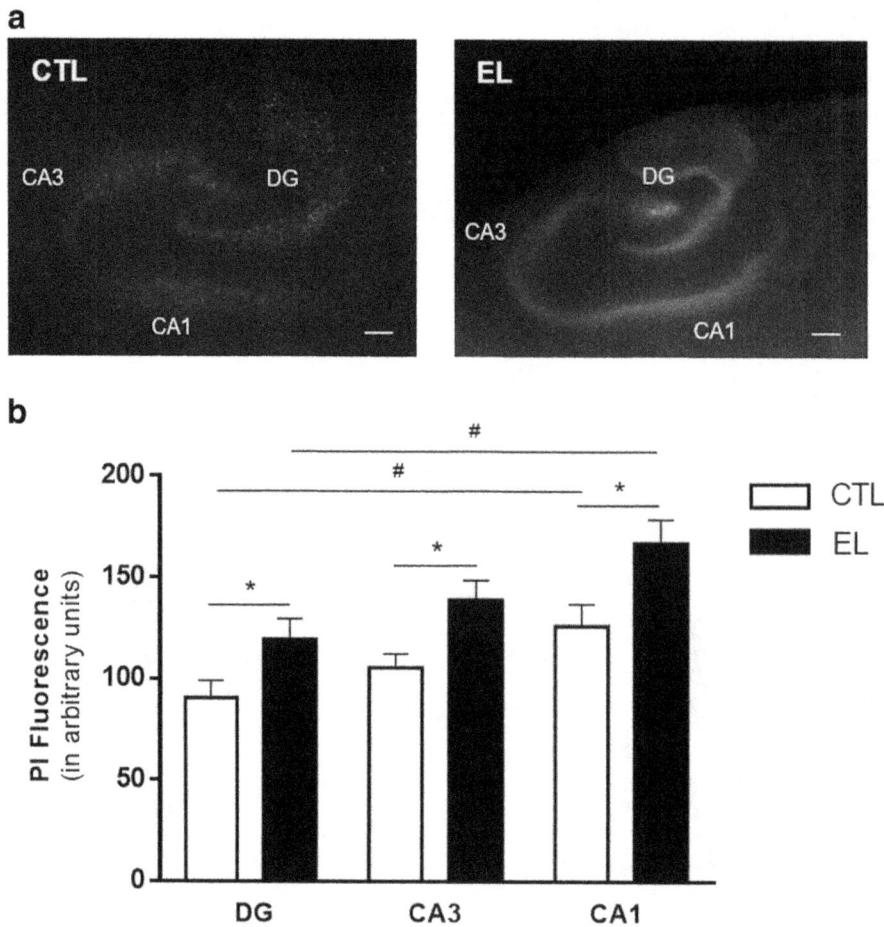

Fig. 4 Propidium iodide uptake of organotypic slices control (CTL) and with spontaneous epileptiform activity (EL). **a** Representative fluorescence photomicrographs of PI uptake in CTL and EL slices. **b** Quantification of PI uptake by each hippocampal region, expressed in arbitrary units of fluorescence intensity, was performed with ImageJ software. In both conditions, the highest PI uptake was observed in CA1 pyramidal region. However, EL slices have a higher PI incorporation in all hippocampal areas when compared to CTL ones. All values are mean ± SEM. $n = 17$–29 slices per condition, from 3 to 4 independent cultures. Statistical tests were performed with one-way ANOVA, followed by Bonferroni's comparison test, *$p < 0.05$, for comparisons within the same hippocampal area, #$p < 0.05$, for comparisons within the same group, as depicted by the lines above the bars. Scale bar, 200 μm

proposed as potential therapeutic targets for new antiepileptic drugs [56, 57].

After showing the occurrence of gliosis in EL slices, it was pertinent to evaluate alterations in the expression of proinflammatory cytokines, namely IL-1β, TNF-α, and IL-6, which are expressed at very low levels in the normal brain, but undergo a fast increase in expression after the induction of seizures [58, 59].

Thus, the expression of these proinflammatory cytokines was evaluated at the mRNA and protein level in CTL and EL slices at 14 DIV.

The transcript expression was evaluated by RT-qPCR, and the results are depicted in Fig. 8a. As can be observed, the mRNA expression of IL-1β, TNF-α, and IL-6 is significantly upregulated in EL slices (*$p < 0.05$, t test).

The protein concentration of these cytokines in the tissue, Fig. 8b, was calculated by an ELISA assay. At the

time point evaluated, protein levels of IL-1β and IL-6 were found to be increased in EL slices (*$p < 0.05$, t test), but TNF-α change at the protein level did not reach statistical significance ($p > 0.05$, t test).

NLRP3 expression is increased in EL slices

Recently, studies indicate a correlation between enhanced NLRP3 inflammasome expression and several neurological-related disorders [30]. NLRP3 activation leads to the processing of pro-IL-1β and pro-IL-18 by caspase-1, with the consequent increased production of the mature cytokines. Since IL-1β was upregulated in EL slices, it was relevant to evaluate if NLRP3 expression was altered in these slices.

To evaluate the differential expression of NLRP3 inflammasome between CTL and EL slices, a western blot was carried out with 14 DIV hippocampal lysates.

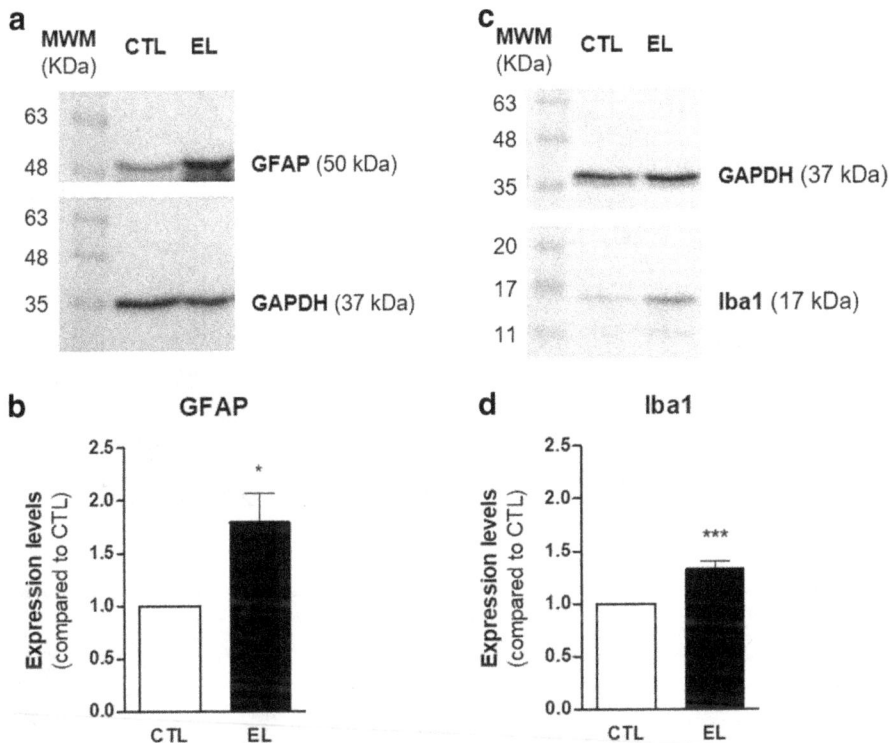

Fig. 5 Western blot analysis of GFAP and Iba1 in organotypic slices control (CTL) and with spontaneous epileptiform activity (EL) at 14 DIV. **a, c** Representative immunoblots for GFAP (50 kDa), Iba1 (17 kDa), and GAPDH (37 kDa). **b, d** Densitometry analysis was performed with ImageJ software using GAPDH as internal control. GFAP and Iba1 expression are significantly upregulated in EL slices. All values are mean ± SEM. $n = 4$, $*p < 0.05$, $***p < 0.001$, unpaired t test

The immunoblot (Fig. 9a) shows that NLRP3 expression was increased in EL slices. This result was confirmed by the densitometric analysis (Fig. 9b), which indicated a statistical significant increase ($*p < 0.05$, t test) in NLRP3 expression in EL slices.

Discussion

This work compares "healthy" organotypic slices with those displaying epileptiform activity, in terms of inflammatory features. We herein show that slices, which exhibit spontaneous epileptiform activity resembling in vivo epilepsy, also depict inflammatory features found in animal models of epilepsy and in TLE patients. We describe increased neuronal death, activation of astrocytes and microglia, and enhanced expression of proinflammatory cytokines, namely IL-1β, TNF-α, and IL-6. We also show that NLRP3 inflammasome expression is increased in slices depicting spontaneous activity. By recapitulating key inflammatory features of epilepsy, the proposed system is of value for mechanistic studies of this disease and can be used as a tool for evaluating potential therapeutic approaches.

Our work confirms the development of interictal-like spikes in combined entorhinal-hippocampus organotypic slices. It was already reported that epileptiform activity

developed in organotypic slices later than 7 DIV, with primarily interictal-like spikes and bursts of activity at 14 to 17 DIV which preceded ictal-like discharges after 21 DIV [42]. These authors suggested that the reorganization of the local network caused by deafferentation and deefferentation occurring during tissue slicing could be the cause of spontaneous activity in organotypic hippocampal slice cultures. However, as we now demonstrate, slices maintained in a serum containing medium, herein denominated CTL slices, do not display spontaneous activity, precluding the possibility that slice preparation per se could be the only cause for spontaneous activity. In our work, CTL slices only depicted a regular activity (Fig. 2a–CTL), whereas slices progressively depleted of serum in the growth medium revealed interictal-like events (Fig. 2a–EL). Interictal spikes in electroencephalographic recordings from epilepsy patients are brief paroxysmal discharges observed between spontaneous recurrent seizures and have been regarded as markers for ongoing epileptogenesis [60]. Hence, according to our recordings, slices gradually deprived of serum in the growth medium mimic some aspects of epileptogenesis, while slices maintained in serum-based conditions do not. To our knowledge, such assessment was never carried out.

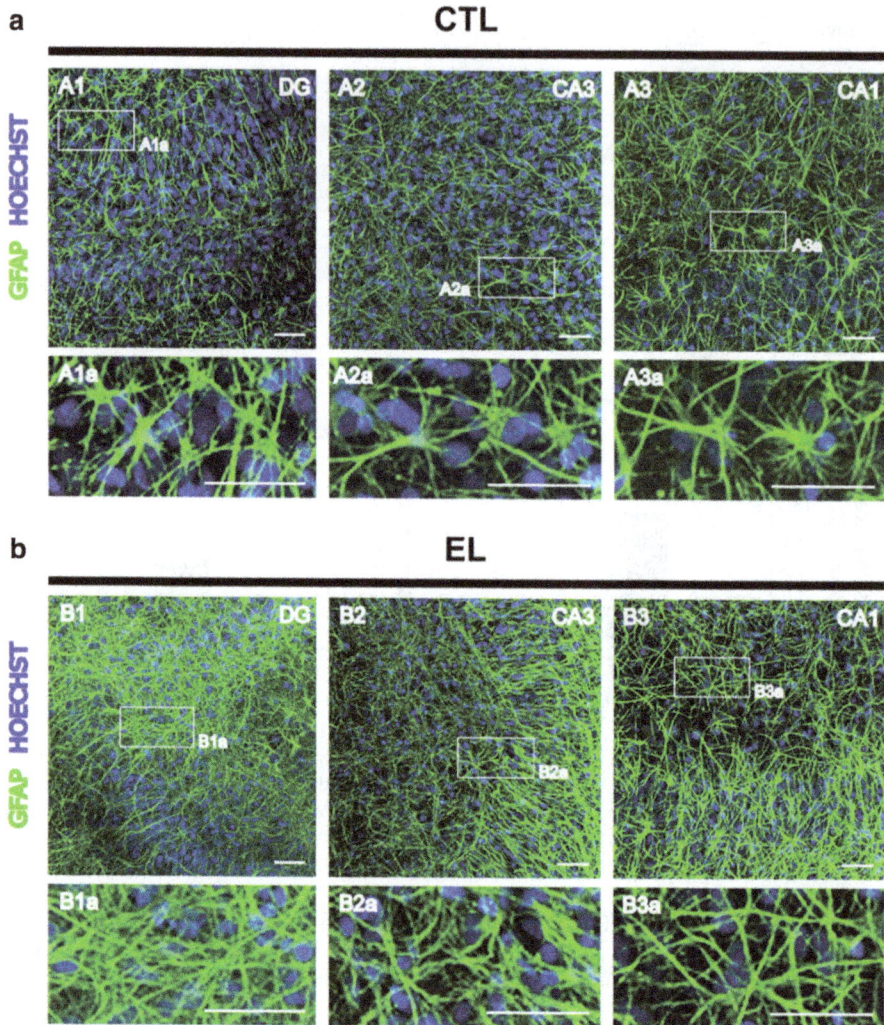

Fig. 6 Representative morphology of astrocytes in organotypic slices control (CTL) and with spontaneous epileptiform activity (EL) at 14 DIV. Images of GFAP-stained astrocytes (green) and Hoechst-stained nuclei (blue) were acquired on a confocal laser microscope (Zeiss LSM 710) with a 20x objective. Magnified images of the dashed areas are shown. **a** In CTL slices, most astrocytes show thin processes with preservation of singular domains. **b** In EL slices, astrocytes have hypertrophic cell bodies, with extensive overlap of astrocytic processes and disruption of individual domains. Scale bars, 50 μm

Serum-free and serum-replacement medium formulations have become essential for biotechnology industries. The elimination of animal components aims standardization, consistency, and reduced risks of contamination in cell culture processes. Furthermore, serum-free medium mimics the serum-free environment found in CNS parenchyma.

However, serum withdrawal from the maintenance medium may play a role in excitability since it affects hippocampal circuitry. It was reported that dendritic spine density and morphology in organotypic slices depend on the presence of serum in the culture media [61] and granule layer cell density was also decreased in the absence of serum [62]. It is therefore plausible to foresee that serum deprivation leads to

persistent changes in the hippocampal circuitry that ultimately decrease the threshold for spikes. Furthermore, recent evidences have shown that serum deprivation increases reactive oxygen species (ROS) production [63]. Although ROS are removed by the antioxidant systems to maintain redox homeostasis, situations of excessive ROS production occur and have been implicated in many pathological disorders including cancer, aging, and neurological diseases [64]. Indeed, ROS generation was suggested to be one of the critical elements for NLRP3 activation [65, 66], one of the features that we observe in our system. Yet, the detailed mechanism through which serum deprivation contributes to epileptiform activity in organotypic slices was not matter of this work and is

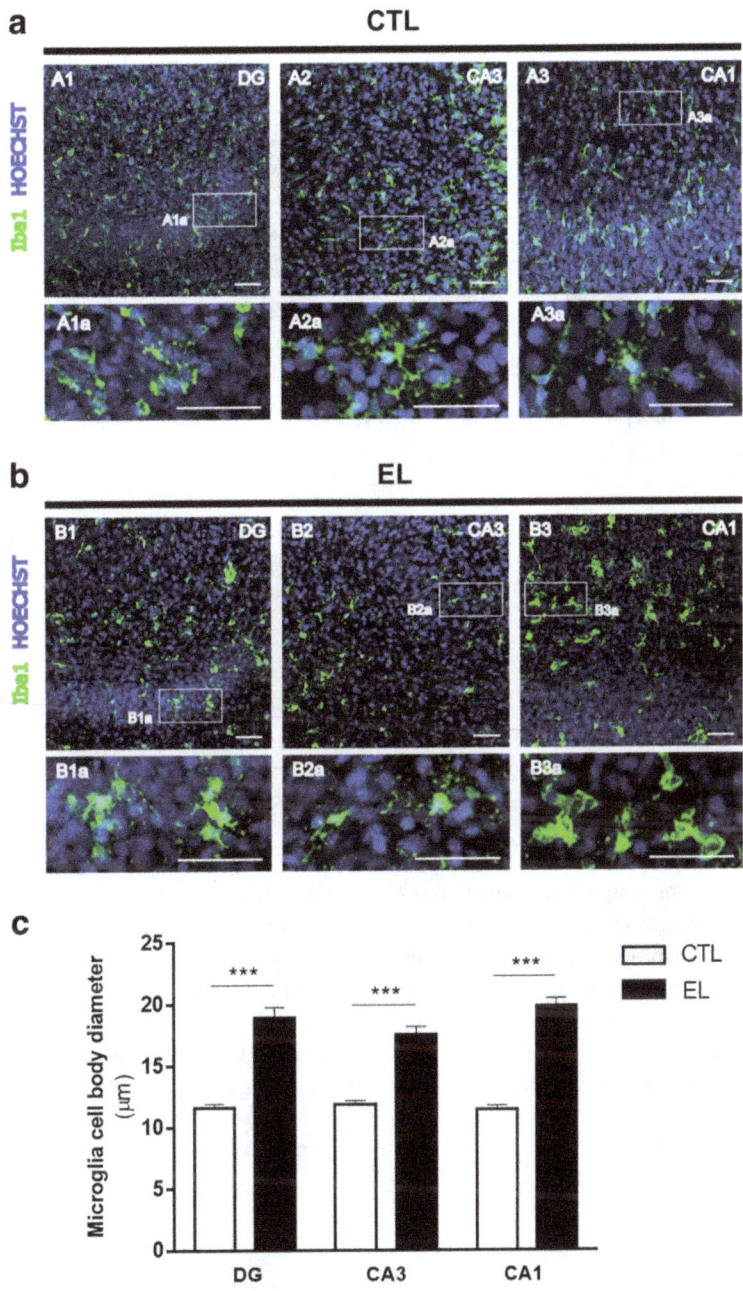

Fig. 7 Representative morphology of microglia in organotypic slices control (CTL) and with spontaneous epileptiform activity (EL) at 14 DIV. Images of Iba1-stained microglia (green) and Hoechst-stained nuclei (blue) were acquired on a confocal laser microscope (Zeiss LSM 710) with a 20x objective. Magnified images of the dashed areas are shown. **a** Most microglia in CTL slices have a ramified morphology, characteristic of a resting state. **b** EL slices depict microglia with a large cell body and retracted processes, corroborating an activated "bushy-like" state. **c** The diameter of microglia cell body was quantified with ImageJ software. In EL slices, microglia show a significant increase in cell body diameter in all hippocampal areas. All values are mean ± SEM. $n = 50$–70 microglia cells per hippocampal area per condition, from 3 independent cultures, ***$p < 0.001$, one-way ANOVA, followed by Bonferroni's comparison test. Scale bars, 50 μm

difficult to address due to the lack of detailed knowledge of the serum and culture media composition.

The hippocampus has become one of the most extensively studied area of the mammalian brain and is considered the most vulnerable brain region for damage. Indeed, its impaired function has been reported in many human brain diseases, such as hypoxia, ischemia, and epilepsy [36].

An association between neuronal death and epileptogenesis has been intensely debated [4]. This work assessed cell death by necrosis and apoptosis, using αII-spectrin cleavage, a major substrate of calpains and

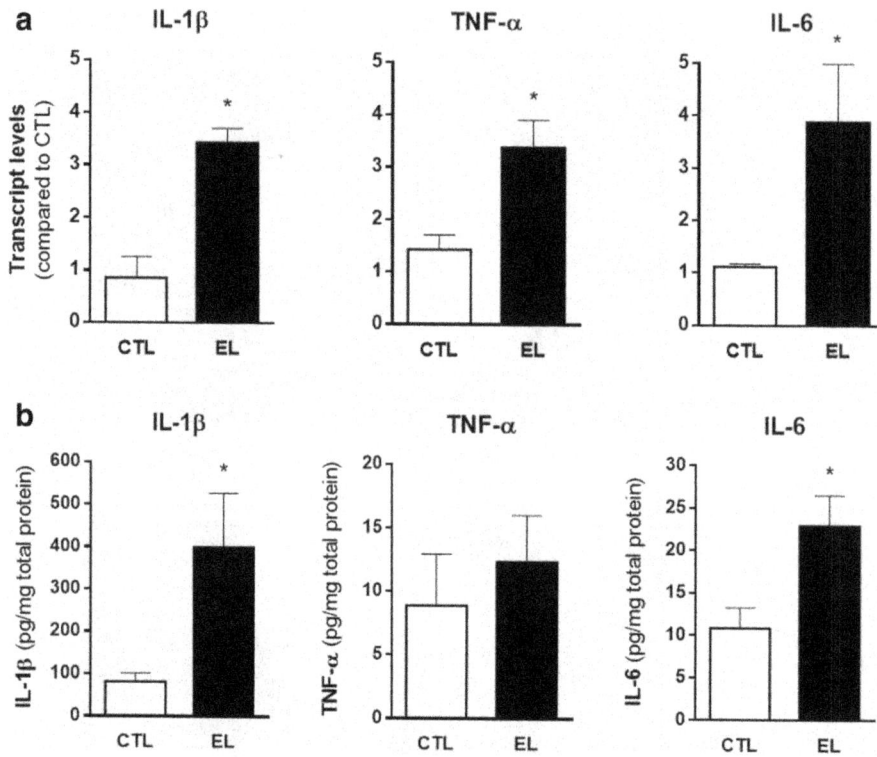

Fig. 8 Expression of proinflammatory cytokines in organotypic slices control (CTL) and with spontaneous epileptiform activity (EL) at 14 DIV. **a** RT-qPCR analysis of IL-1β, TNF-α, and IL-6 shows a transcript upregulation for all cytokines in EL slices. **b** IL-1β and IL-6 protein concentration in tissue, assessed by ELISA, is also significantly increased in EL slices. All values are mean ± SEM. $n = 3–4$, $*p < 0.05$, unpaired t test

caspases, for that purpose. The calpain-mediated fragments of αII-spectrin cleavage (SBDP145/150) were found in slices with epileptiform activity (Fig. 3a), while the caspase-3-mediated apoptotic-specific fragment (SBDP120) was not. This result points to the occurrence of necrosis, which is associated with massive Na^+ and Ca^{2+} influxes and thus with excitotoxicity. Nevertheless, a cross-talk between apoptosis and necrosis cascades [67], as well as caspase-independent cell death processes [68], is gaining recognition among the scientific community and cannot be discarded. Moreover, novel mechanisms of cell death [69, 70], beyond the traditional concepts of necrosis and apoptosis, including autophagy, phagoptosis, necroptosis, and pyroptosis, are nowadays

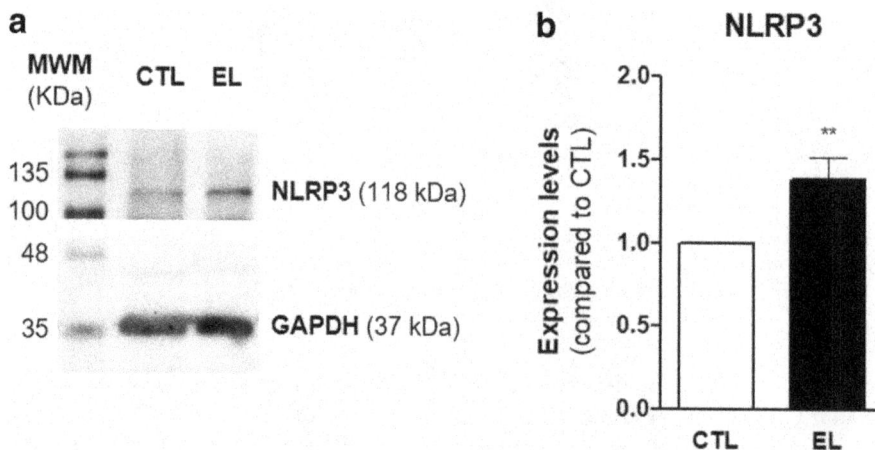

Fig. 9 Protein levels of NLRP3 in organotypic slices control (CTL) and with spontaneous epileptiform activity (EL) at 14 DIV. **a** Representative immunoblot for NLRP3 (118 kDa) and GAPDH (37 kDa). **b** Densitometry analysis was performed with ImageJ software using GAPDH as internal control. NLRP3 expression is significantly upregulated in EL slices. All values are mean ± SEM. $n = 4$, $**p < 0.01$, unpaired t test

being considered to have a role in epileptogenesis [71]. Indeed, the increased NLRP3 expression and activation observed in slices with epileptiform activity point to pyroptosis as one of those mechanisms. But only a complete evaluation of cell death throughout time in culture will fully clarify the cell death mechanisms relevant in this system.

Region-specific neuronal death, across the different regions of the hippocampus, was also explored by the PI uptake assay. PI is a nucleic acid dye that is excluded from viable cells, but can enter in dying or dead cells with compromised membranes and stain their nuclei [49]. We found some PI incorporation in all slices, regardless of culture condition, reflecting cell death as a consequence of the massive deafferentation and deefferentation which occurs during tissue slicing. Truly, although after a few DIV the development of synapses in organotypic slices matches synaptogenesis in vivo, it is known that the density of synaptic contacts decreases immediately after explantation [72]. Nevertheless, at 14 DIV, slices with epileptiform activity display a stronger incidence of PI uptake, and thus cell loss, than control slices (Fig. 4). Stronger PI staining was largely confined to the main neuronal cell layers of the hippocampus, such as DG granular layer and CA1 and CA3 pyramidal layers, suggesting that the dying cells were neurons and thus corroborating neuronal loss, as concluded by the results obtained from αII-spectrin cleavage.

An increased neurogenesis was found in the DG of the slices which display epileptiform activity, corroborating what is reported in many animal models of epilepsy [14]. However, the impact of the newly born granule cells in the progression of the epileptiform activity was not addressed in this study.

Alterations in glial cells near or at the site of a lesion, named as gliosis, constitute a pathological hallmark of damaged CNS tissue, but the way in which gliosis influences a specific neuropathological condition is determined by many factors, including type of disease, injury severity, time after insult, damage location, and cellular changes [53].

Many cellular and molecular processes have been associated with epileptogenesis. Neuroinflammation, which includes the synthesis/release of proinflammatory mediators by activated astrocytes and microglia is one of them. In fact, inflammatory events have been extensively discussed in the context of epilepsy and have been proposed as having a role in the pathophysiology of this neurological disorder [73, 74]. Nowadays, brain inflammation is pointed out as a potential biomarker in epilepsy [75]. In our system, slices with epileptiform activity show noticeable signs of inflammation when compared to control slices, specifically activation of astrocytes and microglia, increased expression of proinflammatory

cytokines, namely IL-1β, and NLRP3 overexpression and activation.

Our results clearly point to the loss of individual domains and extensive overlap of astrocytic processes in slices with epileptiform activity (Fig. 6). It is important to point out that the understanding about the functions and effects of reactive astrogliosis, and their impact on neural function, are still at an early stage. Nowadays, researchers still have a prevalent negative view of reactive astrogliosis and ultimately of glial scar formation, but new lines of evidence point towards its beneficial functions, particularly concerning neural protection and repair, and regulation of CNS inflammation [20]. In this paradoxical view, reactive astrocytes act not only to activate inflammation, at early times after insults, but also to form cell migration barriers that delineate areas of intense inflammation, thereby restricting the spread of inflammatory cells into nearby healthy tissue [76].

Together with reactive astrogliosis, increased microglia proliferation and microglia morphological changes were also observed in slices with epileptiform activity (Fig. 7). In contrast to the resting microglia state observed in control slices, microglia exhibit an activated "bushy-like" appearance in slices with epileptiform activity. We anticipated the occurrence of some amoeboid fully functional phagocytic microglial cell to clear up the cellular debris derived from neuronal death, but amoeboid microglia was not detected at the time point under evaluation.

Interestingly, this work has shown that slices with epileptiform activity demonstrated an increased mRNA expression of proinflammatory cytokines, namely IL-1β, TNF-α, and IL-6 (Fig. 8). Indeed, these cytokines exhibit a low expression level in healthy brain, but their messenger RNA (mRNA) and protein levels were reported to be rapidly increased after the induction of seizures [59]. At the protein level, only IL-1β and IL-6 show an increase in EL slices. TNF-α protein levels remain unchanged between CTL and EL slices, which can be attributed to regulatory processes occurring after TNF-α mRNA production [77] or to the time point under evaluation. In face of the gliosis herein detected, we anticipate that reactive astrocytes and activated microglia are the major contributors for the increased expression of proinflammatory cytokines, as described by others [58, 78].

Furthermore, NLRP3 overexpression in slices with epileptiform activity, together with the increased production of IL-1β, points to a role for NLRP3 inflammasome signaling in epileptogenesis and corroborates that NLRP3 may represent a potential therapeutic target for the treatment of epilepsy, as suggested [31]. Indeed, NLRP3 is nowadays considered a promising therapeutic target for the treatment of neuroinflammation-associated neurological diseases [79].

It is worthwhile to notice that organotypic slice cultures have become a powerful tool to study physiological and pharmacological properties of tissues, since they reproduce the in vivo environment, maintaining the cytoarchitecture of the original tissue. Also, they are relatively inexpensive, markedly reduce the number of animals, and are easy to prepare with no requirements for lengthy animal surgery nor arduous monitorization of physiological parameters, complying with the 3Rs (reduce, refine, replace). In OHSC, the effects of compounds and drugs can be examined without concern about their ability to pass through the BBB and most molecular biology techniques can be applied. However, some drawbacks are still pointed to these types of cultures, namely RNA/protein extraction from few slices, cell morphology assessment with 5–7 cell layers, and the variability in PI staining.

Organotypic slice cultures are established in the study of brain disorders [80]. The most explored brain area in organotypic slice cultures is the hippocampus. Hippocampal organotypic slice cultures are considered adequate to explore the basic mechanisms of epileptogenesis [40, 41], to study stroke and trauma brain injury [81], to study beta-amyloid toxicity, as a model for Alzheimer's disease, and other neurodegenerative diseases [40], and are described to be suitable for neuroprotection studies [39]. Ventral mesencephalon and striatum, as well as cortex-corpus callosum-striatum-SN, organotypic slices, were explored to study Parkinson's disease [80, 82], and organotypic cerebellar slice cultures, which mimic many aspects of axon myelination and cerebellar functions, appear to be the best alternative to in vivo experiments and the most commonly used model for investigating novel therapeutic strategies in multiple sclerosis [83]. It was also reported that organotypic brain slices are an excellent tool to address the therapeutic potential of stem cells, since they allow to study the effect of cell grafts, alone or combined with biomaterials, and to assess the responses of endogenous and implanted cells, as well as their interaction [82]. Nevertheless, although organotypic slice cultures are considered an excellent screening tool, they cannot replace in vivo models, which remain indispensable to evaluate the functional outcome of any therapeutic strategy.

The system herein described, which uses entorhinal cortex-hippocampus organotypic slices, opens a new window to explore neuroinflammation as a cause/consequence of epileptogenesis and reinforces the value of organotypic brain slice cultures as a platform to study brain function.

Conclusions

In conclusion, this system is an excellent tool for monitoring epileptogenesis and the dynamics of spontaneous activity. It also mimics the inflammatory events associated with in vivo epilepsy and allows to interfere pharmacologically with inflammatory pathways, such as the NLRP3 inflammasome signaling, before and after the onset of epileptic-like events, prompting the screening of potential targets for antiepileptic drugs.

Additional files

Additional file 1: Figure S1. Melting curves obtained by RT-qPCR of IL-1β, TNF-α, IL-6 and GAPDH transcripts. Y axis represents the first derivate of raw fluorescence and X axis corresponds to temperature. Each curve has a single melting peak, which indicates that a single PCR product is being amplified.

Additional file 2: Figure S2. Neuronal differentiation in the DG of organotypic slices control (CTL) and with spontaneous epileptiform activity (EL) at 14 DIV. **a** Images of Doublecortin (DCX) stained immature neurons (red) and Hoechst stained nuclei (blue) were acquired on a confocal laser microscope (Zeiss LSM 710) with a 20x objective. **b** Doublecortin fluorescence intensity, quantified with ImageJ software, is significantly higher in EL slices. All values are mean ± SEM. $n = 8$ slices per condition, from 3 independent cultures, $*p < 0.05$, unpaired t-test. Scale bars, 50 μm.

Abbreviations

aCSF: Artificial cerebrospinal fluid; AEDs: Antiepileptic drugs; AP: Action potential; BBB: Blood-brain barrier; BSA: Bovine serum albumin; CA: Cornus ammonis; Ct: Threshold cycle; CTL: Control slices; DCX: Doublecortin; DG: Dentate gyrus; DIV: Days in vitro; EC: Entorhinal cortex; EL: Slices with spontaneous epileptiform activity; GAPDH: Glyceraldehyde-3-phosphate dehydrogenase; GFAP: Glial fibrillary acidic protein; HBSS: Hanks' balanced salt solution; HS: Horse serum; Iba1: Ionized calcium-binding adapter molecule 1; IL-1β: Interleukin-1β; IL-6: Interleukin-6; mRNA: Messenger RNA; MWM: Molecular weight marker; NLRP3 inflammasome: Nucleotide-binding, leucine-rich repeat, pyrin domain containing 3; OHSC: Organotypic hippocampal slice cultures; PBS: Phosphate-buffered saline; PC: Perirhinal cortex; PFA: Paraformaldehyde; PI: Propidium iodide; PVDF: Polyvinylidene difluoride; RMP: Resting membrane potential; ROS: Reactive oxygen species; RT-qPCR: Quantitative real-time PCR; SBDP: Spectrin breakdown products; SDS: Sodium dodecyl sulfate; TLE: Temporal lobe epilepsy; TNF-α: Tumor necrosis factor-α

Acknowledgements

The authors would like to acknowledge Sara Xapelli for all the suggestions concerning organotypic cultures.

Funding

The funding reference is LISBOA-01-0145-FEDER-007391, and the project was cofunded by FEDER, through POR Lisboa 2020–Programa Operacional Regional de Lisboa, PORTUGAL 2020, and Fundação para a Ciência e a Tecnologia. Diogo M. Rombo was in receipt of a fellowship from Fundação para a Ciência e a Tecnologia, SFRH/BD/60386/2009.

Authors' contributions

NP, DMM prepared the organotypic cultures. NP, DMM, DMR, and CBC performed the experiments. AMS acquired the funding. CAV was responsible for the design of the study, provided research supervision, interpreted the data, and wrote the manuscript. All authors contributed to a critical revision of the manuscript and approved the final version.

Consent for publication

Not applicable.

Competing interests

The authors declare that they have no competing interests.

References

1. Engel J, Pedley TA, Aicardi J. Epilepsy: a comprehensive textbook. 2nd ed. Philadelphia: Lippincott Williams & Wilkins; 2007.
2. Fisher RS, et al. Epileptic seizures and epilepsy: definitions proposed by the International League Against Epilepsy (ILAE) and the International Bureau for Epilepsy (IBE). Epilepsia. 2005;46(4):470–2.
3. Lukasiuk K, Becker AJ. Molecular biomarkers of epileptogenesis. Neurotherapeutics. 2014;11(2):319–23.
4. Meldrum BS. Concept of activity-induced cell death in epilepsy: historical and contemporary perspectives. Prog Brain Res. 2002;135:3–11.
5. Wang KK. Calpain and caspase: can you tell the difference? Trends Neurosci. 2000;23:20–6.
6. Brentnall M, Rodriguez-Menocal L, De Guevara RL, Cepero E, Boise LH. Caspase-9, caspase-3 and caspase-7 have distinct roles during intrinsic apoptosis. BMC Cell Biol. 2013;14:32.
7. McIlwain DR, Berger T, Mak TW. Caspase functions in cell death and disease. CSH Perspect Biol. 2013;5:a008656.
8. Pike BR, et al. Accumulation of non-erythroid alpha II-spectrin and calpain-cleaved alpha II-spectrin breakdown products in cerebrospinal fluid after traumatic brain injury in rats. J Neurochem. 2001;78(6):1297–306.
9. Pike BR, et al. Accumulation of calpain and caspase-3 proteolytic fragments of brain-derived alphaII-spectrin in cerebral spinal fluid after middle cerebral artery occlusion in rats. J Cereb Blood Flow Metab. 2004;24(1):98–106.
10. Parent JM, Yu TW, Leibowitz RT, Geschwind DH, Sloviter RS, Lowenstein DH. Dentate granule cell neurogenesis is increased by seizures and contributes to aberrant network reorganization in the adult rat hippocampus. J Neurosci. 1997;7:3727–38.
11. Jessberger S, Romer B, Babu H, Kempermann G. Seizures induce proliferation and dispersion of doublecortin-positive hippocampal progenitor cells. Exp Neurol. 2005;196:342–51.
12. Parent JM, Valentin VV, Lowenstein DH. Prolonged seizures increase proliferating neuroblasts in the adult rat subventricular zone-olfactory bulb pathway. J Neurosci. 2002;22:3174–88.
13. Parent JM, Murphy GG. Mechanisms and functional significance of aberrant seizures-induced hippocampal neurogenesis. Epilepsia. 2008;49(Suppl. 5):19–25.
14. Jessberger S, Parent JM. Epilepsy and adult neurogenesis. Cold Spring Harb Perspect Biol. 2015;7:a020677.
15. Devinsky O, Vezzani A, Najjar S, De Lanerolle NC, Rogawski MA. Glia and epilepsy: excitability and inflammation. Trends Neurosci. 2013;36:174–84.
16. Araque A, Parpura V, Sanzgiri RP, Haydon PG. Tripartite synapses: glia, the unacknowledged partner. Trends Neurosci. 1999;22:208–15.
17. Perea G, Navarrete M, Araque A. Tripartite synapses: astrocytes process and control synaptic information. Trends Neurosci. 2009;32:421–31.
18. Hamilton NB, Attwell D. Do astrocytes really exocytose neurotransmitters? Nat Rev Neurosci. 2010;11:227–38.
19. Pekny M, Nilsson M. Astrocyte activation and reactive gliosis. Glia. 2005;50:427–34.
20. Sofroniew MV. Molecular dissection of reactive astrogliosis and glial scar formation. Trends Neurosci. 2009;32:638–47.
21. Sofroniew MV, Vinters HV. Astrocytes: biology and pathology. Acta Neuropathol. 2010;119:7–35.
22. Block ML, Hong JS. Microglia and inflammation-mediated neurodegeneration: multiple triggers with a common mechanism. Prog Neurobiol. 2005;76:77–98.
23. Mirrione MM, Tsirka SE. A functional role for microglia in epilepsy. In: Afawi Z, editor. Clinical and genetic aspects of epilepsy. London: IntechOpen; 2011.
24. Tambuyzer BR, Ponsaerts P, Nouwen EJ. Microglia: gatekeepers of central nervous system immunology. J Leukoc Biol. 2009;85(3):352–70.
25. Kettenmann H, Hanisch UK, Noda M, Verkhratsky A. Physiology of microglia. Physiol Rev. 2011;91:461–553.
26. Prinz M, Mildner A. Microglia in the CNS: immigrants from another world. Glia. 2011;59:177–87.
27. Vezzani A, Viviani B. Neuromodulatory properties of inflammatory cytokines and their impact on neuronal excitability. Neuropharmacology. 2015;96:70–82.
28. Guo H, Callaway JB, Ting JP. Inflammasomes: mechanism of action, role in disease, and therapeutics. Nat Med. 2015;21(7):677–87.
29. Singhal G, Jaehne EJ, Corrigan F, Toben C, Baune BT. Inflammasome in neuroinflammation and chances in brain function: a focused review. Front Neurosci. 2014;8:315.
30. Walsh JG, Muruve DA, Power C. Inflammasomes in the CNS. Nat Rev. 2014;15:84–97.
31. Edye ME, Walker LE, Sills GJ, Allan SM, Brough D. Epilepsy and the inflammasome: targeting inflammation as a novel therapeutic strategy for seizure disorders. Inflammasome. 2014;1:36–43.
32. Meng X-F, Tan L, Tan M-S, Jiang T, Tan C-C, Li M-M, Wang H-F, Yu J-T. Inhibition of the NLRP3 inflammasome provides neuroprotection in rats following amygdala kindling-induced status epilepticus. J Neuroinflammation. 2014;11:212.
33. Sarkisian MR. Overview of the current animal models for human seizure and epileptic disorders. Epilepsy Behav. 2001;2:201–16.
34. Williams PA, et al. Development of spontaneous recurrent seizures after kainate-induced status epilepticus. J Neurosci. 2009;29:2103–12.
35. Loscher W. Animal models of epilepsy for the development of antiepileptogenic and disease-modifying drugs. A comparison of the pharmacology of kindling and post-status epilepticus models of temporal lobe epilepsy. Epilepsy Res. 2002;50:105–23.
36. Holopainen IE. Organotypic hippocampal slice cultures: a model system to study basic cellular and molecular mechanisms of neuronal cell death, neuroprotection, and synaptic plasticity. Neurochem Res. 2005;30:1521–8.
37. Sundstrom L, Morrison BIII, Bradley M, Pringle A. Organotypic cultures as tools for functional screening in the CNS. Drug Discov Today: Targets. 2005;10:993–1000.
38. De Simoni A, Griesinger CB, Edwards FA. Development of rat CA1 neurones in acute versus organotypic slices: role of experience in synaptic morphology and activity. J Physiol. 2003;550:135–47.
39. Noraberg J, Poulsen FR, Blaabjerg M, et al. Organotypic hippocampal slice cultures for studies of brain damage, neuroprotection and neurorepair. CNS Neurol Disord Drug Targets. 2005;4:435–52.
40. Cho S, Wood A, Bowlby MR. Brain slices as models for neurodegenerative disease and screening platforms to identify novel therapeutics. Curr Neuropharmacol. 2007;5:19–33.
41. Heinemann U, Kann O, Schuma S. An overview of in vitro seizure models in acute and organotypic slices. In: Pitkänen A, Schwartzkroin PA, Moshé SL, editors. Models of seizures and epilepsy. Cambridge: Elsevier Academic Press; 2006. p. 35–44.
42. Dyhrfjeld-Johnsen J, Berdichevsky Y, Swiercz W, Sabolek H, Staley KJ. Interictal spikes precede ictal discharges in an organotypic hippocampal slice culture model of epileptogenesis. J Clin Neurophysiol. 2010;27:418–24.
43. Albus K, Heinemann U, Kovacs R. Network activity in hippocampal slice cultures revealed by long-term in vitro recordings. J Neurosci Methods. 2013;217:1–8.
44. Berdichevsky Y, Dzhala V, Mail M, Staley KJ. Interictal spikes, seizures and ictal cell death are not necessary for post-traumatic epileptogenesis in vitro. Neurobiol Dis. 2012;45:774–85.
45. Stoppini L, Buchs PA, Muller D. A simple method for organotypic cultures of nervous tissue. J Neurosci Methods. 1991;37:173–82.
46. Naundorf B, Geisel T, Wolf F. Action potential onset dynamics and the response speed of neuronal populations. J Comput Neurosci. 2005;18(3):297–309.
47. Aroeira RI, Ribeiro JA, Sebastião AM, Valente CA. Age-related changes of glycine receptor at the rat hippocampus: from the embryo to the adult. J Neurochem. 2011;118:339–53.
48. Pfaffl MW. A new mathematical model for relative quantification in real time RT-PCR. Nucleic Acids Res. 2001;29:2002–7.
49. Noraberg J, Kristensen BW, Zimmer J. Markers for neuronal degeneration in organotypic slice cultures. Brain Res Protocol. 1999;3:278–90.
50. Vismer MS, Forcelli PA, Skopin MD, Gale K, Koubeissi MZ. The piriform, perirhinal, and entorhinal cortex in seizure generation. Front Neural Circuit. 2015;9:27.
51. Yan XX, Jeromin A. Spectrin breakdown products (SBDPs) as potential biomarkers for neurodegenerative diseases. Curr Transl Geriatr Exp Gerontol Rep. 2013;1:85–93.

52. Binder DK, Steinhäuser C. Functional changes in astroglial cells in epilepsy. Glia. 2006;54:358–68.

53. Foresti ML, Arisi GM, Shapiro LA. Role of glia in epilepsy-associated neuropathology, neuroinflammation and neurogenesis. Brain Res Rev. 2011; 66:115–22.

54. Coltman BW, Ide CF. Temporal characterization of microglia, IL-1β-like immunoreactivity and astrocytes in the dentate gyrus of hippocampal organotypic slice cultures. Int J Devl Neuroscience. 1996;14(6):707–19.

55. Wu H, Wu T, Xu X, Wang J, Wang J. Iron toxicity in mice with collagenase-induced intracerebral haemorrhage. J Cereb Blood Flow Metab. 2011;31: 1243–50.

56. Walker L, Sills GJ. Inflammation and epilepsy: the foundations for a new therapeutic approach in epilepsy? Epilepsy Curr. 2012;12:8–12.

57. Vitaliti G, Pavone P, Mahmood F, Nunnari G, Falsaperla R. Targeting inflammation as a therapeutic strategy for drug-resistant epilepsies: an update of new immune-modulating approaches. Hum Vaccin Immunother. 2014;10:868–75.

58. De Simoni MG, Perego C, Ravizza T. Inflammatory cytokines and related genes are induced in the rat hippocampus by limbic status epilepticus. Eur J Neurosci. 2000;12:2623–33.

59. Vezzani A, Granata T. Brain inflammation in epilepsy: experimental and clinical evidence. Epilepsia. 2005;46(11):1724–43.

60. Staley KJ, White A, Dudek FE. Interictal spikes: harbingers or causes of epilepsy? Neurosci Lett. 2011;497(3):247–50.

61. Chapleau CA, Carlo ME, Larimore JL, Pozzo-Miller L. The actions of BDNF on dendritic spine density and morphology in organotypic slice cultures depend on the presence of serum in culture media. J Neurosci Methods. 2008;169(1):182–90.

62. Sadgrove MP, Laskowski A, Gray WP. Examination of granule layer cell count, cell density, and single-pulse BrdU incorporation in rat organotypic hippocampal slice cultures with respect to culture medium, septotemporal position, and time in vitro. J Comp Neurol. 2006;497(3):397–415.

63. Lee SB, Kim JJ, Kim TW, Kim BS, Lee M-S, Yoo YD. Serum deprivation-induced reactive oxygen species production is mediated by Romo1. Apoptosis. 2010;15:204–18.

64. Finkel T. Oxidant signals and oxidative stress. Curr Opin Cell Biol. 2003;15: 247–54.

65. Tschopp J, Schroder K. NLRP3 inflammasome activation: the convergence of multiple signalling pathways on ROS production? Nat Rev Immunol. 2010; 10:210–5.

66. Zhou R, Tardivel A, Thorens B, Choi I, Tschopp J. Thioredoxin-interacting protein links oxidative stress to inflammasome activation. Nat Immunol. 2010;11:136–41.

67. Harwood SM, Yaqoob MM, Allen DA. Caspase and calpain function in cell death: bridging the gap between apoptosis and necrosis. Ann Clin Biochem. 2005;42:415–31.

68. Abraham MC, Shaham S. Death without caspases, caspases without death. Trends Cell Biol. 2004;14(4):184–93.

69. Fink SL, Cookson BT. Apoptosis, pyroptosis, and necrosis: mechanistic description of dead and dying eukaryotic cells. Infect Immun. 2005;73(4): 1907–16.

70. Bergsbaken T, Fink SL, Cookson BT. Pyroptosis: host cell death and inflammation. Nat Rev Microbiol. 2009;7(2):99–109.

71. Dingledine R, Varnel NH, Dudek FE. When and how do seizures kill neurons, and is cell death relevant to epileptogenesis? Adv Exp Med Biol. 2014;813: 109–22.

72. Lossi L, Alasia S, Salio C, Merighi A. Cell death and proliferation in acute slices and organotypic cultures of mammalian CNS. Prog Neurobiol. 2009; 88(4):221–45.

73. Vezzani A, French J, Bartfai T, Baram TZ. The role of inflammation in epilepsy. Nat Rev Neurol. 2011;7(1):31–40.

74. Vezzani A. Epilepsy and inflammation in the brain: overview and pathophysiology. Epilepsy Curr. 2014;14(1 Suppl):3–7.

75. Vezzani A, Friedman A. Brain inflammation as a biomarker in epilepsy. Biomark Med. 2011;5:607–14.

76. Sofroniew MV. Astrocyte barriers to neurotoxic inflammation. Nat Rev Neurosci. 2015;16:249–63.

77. Vogel C, Marcotte EM. Insights into the regulation of protein abundance from proteomic and transcriptomic analyses. Nat Rev Genet. 2012;13(4):227–32.

78. Vezzani A, Moneta D, Richichi C, Aliprandi M, Burrows SJ, Ravizza T, Perego C, De Simoni MG. Functional role of inflammatory cytokines and anti-inflammatory molecules in seizures and epileptogenesis. Epilepsia. 2002;43-S5:30–5.

79. Song L, Pei L, Yao S, Wu Y, Shang Y. NLRP3 inflammasome in neurological diseases, from functions to therapies. Front Cell Neurosci. 2017;11:63.

80. Humpel C. Organotypic brain slice cultures: a review. Neuroscience. 2015; 305:86–98.

81. Li Q, Han X, J W. Organotypic hippocampal slices as models for stroke and traumatic brain injury. Mol Neurobiol. 2016;53(6):4226–37.

82. Daviaud N, Garbayo E, Schiller PC, Perez-Pinzon M, Montero-Menei CN. Organotypic cultures as tools for optimizing central nervous system cell therapies. Exp Neurol. 2013;248:429–40.

83. Doussau F, Dupont JL, Neel D, Schneider A, Poulain B, Bossu JL. Organotypic cultures of cerebellar slices as a model to investigate demyelinating disorders. Expert Opin Drug Discov. 2017;12(10):1011–22.

Inhibition of the NLRP3 inflammasome provides neuroprotection in rats following amygdala kindling-induced status epilepticus

Xiang-Fei Meng[1], Lan Tan[1,2,3*], Meng-Shan Tan[3], Teng Jiang[4], Chen-Chen Tan[1], Meng-Meng Li[1], Hui-Fu Wang[2] and Jin-Tai Yu[1,2,5*]

Abstract

Background: NLRP3 inflammasome is proposed to regulate inflammation in several neurological diseases, but its role in epilepsy remains largely unknown. This study aimed to investigate the role of the NLRP3 inflammasome in neuroinflammation, spontaneous recurrent seizures (SRS) and hippocampal neuronal loss in rat brain following amygdala kindling-induced status epilepticus (SE).

Methods: We detected the protein levels of IL-1β and NLRP3 inflammasome components by Western blot in the hippocampus of shams and SE rats at different time points following SE. To further examine whether the activation of the NLRP3 inflammasome contributes to SE-associated neuronal damage, we employed a nonviral strategy to knock down NLRP3 and caspase-1 expression in brain before undergoing SE. Proinflammatory cytokine levels and hippocampal neuronal loss were evaluated at 12 hours and at 6 weeks following SE respectively in these NLRP3 and caspase-1 deficient rats. Meanwhile, SRS occurrence was evaluated through a 4-week video recording started 2 weeks after SE in these NLRP3 and caspase-1 deficient rats.

Results: IL-1β levels and NLRP3 inflammasome components levels dramatically increased at 3 hours after SE, and reached a maximum at 12 hours after SE compared with the control group. Knock down of NLRP3 or caspase-1 decreased the levels of IL-1β and IL-18 at 12 hours after SE, which was accompanied by a significant suppression in the development and severity of SRS during the chronic epileptic phase. Meanwhile, knock down of NLRP3 or caspase-1 led to a remarkable reduction of hippocampal neuronal loss in the CA1 and CA3 area of the hippocampus at 6 weeks after SE.

Conclusions: Our study provides the first evidence that the NLRP3 inflammasome was significantly up-regulated following SE. More importantly, we show that inhibition of the NLRP3 inflammasome provides neuroprotection in rats following SE. These findings suggest that NLRP3 may represent a potential target for the treatment of epileptogenesis

Keywords: NLRP3, Inflammasome, Status epilepticus, Cytokine, IL-1β, IL-18, Caspase-1, Neuroinflammation, Spontaneous recurrent seizures, Hippocampal neuronal loss

* Correspondence: dr.tanlan@163.com; yu-jintai@163.com
[1]Department of Neurology, Qingdao Municipal Hospital, School of Medicine, Qingdao University, Qingdao, PR China
[2]Department of Neurology, Qingdao Municipal Hospital, Nanjing Medical University, Nanjing, PR China
Full list of author information is available at the end of the article

Background

Status epilepticus (SE), which is one of the most serious manifestations of epilepsy, can be defined as 'a condition characterized by an epileptic seizure that is so frequent or so prolonged as to create a fixed and lasting condition' [1]. Brain inflammation promotes increased neuronal excitability, decreases seizure threshold and is likely to be involved in the molecular, structural and synaptic changes characterizing epileptogenesis [2]. Among all the enhanced proinflammatory cytokines following SE, IL-1β is regarded as a pivotal therapeutic target in SE, as observations have demonstrated IL-1β as being an important inflammation-related epileptogenic factor [3 5]. Many anti-seizure drugs are known to decrease IL-1β levels [6,7]. Moreover, the inhibition or deletion of caspase-1, the enzyme which cleaves pro-IL-1β producing the mature and biologically active form of IL-1β, attained significant seizure reduction [8,9]. However, the mechanisms by which the production of IL-1β is regulated have not been established.

The nucleotide binding and oligomerization domain-like receptor family pyrin domain-containing 3 (NLRP3) inflammasome is a multiprotein complex that mediates the activation of caspase-1, which in turn cleaves pro-IL-1β to form the mature IL-1β and is found to be a pivotal mediator of IL-1β function [10]. The NLRP3 inflammasome [11], composed of NLR family, pyrin domain containing 3 (NLRP3), apoptosis-associated speck-like protein containing a caspase recruitment domain (ASC) and caspase-1, mediates IL-1β transcription and functions via coupling with the NF-κB inflammatory pathway [12]. The NLRP3 inflammasome has been demonstrated as being associated with the innate immunity and inflammatory regulation of the central nervous system (CNS) [13 15]. It should be noted that the high concentrations of extracellular ATP and K^+ ions, the generation of reactive oxygen species (ROS), the increased intracellular Ca^{2+} concentration, acidosis, hypoxia and cell swelling can activate NLRP3 [16 18]. Actually, all of the above factors underlie the generation of SE [19 22]. We hypothesized that this inflammasome may have potential to induce IL-1β-related neuroinflammation in SE. Therefore, it is intriguing to investigate the role of the NLRP3 inflammasome in SE-associated pathology and functional outcomes.

To test this hypothesis, we first investigated the expression profiles of IL-1β and NLRP3 inflammasome components, including NLRP3 and caspase-1 after SE. Next, we applied small interfering RNAs (siRNAs) to knock down NLRP3 and caspase-1 in vivo, and measured the alteration in proinflammatory cytokine and NLRP3 inflammasome components as well as the effects on functional outcomes.

Methods
Animals and experiments groups

To avoid the interference of estrogen on microglial activation, neuroinflammation and cognitive function [23], only male rats were used in this study. Adult male Sprague-Dawley (SD) rats weighing 260 to 300 g were obtained from the Experimental Animal Center of Qingdao University. The rats were specific-pathogen free rats, regularly checked to ensure the status, and housed in a pathogen-free room with a 12-hour light/dark cycle and given free access to food and water. All experiments were performed in strict accordance with the National Institute of Health Guide for the Care and Use of Laboratory Animals. Animal care and sacrifice were conducted according to methods approved by the Qingdao University Animal Experimentation Committee, and all efforts were made to minimize the number of animals used and their suffering. Experimental group allocation and experimental design are shown in Additional file 1: Figure S1.

siRNA administration in rat brain

The NLRP3 siRNA was designed and synthesized by Invitrogen (Carlsbad, CA, USA). Caspase-1 siRNA and control siRNA were purchased from Santa Cruz Biotechnology (Santa Cruz, CA, USA). Entranster -in vivo transfection reagent was purchased from Engreen Biosystem Co, Ltd (Beijing, China). We prepared the Entranster -in vivo-siRNA mixture according to the manufacturer s instructions. Briefly, 50 μg siRNA were resuspended in 50 μL RNase-free water to make a siRNA solution. Then, 50 μL of siRNA solution were mixed with 50 μL of Entranster -in vivo transfection reagent and 100 μL artificial cerebrospinal fluid (aCSF, composition in mmol/L: NaCl 130, KCl 2.99, $CaCl_2$ 0.98, $MgCl_2$ $6H_2O$ 0.80, $NaHCO_3$ 25, Na_2HPO_4 $12H_2O$ 0.039, NaH_2PO_4 $2H_2O$ 0.46) to obtain a 200 μL Entranster -in vivo transfection mixture. Then, the 200 μL Entranster -in vivo transfection mixture (containing NLRP3 or caspase-1 siRNA, control siRNA, no siRNA (aCSF only)) was filled into an osmotic pump (Model 2006; ALZET, Cupertino, CA, USA). Meanwhile, rats were anesthetized with 10% chloral hydrate (0.3 mL/100 g, intraperitoneal) and were placed in a stereotaxic apparatus (Stoelting, Wood Dale, IL, USA). A brain-infusion cannula (Brain Infusion Kit 2; ALZET, Cupertino, CA, USA) coupled via vinyl tubing to the osmotic pump was implanted into the dorsal third ventricle (AP: −1.8 mm; L: −0 mm; V: −5 mm). The osmotic pump was placed subcutaneously between the rat scapulae, and the siRNAs were continuously infused into the brain over a 6-week duration at a flow rate of 0.15 μL/hour. This dose of NLRP3 siRNA or caspase-1 siRNA infusion was well tolerated, and no signs of neurotoxicity including hind-limb paralysis, vocalization, food intake, or neuro-anatomical damage were observed in preliminary study.

Incidentally, the behavioral and biochemical data between control siRNA-treated and non-siRNA-treated rats do not differ. All of the operations were carried out with aseptic techniques.

Electrode implantation and SE induction

SE was triggered following the methods of our previous work [24]. Briefly, rats were fixed in a stereotactic apparatus (Stoelting, Wood Dale, IL, USA) under deep anesthesia (10% chloral hydrate, 0.3 mL/100 g, intraperitoneal). The electrodes were permanently implanted into the right basolateral amygdala (AP: −3.0 mm; L: −4.8 mm; V: −8.8 mm) and were connected to a miniature receptacle, embedding in the skull with screws and dental acrylic cement. After electrode implantation, the animals were allowed to recover from surgery for 2 weeks. SE was induced by continuous delivery of 100-ms trains, consisting of 60 Hz 400 μA (peak-to-peak) bipolar 1-ms square-wave pulses, delivered at 60 Hz every 0.5 seconds using a ML1101 electronic stimulator (Nihon Kohden) via the implanted electrode for up to 20 minutes. Electroencephalograms (EEGs) of the right amygdala were recorded with a digital amplifier (AD Instrument, Bio Amp (Shanghai, China), USA). After 20 minutes of continuous stimulation the stimulation was interrupted and the behavioral and electrographic activity of the animals was observed for 60 seconds. If the behavior of the animals indicated the presence of epileptic activity (head nodding or limb clonus), observation was continued for another 5 minutes. If an animal did not meet the criteria of clonic SE (continuous EEG epileptiform spiking and recurrent clonic seizures), stimulation was resumed and the behavior of the animal was checked again after 5 minutes. Once the criteria of SE were achieved, no further stimulation was given. Stimulation period never exceeded 40 minutes. All of the operations were carried out with aseptic techniques. Sham rats were handled in the same manner but without receiving any electrical stimulation. Moreover, our preliminary experiments also show that this amygdala stimulation model is effective.

Monitoring of SRS

SRS occurrence was evaluated through a 4-week video monitoring started 2 weeks after SE. All recordings for SRS were done during the light period. Epileptic rats were video-recorded for at least 12 hours daily. The frequency and duration of stage 4/5 seizures were recorded, and the severity of SRS was scored according to Racines scale [25]. The recordings were analyzed by observers who were blind to the results of group allocation.

Brain tissue preparation

Rats were sacrificed under deep anesthesia and were handled as follows: For Western blot analysis, quantitative real-time PCR, and ELISA, rats were perfused transcardially with 0.9% saline (pH 7.4) only. The brains were removed rapidly and stored in liquid nitrogen until use. For cresyl violet staining and terminal deoxynucleotidyl transferase-mediated dUTP end-labeling assay (TUNEL) analysis, rats were perfused transcardially with 0.9% saline (pH 7.4), followed by a fixative solution containing 4% paraformaldehyde in 0.9% saline (pH 7.4). The brains were removed and fixed in the same fixative at 4C until use. For double immunofluorescence staining, rat brain was removed without perfusion, embedded in tissue freezing medium, and immediately frozen at −4C. Frozen tissue was stored at −80C until sectioning.

Western blotting

Tissues samples were digested with radio immunoprecipitation assay (RIPA) lysis buffer (50 mmol/L Tris-HCl, 150 mmol/L NaCl, 1% Nonidet-40, 0.5% sodium deoxycholate, 1 mmol/L EDTA, 1 mmol/L PMSF) with protease inhibitors (pepstatin 1 μg/mL, aprotinin 1 μg/mL, leupeptin 1 μg/mL) for 30 minutes and centrifuged at 12,000 g for 15 minutes at 4C. The protein concentration was determined using the Bradford assay kit (Bio-Rad Laboratories, Hercules, CA, USA). The equal amount of protein from different samples was separated using 8 to12% sodium dodecyl sulfate (SDS) polyacrylamide gels and transferred to polyvinylidene fluoride (PVDF) membranes. The membranes were blocked with 10% non-fat milk in Tween-TBS (TBST) and incubated at 4C overnight, with the primary antibodies against NLRP3 (1:200; Santa Cruz Biotechnology, Santa Cruz, CA, USA), cleaved IL-1β (1:200; Santa Cruz Biotechnology, Santa Cruz, CA, USA), cleaved caspase-1 (1:200; Biorbyt, San Francisco, CA, USA), and β-actin (1:1,000; Santa Cruz Biotechnology, Santa Cruz, CA, USA). After rinsing, the membranes were appropriately incubated with horseradish peroxidase (HRP)-conjugated suitable secondary antibodies (1:5,000; Zhongshan Inc., Beijing, China) for 2 hours at room temperature. Cross-reactivity was visualized using electrochemiluminescence (ECL) Western blotting detection reagents and analyzed by scanning densitometry using a UVP BioDoc-It Imaging System (UVP, Upland, CA, USA).

Quantitative Real-Time PCR

Total RNA was extracted using TRIzol reagent (Invitrogen, Carlsbad, CA, USA), using the protocol supplied by the manufacturer. The cDNA was synthesized using Reverse Transcription System (Bio-Rad, Hercules, CA, USA). The reaction was performed at 42 C for 50 minutes, 95C for 5 minutes, and 5C for 5 minutes, then the cDNA was stored at −20C. Amplification was carried out using the Stratagene Mx3000P real-time PCR system (Stratagene, La Jolla, CA, USA) and real-time SYBR Green PCR technology (Takara Bio, Inc., Shiga,

Japan). Reverse transcription was performed in a final volume of 20 μL containing 2 μL cDNA, 10 μL SYBR Green, 0.4 μL ROX Reference Dye, 0.4 μL forward and reverse primer (1 mol/L), and 6.8 μL nuclease-free water. The optimal conditions were 40 cycles of 95C for 30 seconds, 60C for 32 seconds, and 72C for 30 seconds. All reactions were run in duplicates and the mean values are used. Total RNA concentrations from each sample were normalized by quantity of β-actin mRNA, and the target genes expression was evaluated by ratio of the number of target mRNA to β-actin mRNA. Relative expression of genes was obtained by the $2^{-\triangle\triangle CT}$ method. Primers were purchased from Invitrogen (Carlsbad, CA, USA) as follows (name: forward primer, reverse primer): nlrp3: 5 -cc agggctctgttcattg-3 , 5 -ccttggctttcacttcg-3 ; caspase-1: 5 -ag gagggaatatgtggg-3 , 5 -aaccttgggcttgtctt-3 ; β-actin: 5 -agg gaaatcgtgcgtgac3 , 5 -cgctcattgccgatagtg-3 .

Cytokine measurement
The cytokine analysis was performed in duplicate using commercial ELISA assay kits according to the manufacturers instructions. IL-1β was measured in ELISAs from R&D Systems (Minneapolis, MN, USA). IL-18 was measured in ELISAs from Invitrogen (Carlsbad, CA, USA). The results are expressed in pg/mL.

Nissl staining (cresyl violet staining) and TUNEL staining
The brains were embedded in paraffin and cut into 7-μm sections. Nissl staining was employed to detect surviving neurons. Briefly, the paraffin-embedded sections were dewaxed and rehydrated according to the standard protocols, and immersed in 1% cresyl violet at 50C for 5 minutes. After being rinsed with water, the sections were dehydrated in increasing concentrations of ethanol, mounted on the slides, and examined with a light microscope. Only the neurons with a violet nucleus and intact morphology were counted as surviving neurons. The TUNEL staining, which detects DNA fragmentation resulting from apoptotic signaling cascades, was performed to label apoptotic neurons. It may also label cells that have suffered severe DNA damage. Therefore, the TUNEL assay is helpful in identifying seizure-induced neuronal loss in our experiment. We employed the TUNEL assay via a commercial kit according to the manufacturer's instructions (Roche Co., Mannheim, Germany). TUNEL-positive neurons with condensed nuclei were identified as dead neurons. Cell counting was performed on six randomly selected non-overlapping fields in the CA1 and CA3 regions of the hippocampus per slide. The densities of surviving neurons or TUNEL-positive neurons in the hippocampus of the scanned digital images were calculated using Image-Pro Express software (Media Cybernetics, Silver Spring, MD, USA). The total cell counts were averaged from six sections per animal. The survival index was defined as:

$$Surviving\ index\ \% \\ 100 \times Number\ of\ survivng\ neurons \\ /Total\ numbers\ of\ neurons$$

Furthermore, the TUNEL-positive neuron index was defined as:

$$TUNEL-positive\ neurons\ index\ \% \\ 100 \times Count\ of\ TUNEL-positive\ neurons \\ /Total\ count\ of\ neurons$$

Double immunofluorescence staining
In brief, frozen tissue sections of hippocampus area (20 μm thick) from epileptic rats at 12 hours following amygdala stimulation and time-matched shams were used for double staining of NLRP3/ionized Ca^+ binding adaptor molecule 1 (Iba1). The sections were obtained by cryosectioning at −20C, mounted on a glass slide, and incubated at room temperature for 1 hour. Afterward, the sections were fixed in ice-cold acetone for 10 minutes and then dried on a heater for 10 minutes at 40C. The sections were then blocked with 5% BSA and 0.1% Triton X-100 for 2 hours at room temperature. After a single wash with PBS, sections were incubated overnight at 4C with a goat polyclonal antibody against Iba1 (1:100, Abcam, Cambridge, UK) as well as a rabbit polyclonal antibody against NLRP3 (1:50; Santa Cruz Biotechnology, Santa Cruz, CA, USA)). Sections were rinsed in PBS and washed 3 times, and then incubated respectively with tetramethylrhodamine (TRITC)-conjugated anti-goat IgG (1:200; Zhongshan Inc., Beijing, China) and fluorescein isothiocyanate (FITC)-conjugated anti-rabbit IgG (1:200; Santa Cruz Biotechnology) for 2 hours at room temperature in a dark and humidified container. After that, the sections were washed with PBS and sealed with a coverslip. The slides were analyzed with a fluorescence microscopy (Olympus, Tokyo, Japan). For nuclear staining we used 4',6-diamidino-2-phenylindole (DAPI). To ensure the specificity of the immunoblotting procedure, control experiments were performed in which the corresponding primary antibody was omitted. Under these conditions, no signal was observed.

Statistical analysis
Statistical analysis was carried out by SPSS software 17.0 (IBM Inc., Chicago, IL, USA). After confirming normal distribution with skewness and kurtosis statistic test, independent sample t-test or one-way analysis of variance (ANOVA) followed by the Bonferroni post hoc test used to analyze differences among groups. All data were presented as mean standard deviation (SD). $P < 0.05$ was considered statistically significant.

Results

Cleaved IL-1β, NLRP3 and cleaved caspase-1 were up-regulated in SE rat

We first investigated whether the expression of IL-1β was altered in rat brain after SE which was induced by amygdala stimulation. Total proteins were extracted from the hippocampal regions of SE rats at different time points (including 3, 6, 12, 24 hours following SE) and of shams, and subjected to Western blot analysis. Because there was no significant difference in all detected variables among different sham groups according to our preliminary analysis, the samples of sham group were collected at 12 hours

after the sham operation of amygdala stimulation (without any electrical stimulation). We found that the cleaved IL-1β levels of SE rats were significantly elevated compared to control samples during all time points studied (Figure 1A). In the SE group, cleaved IL-1β levels dramatically increased at 3 hours and reached a maximum at 12 hours (about 4 those of the sham group) after SE ($P < 0.05$; n = 6). Following this maximum, no statistically significant difference was observed in expression level of cleaved IL-1β among rat brains at 24 hours compared with that at 12 hours ($P = 1.000$; n = 6). Next, we analyzed the expression of hippocampal NLRP3

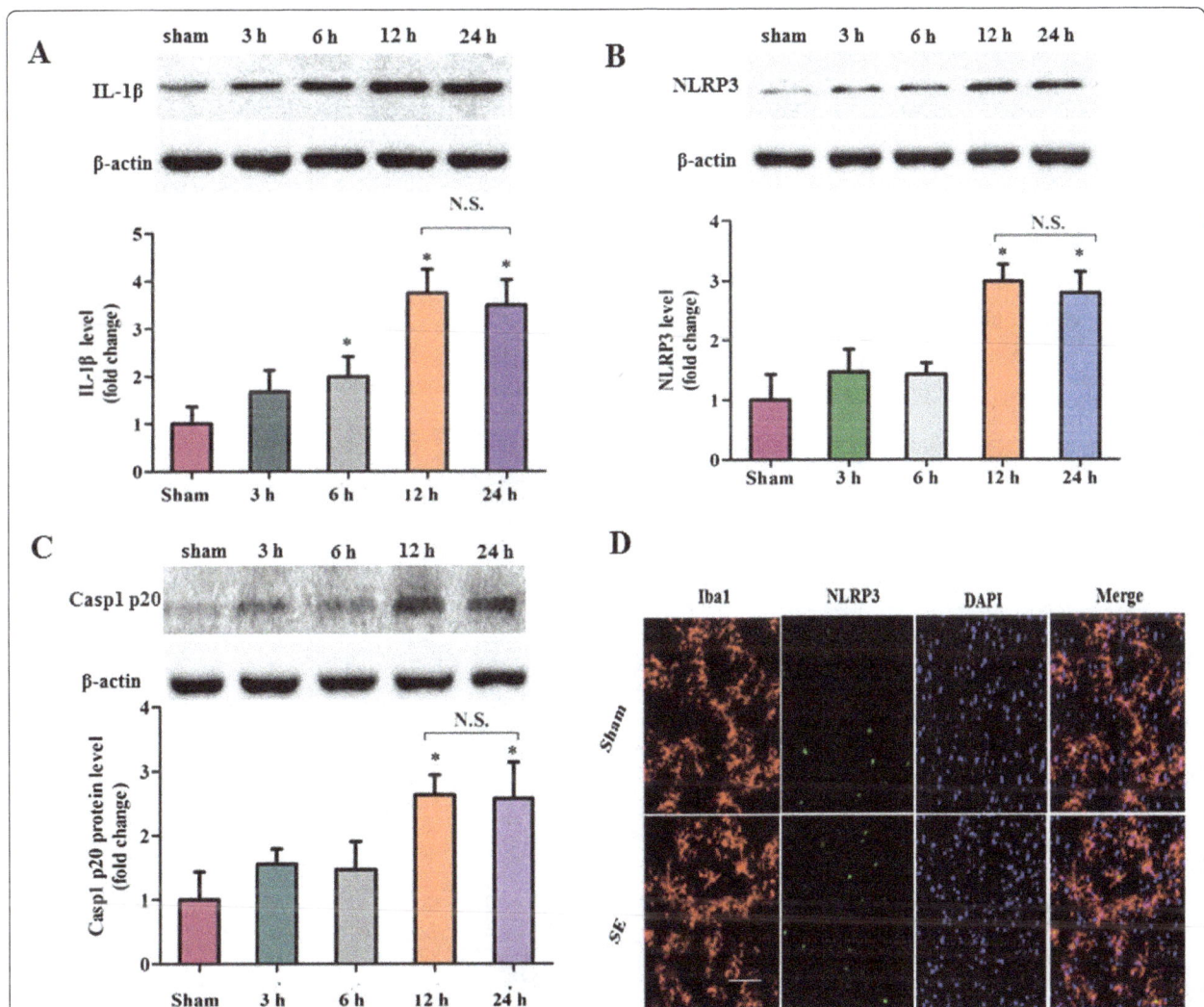

Figure 1 Expression profiles of the nucleotide binding and oligomerization domain-like receptor family pyrin domain-containing 3 (NLRP3) inflammasome components following status epilepticus (SE). (A-C) Western blot assay for the expression profiles of cleaved IL-1β (18 kDa) (A), NLRP3 (106 kDa) (B) and cleaved caspase-1 (20 kDa) (C) in the hippocampus of sham rat at 12 hours following the sham operation of amygdala stimulation (without any electrical stimulation) and SE rat at 3, 6, 12, and 24 hours following amygdala stimulation. Data are expressed as a fold change relative to sham group. n = 6 rat per group and per time point. Error bars represent mean standard deviation. *$P < 0.05$ versus sham control group. NS: not significant versus 12 hours following SE. (D) Representative photographs of immunofluorescence staining for NLRP3 (green) expression in microglia (Iba-1, red) in the hippocampal area 12 hours following SE. Scale bars: 100 μm.

inflammasome components in SE rats. Importantly, the levels of hippocampal NLRP3 protein, and caspase-1 p20, the products of NLRP3 inflammasome activation, were significantly increased at 3 hours and reached a maximum at 12 hours after SE (both $P < 0.05$; n = 6, Figure 1B, C). Accordingly, no significant differences were observed in NLRP3 levels ($P = 1.000$; n = 6), and cleaved caspase-1 levels ($P = 1.000$; n = 6) among rat brains at 24 hours compared with that at 12 hours after SE. Using double immunofluorescence staining to colocalize NLRP3 with microglia marker Iba1, our result further demonstrated the increased expression of NLRP3 in the Iba1-positive microglia of hippocampus at 12 hours following SE (Figure 1D).

Downregulation of NLRP3 by siRNA led to significant reduction in proinflammatory cytokines and cleaved caspase-1 expression levels in SE rat

To directly study the potential impact of increased NLRP3 expression levels on the maturation and secretion of IL-1β in SE rats, we knocked down brain NLRP3 expression in animals before undergoing SE by using *in-vivo* nonviral RNA interference methodology [26]. To evaluate the silencing efficiency of siRNA infusion, the gene expression and protein level of NLRP3 protein were detected by quantitative real-time PCR and Western blotting, respectively. This approach of using NLRP3 siRNA infusion could produce a significant down-regulation of NLRP3 mRNA (by 60%) and protein levels (by 51%) in the

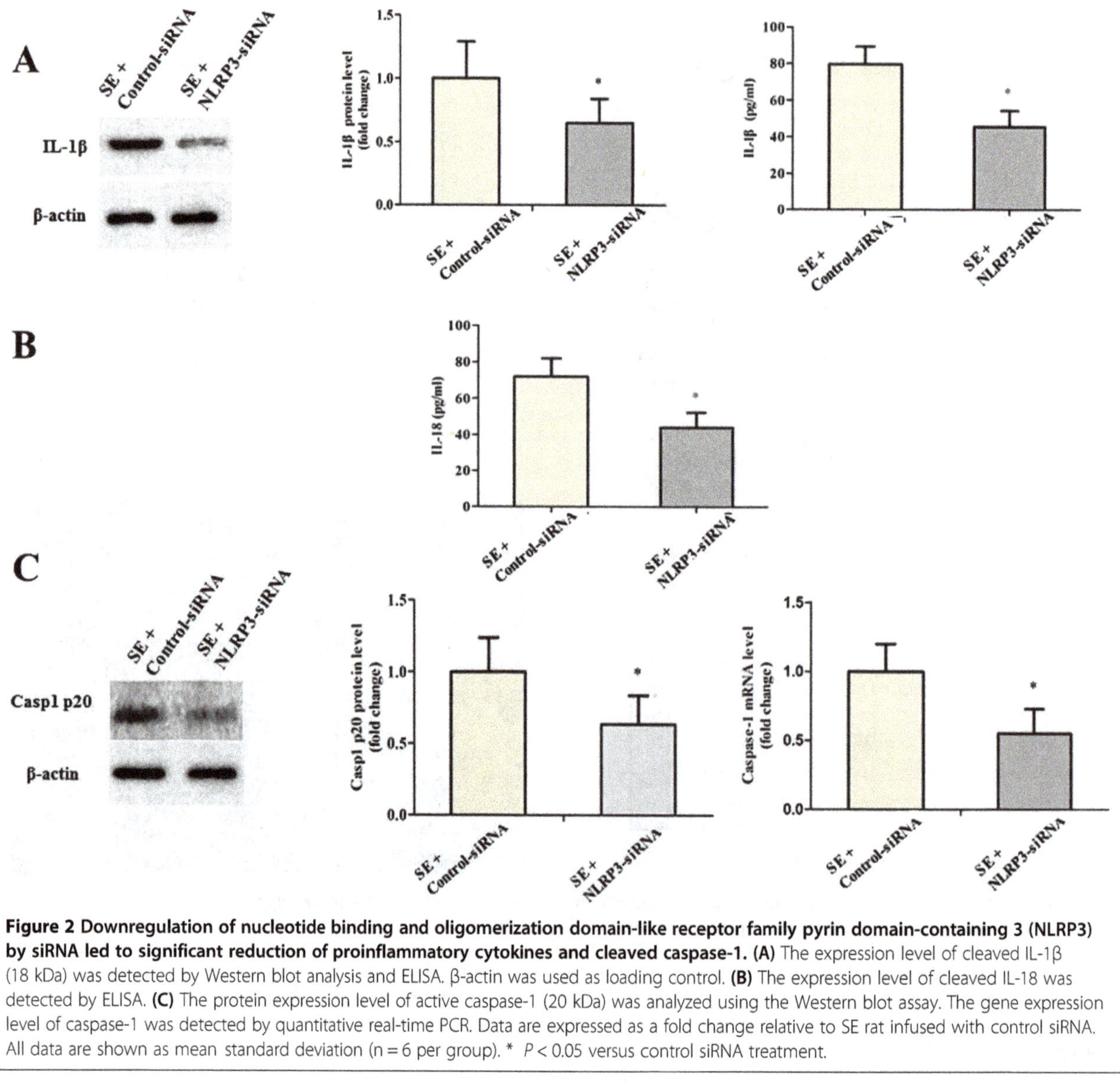

Figure 2 Downregulation of nucleotide binding and oligomerization domain-like receptor family pyrin domain-containing 3 (NLRP3) by siRNA led to significant reduction of proinflammatory cytokines and cleaved caspase-1. (A) The expression level of cleaved IL-1β (18 kDa) was detected by Western blot analysis and ELISA. β-actin was used as loading control. **(B)** The expression level of cleaved IL-18 was detected by ELISA. **(C)** The protein expression level of active caspase-1 (20 kDa) was analyzed using the Western blot assay. The gene expression level of caspase-1 was detected by quantitative real-time PCR. Data are expressed as a fold change relative to SE rat infused with control siRNA. All data are shown as mean standard deviation (n = 6 per group). * $P < 0.05$ versus control siRNA treatment.

brain compared with control siRNA under epileptic conditions (all $P < 0.05$; Additional file 2: Figure S2 A, B). Incidentally, the NLRP3 levels and gene expression between control-siRNA treated and non-siRNA-treated tissues under epileptic conditions or under control conditions do not differ (all $P > 0.05$; n = 6, Additional file 2: Figure S2 A, B, and E), excluding potential indirect siRNA-effects on gene expression or the protein level of NLRP3.

Next, we determined the effects of NLRP3 knock down on SE-induced neuroinflammation. The proinflammatory cytokines expression levels were then assessed by Western blot analysis and ELISA assay. Compared to the control-siRNA group, the elevated expression level of cleaved IL-1β in the brain tissues of SE rats could be inhibited by NLRP3 siRNA treatment ($P < 0.05$; n = 6; Figure 2A). In addition, SE rats infused with NLRP3 siRNA showed a dramatic reduction in brain IL-18 protein levels ($P < 0.05$; n = 6; Figure 2B). We further examined the changes in caspase-1, which has been known to play a central role in the cleavage of IL-1β and IL-18. The gene expression and protein level of caspase-1 protein were detected by quantitative real-time PCR and Western blotting, respectively. As indicated in Figure 2C, the NLRP3 siRNA treatment could reduce the active caspase-1 protein levels and gene expression in SE rats (both $P < 0.05$; n = 6).

Downregulation of NLRP3 by siRNA attenuated the development and severity of spontaneous recurrent seizures following SE

In above work, we demonstrated that NLRP3 mediated IL-1β over-expression and inflammatory signal activation in the SE rat hippocampus. Accumulating data suggest that inflammation may contribute to epileptogenesis

in experimental models as well as in humans. However, whether anti-inflammatory treatments can prevent epileptogenesis remains controversial. Here, we examined the anti-epileptogenic effect of NLRP3 inhibition.

To determine the effect of NLRP3 siRNA on the development and severity of SRS in the chronic phase, SRS were observed from a 4-week video recording, which started 2 weeks after SE. The severity of SRS between siRNA (non or control)-treated SE rats and SE rats do not differ (all $P > 0.05$; n = 18, Additional file 3: Table S1), excluding an effect of siRNA transfection on status severity.

As revealed by Table 1(A), all rats (18/18) in the control siRNA-treated SE group had SRS during the monitoring period, whereas 66% (12/18) of the rats in the NLRP3 siRNA-treated SE group had SRS. The time to development of SRS was longer in the NLRP3 siRNA-treated SE group compared with the control siRNA-treated SE group (SE + control siRNA group: 14.8 5.5 days; SE + NLRP3 siRNA group: 27.5 9.3 days, Table 1A). The mean number of seizures (total number of seizures/number of recording days, calculated separately for each animal) in the control siRNA-treated SE group and NLRP3 siRNA-treated SE group was 7.58 1.09 and 1.34 0.44 seizures/day respectively. NLRP3 siRNA treatment also dramatically reduced the duration of observed seizures during the chronic epileptic phase (control siRNA, 26.62 6.94 seconds; NLRP3 siRNA, 10.48 2.76 seconds, Table 1A). The differences between the two groups were significant ($P < 0.05$, Table 1A).

NLRP3, nucleotide binding and oligomerization domain-like receptor family pyrin domain-containing 3; SE, status epilepticus; sec, seconds; SRS, spontaneous recurrent seizures.

Table 1 The development and severity of animals with spontaneous recurrent seizures (SRS) during the 4-week video monitoring in experimental groups

(A) Results from rats after 6 weeks of treatment with NLRP3 siRNA or control siRNA

	The number of rats developing SRS	The time to development of SRS (days)	The mean number of seizures (seizures/day)	The mean seizure duration (sec/seizure)
Control siRNA + sham	0 (18)	0	0	0
NLRP3 siRNA+ sham	0 (18)	0	0	0
Control siRNA + SE	18 (18)	14.8 5.5	7.58 1.09	26.62 6.94
NLRP3 siRNA+ SE	12 (18)[a]	27.5 9.3 [a]	1.34 0.44 [a]	10.48 2.76 [a]

(B) Results from rats after 6 weeks of treatment with caspase-1 siRNA or control siRNA

	The number of rats developing SRS	The time to development of SRS (days)	The mean number of seizures (seizures/day)	The mean seizure duration (sec/seizure)
Control siRNA + sham	0 (18)	0	0	0
Caspase-1 siRNA + sham	0 (18)	0	0	0
Control siRNA+ SE	17 (18)	16.6 6.1	9.02 1.56	23.67 5.90
Caspase-1 siRNA+ SE	11 (18)[a]	26.8 9.1 [a]	2.40 0.78 [a]	8.21 2.66 [a]

All data are shown as mean ? standard deviation (n = 18 per group). [a]$P < 0.05$ versus control siRNA treatment.

Downregulation of NLRP3 by siRNA inhibited hippocampal neuronal loss in SE rat

If left untreated, SE can cause irreversible brain damage. On this basis, we next investigated the effects of NLRP3 inhibition on neuronal loss in the CA1 and CA3 area of the hippocampus at 6 weeks after SE. Nissl staining was firstly used to detect surviving neurons in the hippocampus. As shown by Figure 3A, a significant increase in neuronal survival rate was noted in CA1 and CA3 regions in the hippocampus of SE rats treated with NLRP3 siRNA compared to the control-siRNA group (CA1: 77.34 5.7% versus 59.57 5.8%, $P < 0.05$; CA3: 83.43 7.3% versus 62.1 6.5%, $P < 0.05$). The TUNEL staining assay was then used. As indicated by Figure 3B, a dramatic reduction of the TUNEL-positive neurons index was observed in CA1 and CA3 regions of the hippocampus of SE rats treated

with NLRP3 siRNA compared to the control-siRNA group (CA1: 11.41 2.4% versus 15.95 3.3%, $P < 0.05$; CA3: 9.9 1.9% versus 13.29 2.8%, $P < 0.05$).

Downregulation of caspase-1 by siRNA alleviated neuroinflammation, spontaneous recurrent seizures and hippocampal neuronal loss following SE

Considering the central role of caspase-1 in the process of IL-1β maturation and secretion, we also successfully knocked down brain caspase-1 in SE rat by in-vivo nonviral RNA interference methodology for 6 weeks (Additional file 2: Figure S2 C, D, and F). We found a significant reduction of IL-1β levels after infused with caspase-1 siRNA ($P < 0.05$; n = 6, Figure 4A). Furthermore, caspase-1 silencing attenuated the development and severity of SRS in the chronic phase ($P < 0.05$; n = 18, Table 1B). A marked

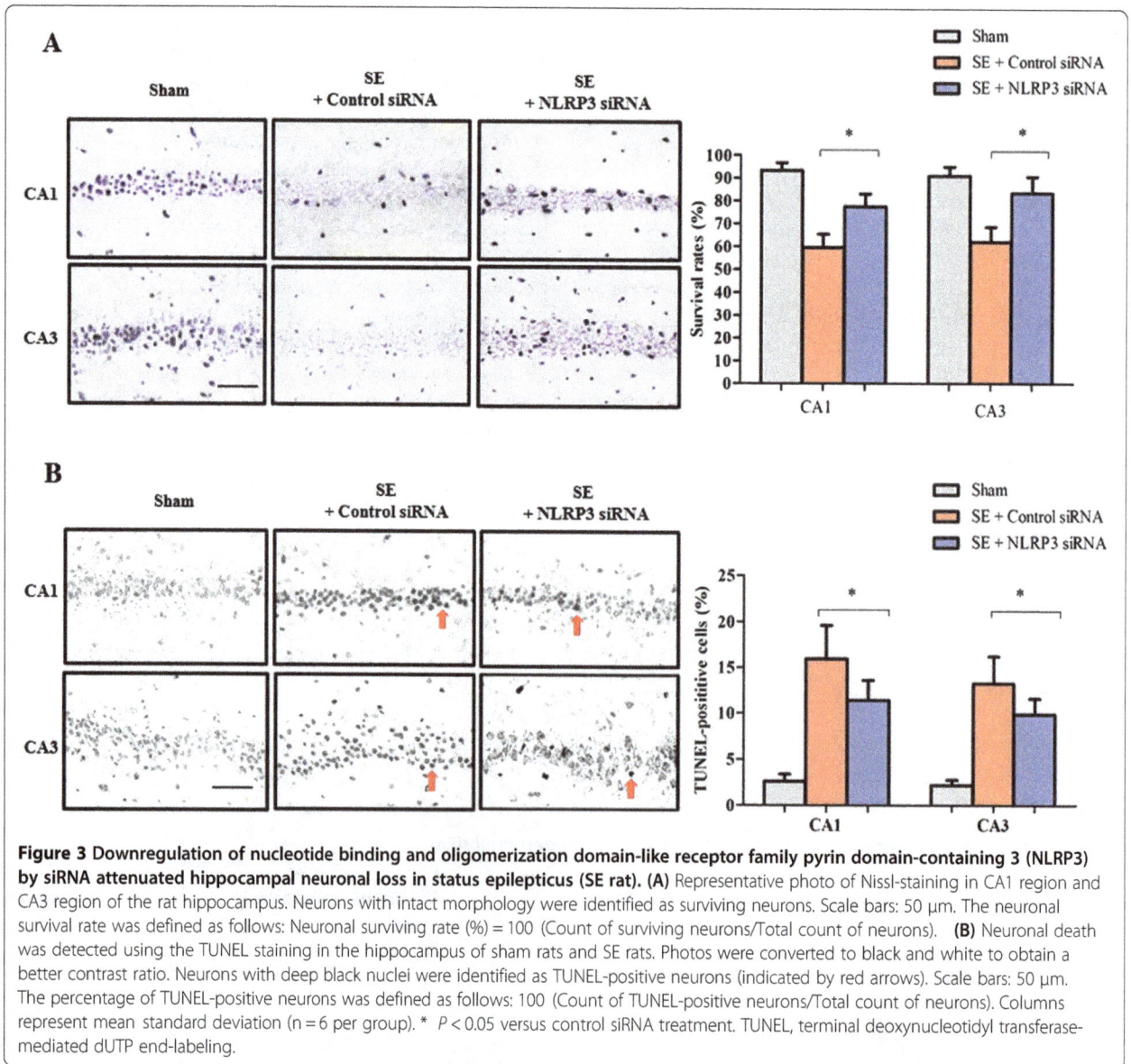

Figure 3 Downregulation of nucleotide binding and oligomerization domain-like receptor family pyrin domain-containing 3 (NLRP3) by siRNA attenuated hippocampal neuronal loss in status epilepticus (SE rat). **(A)** Representative photo of Nissl-staining in CA1 region and CA3 region of the rat hippocampus. Neurons with intact morphology were identified as surviving neurons. Scale bars: 50 μm. The neuronal survival rate was defined as follows: Neuronal surviving rate (%) = 100 (Count of surviving neurons/Total count of neurons). **(B)** Neuronal death was detected using the TUNEL staining in the hippocampus of sham rats and SE rats. Photos were converted to black and white to obtain a better contrast ratio. Neurons with deep black nuclei were identified as TUNEL-positive neurons (indicated by red arrows). Scale bars: 50 μm. The percentage of TUNEL-positive neurons was defined as follows: 100 (Count of TUNEL-positive neurons/Total count of neurons). Columns represent mean standard deviation (n = 6 per group). * $P < 0.05$ versus control siRNA treatment. TUNEL, terminal deoxynucleotidyl transferase-mediated dUTP end-labeling.

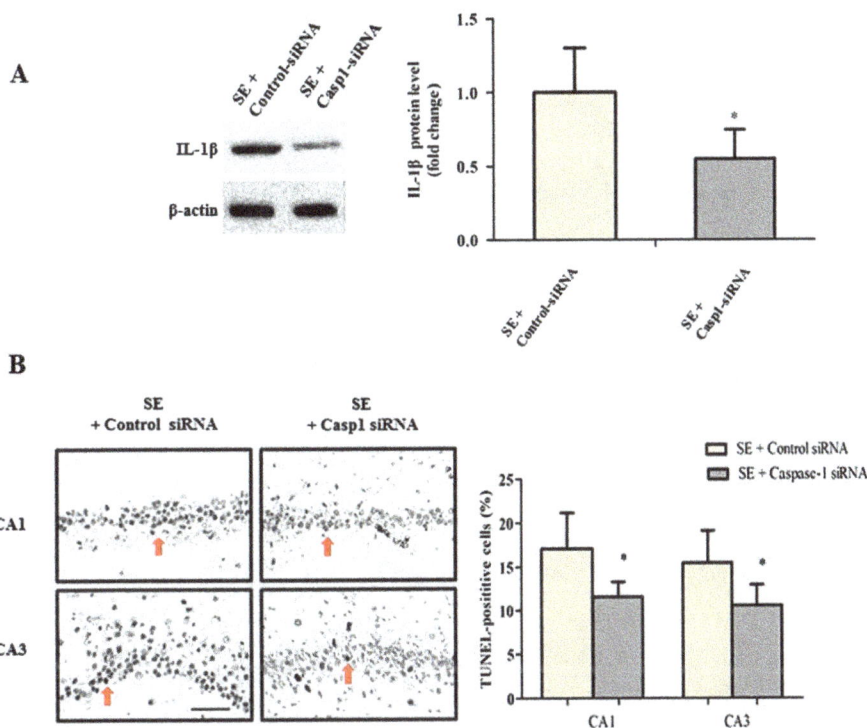

Figure 4 Caspase-1 inhibition ameliorated neuroinflammation and hippocampal neuronal loss in status epilepticus (SE) rat. (A) The expression level of cleaved IL-1β (18 kDa) was detected by Western blot. β-actin was used as loading control. Data are expressed as a fold change relative to SE rat infused with control siRNA. *$P < 0.05$ versus control siRNA treated group. **(B)** Neuronal death was detected using the TUNEL staining in the CA1 and CA3 region of the hippocampus. Photos were converted to black and white to obtain a better contrast ratio. Neurons with deep black nuclei were identified as TUNEL-positive neurons (indicated by red arrows). Scale bars: 50 µm. The percentage of TUNEL-positive neurons was defined as follows: 100 (Count of TUNEL-positive neurons/Total count of neurons). All data are shown as mean standard deviation (n = 6 per group). *$P < 0.05$ versus control siRNA-treated group. TUNEL, terminal deoxynucleotidyl transferase-mediated dUTP end-labeling.

reduction of TUNEL-positive cell densities in the CA1 and CA3 region of the hippocampus in the SE rat treated with caspase-1 siRNA was also observed ($P < 0.05$; n = 6, Figure 4B).

Discussion

Experimental evidence supports a role for inflammatory processes in the precipitation and recurrence of seizures and neuronal damage. The involvement of proinflammatory cytokine IL-1β in the development of seizure is strongly supported by pharmacological and genetic studies in animal models, showing that interference with IL-1β reduces the incidence of SE or attenuates recurrent seizures [8,27,28], whereas its amplification exacerbates seizures [27,29,30] as well as lowers the seizure threshold [15,31]. Accordingly, selective blockade [8,9], or gene deletion [9] of caspase-1, the enzyme which cleaves pro-IL-1β producing the mature and biologically active form of IL-1β, reduces seizures significantly. IL-1β could also affect neuronal excitability at different levels [32 34]. Both hyperexcitability and excitotoxicity are required and need to be sufficient for the contributory effect of IL-1β to the generation of SRS. Moreover, specific cytokines, including

IL-1β, have been shown to contribute to neuronal death [35], perhaps in part via enhanced excitability [5]. Conversely, SE, in the absence of pre-existing or concomitant systemic or CNS inflammation, induce proinflammatory reactions in the brain (that is sterile inflammation), which in turn contribute to seizure recurrence and severity [36].

Therefore, inflammation is both a cause and a consequence of SE. Experimental studies show that once SE develop, it can contribute to perpetuate inflammation in the brain, thus activating a vicious cycle that in turn fosters aberrant hyperexcitability (Figure 5). Thus, a prolonged condition of ongoing seizures with SE can be generated.

Our study was to examine for first time whether the NLRP3 inflammasome is a potential mechanism in neuroinflammation of SE rats. We compared expression of proinflammatory cytokine IL-1β, NLRP3 and caspase-1 in hippocampus from SE rats model evoked by amygdala stimulation to matched sham samples. The present study detected up-regulated IL-1β, NLRP3 and caspase-1 levels within SE samples than controls. All protein levels reach a maximum at 12 hours following SE. Meanwhile, the cellular localization of NLRP3 on microglia in SE rat brain was demonstrated by double immunofluorescence

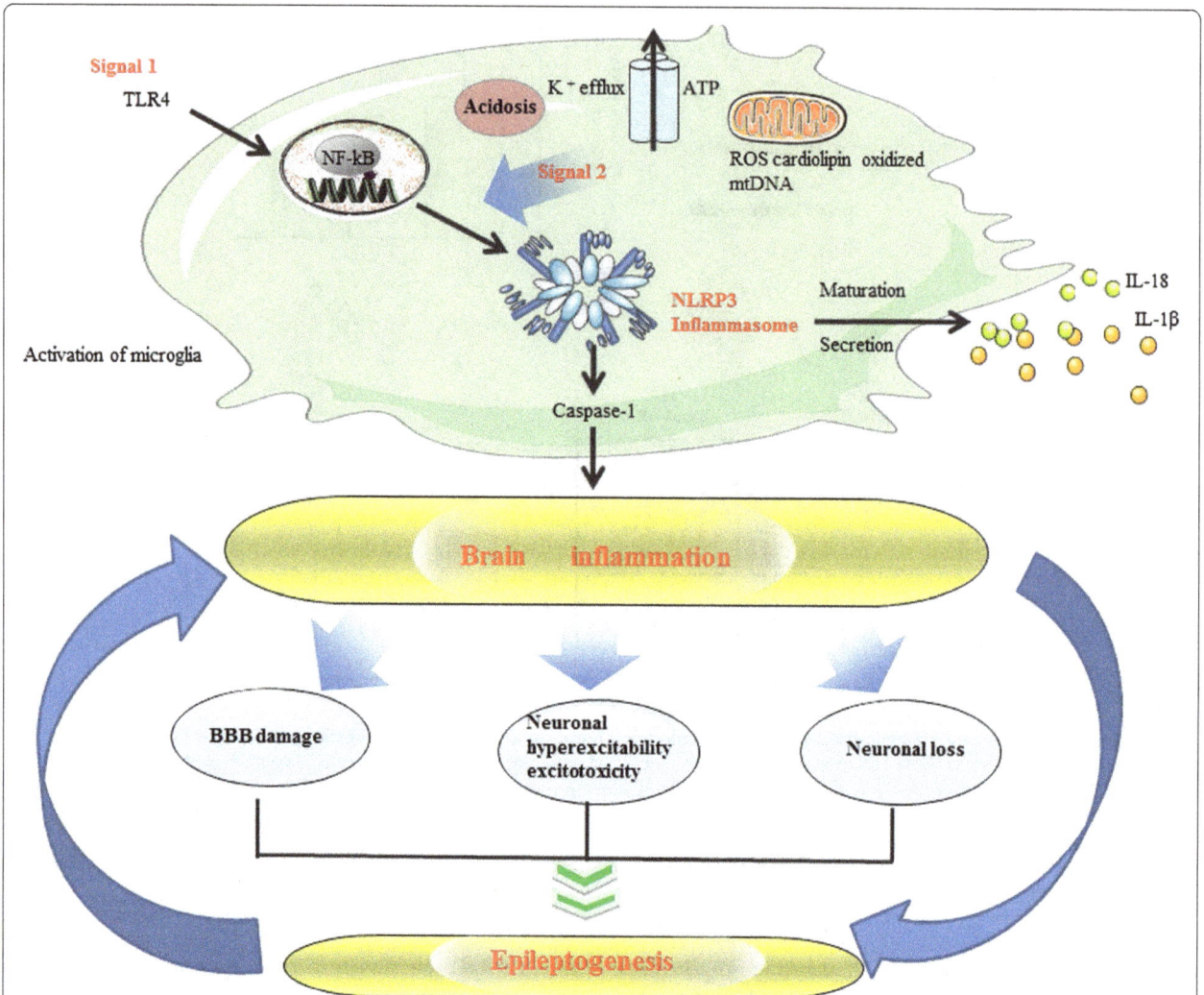

Figure 5 A schematic linking the nucleotide binding and oligomerization domain-like receptor family pyrin domain-containing 3 (NLRP3) inflammasome activation to status epilepticus (SE) pathogenesis. Activation of the NLRP3 inflammasome typically requires a bimodal signaling pathway. A Toll-like receptor (TLR)-dependent priming step activates the NF-κB-dependent transcription of NLRP3 and the pro-forms of the proinflammatory cytokines (which are IL-1β and IL-18). NLRP3-activating stimulation agents provide a second signal in the form of K+ efflux, cytosolic release of mitochondria-derived factors such as reactive oxygen species (ROS), cardiolipin, and oxidized mitochondrial DNA (mtDNA). Note that acidic extracellular pH represents a novel stimulation agent for triggering NLRP3 inflammasome activation. Oligomerization of NLRP3 is followed by recruitment of the adaptor molecule apoptosis-associated speck-like protein containing a caspase recruitment domain (ASC) and the pro-form of caspase-1, leading to the activation (cleavage) of caspase-1. Activated caspase-1 in turn catalyzes the cleavage of IL-1β and IL-18. This event may lead to changes in brain parenchyma such as leakage of the blood-brain barrier (BBB), neuronal hyperexcitability and excitotoxicity as well as neuronal damage which contribute to lowering the threshold for seizure induction and thus to trigger epileptogenesis. Activation of innate immune mechanisms during epileptogenesis can recruit inflammatory cells from the periphery which perpetuate inflammation, thus activating a vicious cycle that in turn fosters aberrant hyperexcitability. The onset of SE can in turn further promote inflammation via the production of proinflammatory cytokines.

staining. Moreover, we knocked down brain NLRP3 expression by implanting mini-osmotic pumps for direct infusion of siRNA to investigate its role on neuroinflammation in the SE rat model. In our study, we found that this approach effectively down-regulated the levels of NLRP3 mRNA and protein in SE rat brain. Meanwhile, compared to non-siRNA-treated SE rat, the treatment with control siRNA did not alter NLRP3 mRNA and protein levels, thus excluding an effect of pump-mediated

infusion on NLRP3 expression levels. For the first time, we revealed that NLRP3 siRNA treatment could significantly reduce proinflammatory cytokine levels and the active caspase-1 expression levels. Meanwhile, NLRP3 inhibition could also suppress SRS, and attenuate hippocampal neuronal loss.

As we know, caspase-1 is a critical pathway by which NLRP3 inflammasomes contribute to the downstream effects. Hence, we also knocked down brain caspase-1 by this *incpyvivo* nonviral RNA interference methodology in SE rats. Consistent biochemical and behavioral results were found between caspase-1 siRNA- and NLRP3 siRNA-treated SE rats, further supporting that NLRP3 exerts the effects of neuroinflammation in rats following SE.

We have determined that the NLRP3 inflammasome contributes to the SE-induced inflammatory response; however, the molecular basis of NLRP3 inflammasome activation in SE-induced brain injury has not been established. Evidence shows that assembly of the NLRP3 inflammasome depends on the activation of NLRP3. This process relies on exposure to whole pathogens, as well as a number of structurally diverse pathogen or danger-associated molecular patterns (PAMPs or DAMPs, respectively) and environmental irritants. It should be noted that, the high concentrations of extracellular ATP and K^+ ions, and the generation of ROS are the most important factors for activating NLRP3 [37]. In fact, all of the factors above can be involved after SE. Additionally, it should be noted that IL-1β may trigger the classical cascade of events which includes the activation of the NF-κB-dependent pathways, thus resulting in the transcription of genes that may contribute to the acquired molecular changes (for example, modifications in ion channels) associated with the epileptogenic process [38]. Interestingly, NLRP3, an important component of the NLRP3 inflammasome complex, is activated by IKKβ/NF-κB [12]. The activation of the NLRP3 inflammasome, results in the secretion of bioactive IL-1β, and subsequently triggers the activation of NF-κB which in turn promotes the secretion of bioactive IL-1β [39]. Local acidosis has been demonstrated at inflammatory sites. Recent data suggest that acidosis is a regulator of inflammatory pathways [16,40]. The study by Edye *et al.* [40] suggested that acidosis promotes alternative DAMP-induced processing of IL-1β independent of caspase-1, and this result seemed to be inconsistent with the findings by Rajamki and colleagues [16], as they found that acidic extracellular pH triggers NLRP3 inflammasome activation and IL-1 secretion in human macrophages (Figure 5).

Conclusions

Our study firstly demonstrates that the expression of the NLRP3 inflammasome was up-regulated in the SE rat. The increase in NLRP3 levels can activate caspase-1 signaling that is responsible for neuroinflammation, neuronal loss and epileptogenesis (Figure 5). Using the pump-mediated *in vivo* infusion of nonviral siRNA to knock down NLRP3 and caspase-1 in the brain of SE rats, our study further indicated that inhibition of the NLRP3 inflammasome may play a neuroprotective role against SE-related neuroinflammation and neuronal damage.

Additional files

Additional file 1: Figure S1. Scheme of the experimental design and the main experimental protocol. The rats were randomly divided into five groups: sham group, SE group, control siRNA + SE group, NLRP3 siRNA + SE group, and caspase-1 siRNA + SE group. siRNA, small interfering RNA; SE, status epilepticus; TUNEL assay, terminal deoxynucleotidyl transferase-mediated dUTP end-labeling assay; Elisa, enzyme-linked immunosorbent assay; qRT-PCR, quantitative real-time PCR.

Additional file 2: Figure S2. Small interfering RNA (siRNA) targeting NLRP3 or caspase-1 effectively downregulated NLRP3 or caspase-1 in status epilepticus (SE) rat. (A) Messenger RNA levels of NLRP3 in brain of SE rats after 6-week infusion of artificial cerebrospinal fluid (aCSF), control siRNA or NLRP3 siRNA. (B) Protein levels of NLRP3 in brain of SE rats after 6-week infusion of artificial cerebrospinal fluid (aCSF), control siRNA, or NLRP3 siRNA. (C) Messenger RNA levels of caspase-1 in brain of SE rats after 6-week infusion of aCSF, control siRNA, or caspase-1 siRNA. (D) Protein levels of caspase-1 in brain of SE rats after 6-week infusion of aCSF, control siRNA or caspase-1 siRNA. Data are expressed as a fold change relative to sham group. Columns represent mean standard deviation. n = 6 rats per group. *$P < 0.05$ versus control siRNA treatment. (E) Protein levels of NLRP3 in brain of sham rats after 6-week infusion of control siRNA, or aCSF. (F) Protein levels of caspase-1 in brain of sham rats after 6-week infusion of control siRNA oraCSF. Data are expressed as a fold change relative to sham group. Columns represent mean standard deviation. n = 6 rats per group. NS: not significant versus sham rats.

Additional file 3: Table S1. Pump-mediated infusion of small interfering RNA (siRNA) prior to status epilepticus (SE) induction has no potential effects directly on the development and severity of spontaneous recurrent seizures (SRS).

Abbreviations

SE: status epilepticus; CNS: central nervous system; NLRP3: nucleotide binding and oligomerization domain-like receptor family pyrin domain-containing 3; ASC: apoptosis-associated speck-like protein containing a caspase recruitment domain; siRNA: small interfering RNA; SDS: sodium dodecyl sulfate; PVDF: polyvinylidene fluoride; TRITC: tetramethylrhodamine; SRS: spontaneous recurrent seizures; PCR: polymerase chain reaction; ELISA: enzyme linked immunosorbent assay; TUNEL: terminal deoxynucleotidyl transferase-mediated dUTP end-labeling; RIPA: radio immunoprecipitation assay; EEG: Electroencephalogram; Iba1: ionized calcium binding adaptor molecule 1; BBB: blood brain barrier.

Competing interests

The authors declare that they have no competing interests.

Authors contributions

XFM, LT, and JTY were the main researchers in this study, and contributed to writing the manuscript. XFM, MML, MST, TJ, HFW and CCT planned the study, wrote the protocol, were involved in the genetic and clinical aspects of data analyses, and revised the manuscript. All authors read and approved the final manuscript for publication.

Acknowledgments

This work was supported by grants from the National Natural Science Foundation of China to LT (81171209, 81371400) and JTY (81000544), grants from the Shandong Provincial Natural Science Foundation to LT (ZR2011HZ001) and JTY (ZR2010HQ004), and the Medicine and Health Science Technology Development Project of Shandong Province to LT (2011WSA02018) and JTY (2011WSA02020).

Author details

[1]Department of Neurology, Qingdao Municipal Hospital, School of Medicine, Qingdao University, Qingdao, PR China. [2]Department of Neurology, Qingdao Municipal Hospital, Nanjing Medical University, Nanjing, PR China. [3]Department of Neurology, Qingdao Municipal Hospital, College of Medicine and Pharmaceutics, Ocean University of China, Qingdao, PR China. [4]Department of Neurology, Nanjing First Hospital, Nanjing Medical University,

Nanjing, PR China. [5]Department of Neurology, Memory and Aging Center, University of California, San Francisco, CA, USA.

References

1. Gastaut H: Clinical and electroencephalographical classification of epileptic seizures. *Epilepsia* 1970, 11:102 113.
2. Vezzani A, French J, Bartfai T, Baram TZ: The role of inflammation in epilepsy. *Nat Rev Neurol* 2011, 7:31 40.
3. Dube C, Vezzani A, Behrens M, Bartfai T, Baram TZ: Interleukin-1beta contributes to the generation of experimental febrile seizures. *Ann Neurol* 2005, 57:152 155.
4. Vezzani A, Friedman A, Dingledine RJ: The role of inflammation in epileptogenesis. *Neuropharmacology* 2013, 69:16 24.
5. Vezzani A, Baram TZ: New roles for interleukin-1 Beta in the mechanisms of epilepsy. *Epilepsy Curr* 2007, 7:45 50.
6. Gomez CD, Buijs RM, Sitges M: The anti-seizure drugs vinpocetine and carbamazepine, but not valproic acid, reduce inflammatory IL-1beta and TNF-alpha expression in rat hippocampus. *J Neurochem* 2014, 130:770 779.
7. Jeon KI, Xu X, Aizawa T, Lim JH, Jono H, Kwon DS, Abe J, Berk BC, Li JD, Yan C: Vinpocetine inhibits NF-kappaB-dependent inflammation via an IKK-dependent but PDE-independent mechanism. *Proc Natl Acad Sci U S A* 2010, 107:9795 9800.
8. Maroso M, Balosso S, Ravizza T, Iori V, Wright CI, French J, Vezzani A: Interleukin-1beta biosynthesis inhibition reduces acute seizures and drug resistant chronic epileptic activity in mice. *Neurotherapeutics* 2011, 8:304 315.
9. Ravizza T, Lucas SM, Balosso S, Bernardino L, Ku G, Noe F, Malva J, Randle JC, Allan S, Vezzani A: Inactivation of caspase-1 in rodent brain: a novel anticonvulsive strategy. *Epilepsia* 2006, 47:1160 1168.
10. Haneklaus M, O'Neill LA, Coll RC: Modulatory mechanisms controlling the NLRP3 inflammasome in inflammation: recent developments. *Curr Opin Immunol* 2013, 25:40 45.
11. Cassel SL, Sutterwala FS: Sterile inflammatory responses mediated by the NLRP3 inflammasome. *Eur J Immunol* 2010, 40:607 611.
12. Bauernfeind FG, Horvath G, Stutz A, Alnemri ES, MacDonald K, Speert D, Fernandes-Alnemri T, Wu J, Monks BG, Fitzgerald KA, Hornung V, Latz E: Cutting edge: NF-kappaB activating pattern recognition and cytokine receptors license NLRP3 inflammasome activation by regulating NLRP3 expression. *J Immunol* 2009, 183:787 791.
13. Liu HD, Li W, Chen ZR, Hu YC, Zhang DD, Shen W, Zhou ML, Zhu L, Hang CH: Expression of the NLRP3 inflammasome in cerebral cortex after traumatic brain injury in a rat model. *Neurochem Res* 2013, 38:2072 2083.
14. Ransohoff RM, Brown MA: Innate immunity in the central nervous system. *J Clin Invest* 2012, 122:1164 1171.
15. Jha S, Srivastava SY, Brickey WJ, Iocca H, Toews A, Morrison JP, Chen VS, Gris D, Matsushima GK, Ting JP: The inflammasome sensor, NLRP3, regulates CNS inflammation and demyelination via caspase-1 and interleukin-18. *J Neurosci* 2010, 30:15811 15820.
16. Rajamaki K, Nordstrom T, Nurmi K, Akerman KE, Kovanen PT, Oorni K, Eklund KK: Extracellular acidosis is a novel danger signal alerting innate immunity via the NLRP3 inflammasome. *J Biol Chem* 2013, 288:13410 13419.
17. Fann DY, Lee SY, Manzanero S, Chunduri P, Sobey CG, Arumugam TV: Pathogenesis of acute stroke and the role of inflammasomes. *Ageing Res Rev* 2013, 12:941 966.
18. Schroder K, Tschopp J: The inflammasomes. *Cell* 2010, 140:821 832.
19. Wasterlain CG, Fujikawa DG, Penix L, Sankar R: Pathophysiological mechanisms of brain damage from status epilepticus. *Epilepsia* 1993, 34 (Suppl 1):S37 S53.
20. Kim JE, Yeo SI, Ryu HJ, Kim MJ, Kim DS, Jo SM, Kang TC: Astroglial loss and edema formation in the rat piriform cortex and hippocampus following pilocarpine-induced status epilepticus. *J Comp Neurol* 2010, 518:4612 4628.
21. Sheen SH, Kim JE, Ryu HJ, Yang Y, Choi KC, Kang TC: Decrease in dystrophin expression prior to disruption of brain-blood barrier within the rat piriform cortex following status epilepticus. *Brain Res* 2011, 1369:173 183.
22. Chen JW, Wasterlain CG: Status epilepticus: pathophysiology and management in adults. *Lancet Neurol* 2006, 5:246 256.
23. Bjorling DE, Wang Z-Y: Estrogen and neuroinflammation. *Urology* 2001, 57:40 46.
24. Sun Z, Yu JT, Jiang T, Li MM, Tan L, Zhang Q: Genome-wide microRNA profiling of rat hippocampus after status epilepticus induced by amygdala stimulation identifies modulators of neuronal apoptosis. *PLoS One* 2013, 8:e78375.
25. Racine RJ: Modification of seizure activity by electrical stimulation. *II Motor seizure Electroencephalogr Clin Neurophysiol* 1972, 32:281 294.
26. Thakker DR, Hoyer D, Cryan JF: Interfering with the brain: use of RNA interference for understanding the pathophysiology of psychiatric and neurological disorders. *Pharmacol Ther* 2006, 109:413 438.
27. Vezzani A, Moneta D, Conti M, Richichi C, Ravizza T, De Luigi A, De Simoni MG, Sperk G, Andell-Jonsson S, Lundkvist J, Iverfeldt K, Bartfai T: Powerful anticonvulsant action of IL-1 receptor antagonist on intracerebral injection and astrocytic overexpression in mice. *Proc Natl Acad Sci U S A* 2000, 97:11534 11539.
28. Marchi N, Fan Q, Ghosh C, Fazio V, Bertolini F, Betto G, Batra A, Carlton E, Najm I, Granata T, Janigro D: Antagonism of peripheral inflammation reduces the severity of status epilepticus. *Neurobiol Dis* 2009, 33:171 181.
29. Balosso S, Maroso M, Sanchez-Alavez M, Ravizza T, Frasca A, Bartfai T, Vezzani A: A novel non-transcriptional pathway mediates the proconvulsive effects of interleukin-1beta. *Brain* 2008, 131:3256 3265.
30. Vezzani A, Conti M, De Luigi A, Ravizza T, Moneta D, Marchesi F, De Simoni MG: Interleukin-1beta immunoreactivity and microglia are enhanced in the rat hippocampus by focal kainate application: functional evidence for enhancement of electrographic seizures. *J Neurosci* 1999, 19:5054 5065.
31. Heida JG, Moshe SL, Pittman QJ: The role of interleukin-1beta in febrile seizures. *Brain Dev* 2009, 31:388 393.
32. Hu S, Sheng WS, Ehrlich LC, Peterson PK, Chao CC: Cytokine effects on glutamate uptake by human astrocytes. *Neuroimmunomodulation* 2000, 7:153 159.
33. Bezzi P, Domercq M, Brambilla L, Galli R, Schols D, De Clercq E, Vescovi A, Bagetta G, Kollias G, Meldolesi J, Volterra A: CXCR4-activated astrocyte glutamate release via TNFalpha: amplification by microglia triggers neurotoxicity. *Nat Neurosci* 2001, 4:702 710.
34. Wang S, Cheng Q, Malik S, Yang J: Interleukin-1beta inhibits gamma-aminobutyric acid type A (GABA(A)) receptor current in cultured hippocampal neurons. *J Pharmacol Exp Ther* 2000, 292:497 504.
35. Loscher W: Animal models of epilepsy for the development of antiepileptogenic and disease-modifying drugs. A comparison of the pharmacology of kindling and post-status epilepticus models of temporal lobe epilepsy. *Epilepsy Res* 2002, 50:105 123.
36. Vezzani A, Balosso S, Ravizza T: The role of cytokines in the pathophysiology of epilepsy. *Brain Behav Immun* 2008, 22:797 803.
37. Walsh JG, Muruve DA, Power C: Inflammasomes in the CNS. *Nat Rev Neurosci* 2014, 15:84 97.
38. Pitkanen A, Sutula TP: Is epilepsy a progressive disorder? Prospects for new therapeutic approaches in temporal-lobe epilepsy. *Lancet Neurol* 2002, 1:173 181.
39. Grant RW, Dixit VD: Mechanisms of disease: inflammasome activation and the development of type 2 diabetes. *Front Immunol* 2013, 4:50.
40. Edye ME, Lopez-Castejon G, Allan SM, Brough D: Acidosis drives damage-associated molecular pattern (DAMP)-induced interleukin-1 secretion via a caspase-1-independent pathway. *J Biol Chem* 2013, 288:30485 30494.

11

Increased expression of the chemokines CXCL1 and MIP-1α by resident brain cells precedes neutrophil infiltration in the brain following prolonged soman-induced status epilepticus in rats

Erik A Johnson[*], Thuy L Dao, Michelle A Guignet, Claire E Geddes, Andrew I Koemeter-Cox and Robert K Kan

Abstract

Background: Exposure to the nerve agent soman (GD) causes neuronal cell death and impaired behavioral function dependent on the induction of status epilepticus (SE). Little is known about the maturation of this pathological process, though neuroinflammation and infiltration of neutrophils are prominent features. The purpose of this study is to quantify the regional and temporal progression of early chemotactic signals, describe the cellular expression of these factors and the relationship between expression and neutrophil infiltration in damaged brain using a rat GD seizure model.

Methods: Protein levels of 4 chemokines responsible for neutrophil infiltration and activation were quantified up to 72 hours in multiple brain regions (i.e. piriform cortex, hippocampus and thalamus) following SE onset using multiplex bead immunoassays. Chemokines with significantly increased protein levels were localized to resident brain cells (i.e. neurons, astrocytes, microglia and endothelial cells). Lastly, neutrophil infiltration into these brain regions was quantified and correlated to the expression of these chemokines.

Results: We observed significant concentration increases for CXCL1 and MIP-1α after seizure onset. CXCL1 expression originated from neurons and endothelial cells while MIP-1α was expressed by neurons and microglia. Lastly, the expression of these chemokines directly preceded and positively correlated with significant neutrophil infiltration in the brain. These data suggest that following GD-induced SE, a strong chemotactic response originating from various brain cells, recruits circulating neutrophils to the injured brain.

Conclusions: A strong induction of neutrophil attractant chemokines occurs following GD-induced SE resulting in neutrophil influx into injured brain tissues. This process may play a key role in the progressive secondary brain pathology observed in this model though further study is warranted.

Background

Soman (pinacolyl methylphosphonofluoridate, GD) is a G-series nerve agent that rapidly and irreversibly binds to acetylcholinesterase, causing excess acetylcholine accumulation in the central and peripheral nervous sys-

tems, which results in cholinergic crisis. A consequence of this cholinergic crisis is rapid induction of status epilepticus (SE) that can continue unabated for many hours [1]. The duration of this seizure activity increases the magnitude of neuropathology [2,3] with the hippocampus, amygdala, thalamus and piriform cortex being the most severely affected [4,5]. Although initial injury occurs rapidly, a robust neuroinflammatory response can exacerbate damage to the brain over time. Neuroinflammation is a key factor in pathology development in

* Correspondence: erik.a.johnson1@us.army.mil
Research Division, Pharmacology Branch, US Army Medical Research Institute of Chemical Defense (USAMRICD), Aberdeen Proving Ground, MD 21010, USA

other models of SE [6,7] as well as following nerve agent-induced seizure [8-11].

An early component of neuroinflammation is the recruitment and activation of circulating neutrophils to areas of injury. Neutrophil infiltration is an important step in the development of neuropathology following seizure [6,12,13]. Once through the blood-brain barrier, the respiratory burst of neutrophils can exacerbate the initial injury through indiscriminate protease damage to surrounding healthy tissues [14]. Infiltrating neutrophils are directed to and activated in injured brain regions by chemokines. For example, the chemokine (C-X-C motif) ligand 1 (CXCL1 or GRO KC) directs neutrophils to injured tissues [15] and propagates the neuroinflammatory response by inducing the synthesis of acute phase response cytokines interleukin (IL)-1, IL-6 and tumor necrosis factor-α in those cells [16]. Similarly, macrophage inflammatory protein (MIP)-1α functions to recruit and activate granulocytes (including neutrophils) in damaged brain regions [17-19]. Because inflammatory chemokines are up-regulated in many SE models [20-22], these factors likely play a role in this model as well.

Most studies of neuroinflammation following seizurogenic nerve agent exposure have centered on transcript changes [8,23,24] or limited protein changes [10]. Recently, however, we have reported the upregulation of multiple acute phase cytokines in this GD model [11]. In this study, we quantified the protein levels of the neutrophil chemoattractant and activating factors CXCL1, MIP-1α, granulocyte colony stimulating factor (G-CSF) and granulocyte-macrophage colony stimulating factor (GM-CSF), using multiplex immunoassays in brain tissue lysates following GD exposure up to 72 hours after SE onset. Additionally, cell-specific chemokine expression and neutrophil infiltration were investigated in damaged brain regions (i.e. piriform cortex, hippocampus and thalamus). CXCL1 and MIP-1α concentrations were significantly increased in all three brain regions investigated, while no change was observed in G-CSF or GM-CSF. CXCL1 and MIP-1α predominantly localized to neurons and either endothelial cells (CXCL1) or microglia (MIP-1α). Expression also preceded and positively correlated to significant neutrophil infiltration in these brain regions. These data are the first to show upregulation and cellular expression of chemokines and the ensuing influx of neutrophils in damaged brain regions following GD-induced SE.

Methods
GD seizure model
This model has been described previously [11,25]. Briefly, adult male Sprague-Dawley rats (Charles River Laboratories, Wilmington, MA; CRL: CD[SD]-BR, 250 - 350 g) were treated with HI-6 dichloride (1-(((4-

(aminocarbonyl)pyridinio) methoxy)methyl)-2-((hydroxyimino)methyl)pyridinium dichloride)(BN44621, Starks Associates, Buffalo, NY; 125 mg/kg, i.p.) 30 minutes prior to GD administration and with atropine methyl nitrate (AMN, Sigma-Aldrich, St. Louis, MO; 2.0 mg/kg, i.m.) 1 minute after GD administration. Vehicle control animals received HI-6, AMN and saline, while naïve animals received no injections. GD (GD-U-2323-CTF-N, purity 98.8 wt%) was diluted in saline at the United States Army Medical Research Institute of Chemical Defense (USAMRICD) and administered subcutaneously (1.6 LD$_{50}$ = 180 µg/kg). The experimental protocol was approved by the Animal Care and Use Committee at USAMRICD, and all procedures were conducted in accordance with the principles stated in the Guide for the Care and Use of Laboratory Animals (National Research Council, 1996), and the Animal Welfare Act of 1966 (P.L. 89-544), as amended. The animal care program at this institute is fully accredited by the Association for Assessment and Accreditation of Laboratory Animal Care International.

Multiplex bead array immunoassay
As previously described [11], piriform cortex, hippocampus and thalamus brain tissue samples were procured from experimental and vehicle control animals at 0.5, 1, 3, 6, 12, 24, 48 or 72 hours after onset of convulsions. Tissue lysates were produced by first rinsing the excised tissue with cold PBS followed by snap freezing in liquid nitrogen. A ratio of 1 ml ice-cold triple detergent lysis buffer containing a Complete™ protease inhibitor cocktail (Roche Biochemicals, Indianapolis, IN) to 50 mg of frozen tissue was used for homogenization. Two 30 sec pulses on a mini Beadbeater (Biospec Products Inc., Bartlesville, OK) using 3.2 mm stainless steel beads were used to homogenize the tissue. Samples were centrifuged at 8000 × g for 5 minutes to separate the lysate from the tissue pellet. Rat cytokine multiplex bead immunoassay kits were used to quantify the concentrations of CXCL1 (GRO KC), MIP-1α, G-CSF and GM-CSF (LINCO Research, St. Charles, MO). Individual standard curves were generated in duplicate using the supplied reference chemokine concentrations according to the manufacturer's instructions. A volume of 25 µl of sample (94 ± 8 µg protein) per well, assayed in duplicate, was used for data generation. The plate was read on a Bioplex™ 100 instrument (Bio-Rad Laboratories, Hercules, CA) and analyzed with either BioRad or STaRStation software (Applied Cytometry, Sacramento, CA). Values that were calculated by the assay to be below the minimum detectable concentration (MinDC) for that particular analyte were conservatively estimated to be the MinDC value minus 0.01 pg/ml for statistical analysis. The number of replicates for the experimental

samples are as follows: piriform cortex, n = 6 for each time point and naïve; hippocampus, n = 6 for each time point except for naïve (n = 5), 6 hr (n = 5) and 24 hr (n = 7); and thalamus, n = 5 for each time point and naïve except for 0.5 hr (n = 6), 6 hr (n = 4), 12 hr (n = 3), 24 hr (n = 6) and 48 hr (n = 6). Time matched vehicle controls (n = 3 per time point) were analyzed individually and condensed into a single vehicle control comparison group when no significant statistical difference was found between these samples over time by analyte or brain region.

Immunohistochemistry (IHC)

Separate from the animals used in the multiplex bead array immunoassay, experimental, vehicle control and naïve animals were deeply anesthetized and perfused with isotonic saline followed by 4% paraformaldehyde via cardiac puncture. Brains were processed and sectioned at 40 microns as previously described [11]. The 12 hour time point was selected based on the peak expression times of the analytes from the multiplex assays. Free float fluorescent IHC labeling was conducted as previously described [26]. The antibodies used were as follows: rabbit anti-Gro α (CXCL1) (1:100; ab9772), rabbit anti-MIP-1α (1:500, ab9781) and mouse anti-rat endothelial cell antigen (RECA,1:1000; ab9774) from Abcam (Cambridge, MA), mouse anti-NeuN to label neurons (1:1000; MAB377) and mouse anti-CD11b to label microglia and macrophages (1:1000; CBL1512) from Chemicon (Temecula, CA), and mouse anti-GFAP to label astrocytes (1:1000; MS-280-P) from NeoMarkers (Fremont, CA). Alexafluor™ fluorescent-tagged secondary and tertiary antibodies (Molecular Probes, Eugene, OR) were used for visualization. Tissue sections labeled with only secondary and tertiary antibodies were used as controls. Sections were viewed and digitally captured with an Olympus BX51 microscope equipped with an Olympus DP-70 high-resolution color CCD digital camera (Opelco, Dulles, VA). An Olympus BX61 equipped with a DSU spinning disk confocal system and DP-70 CCD camera and a Zeiss LSM 700 confocal microscope were used for subsequent IHC micrographs to confirm same cell co-localization. Images of 40-μm tissues were acquired using a z step interval of 1 μm and analyzed using Slidebook™ (Olympus) or Zen 2009 (Zeiss) software. Publication images were compiled using Adobe Photoshop CS digital image software. Color levels and background labeling were reduced and evened using the "levels" tool. All input levels (0-255) were normalized in the RGB channel as follows: highlight input levels were set at the peak of the image histogram, midtone levels were set at 0.8 and shadow levels were set either at the edge of the histogram closest to 255 or at 180, whichever was greater. This technique was successful at reducing background while not oversaturating specific labeling. For all time points, n = 3.

Quantitative Stereology

Sections were labeled with Mayer's hematoxylin/eosin-phloxine stain. Infiltrating neutrophils were visually identified by the user and quantified within the piriform cortex, hippocampus and thalamus using Stereologer 2000 software (Stereology Resource Center, Chester, MD) on an Olympus BX51 microscope equipped with an IK-C44H CCD Toshiba camera (Imaging Planet, Goleta, CA). Four to eight sections from tissue slabs of approximately 1440 to 3300 μm in length were used for counting in each case. Estimates used the optical fractionator method. For each tissue section analyzed, section thickness was assessed empirically and guard zones 2 μm thick were used at the top and bottom of each section. The tissue regions were outlined using 10 × magnification, and cells were counted using 40 × magnification. Approximately 50% of the outlined region was analyzed using a systematic random sampling design with a counting frame size of 175 μm and a disector height of 7 μm. The coefficients of error (CE) were calculated by the software and maximum CE was set at 0.1600.

Statistical Analysis

Immunoassay data were evaluated by one-way ANOVA with a post-hoc Dunnett's analysis and expressed in pg/ml. Neutrophil stereology data were evaluated by one-way ANOVA with a post-hoc Newman-Kuel analysis and expressed as cells/mm³. A Pearson's correlation coefficient using a one measurement time lag between CXCL1 or MIP-1α concentration and neutrophil infiltration was also calculated. The one measurement time lag was used due to the many downstream molecular events that occur following neutrophil exposure to these chemokines that allow the neutrophil to traverse the vasculature into the injured tissue. Values are expressed as mean ± SEM. Differences were considered significant at the level of $p \leq 0.05$.

Results

Brain concentrations of CXCL1 significantly increase in response to GD-induced SE

Temporal and regional changes in CXCL1, MIP-1α, G-CSF and GM-CSF protein concentrations were determined using a bead-based multiplex immunoassay on tissue lysates from the piriform cortex, hippocampus and thalamus. CXCL1 and MIP-1α significantly increased in all brain regions investigated. G-CSF and GM-CSF concentrations did not significantly change and were not analyzed further (data not shown).

CXCL1 concentrations significantly increased in all three brain regions (Figure 1). The highest concentrations were in the hippocampus, where concentrations significantly increased by 6 hours (4674 ± 1504 pg/ml) and peaked by 12 hours (8441 ± 2152 pg/ml vs. 58 ± 6 pg/ml in vehicle controls) following GD-induced SE. In the piriform cortex, CXCL1 levels peaked at 6 hours (1164 ± 195 pg/ml) and remained significantly elevated up to 24 hours (501 ± 176 pg/ml) compared to vehicle controls (49 ± 9 pg/ml). In the thalamus, CXCL1 concentration became significant at 12 hours compared to controls (4571 ± 643 pg/ml vs. 50 ± 3 pg/ml).

CXCL1 is expressed by neurons and endothelial cells
Twelve hours following GD-induced SE, CXCL1 immunolabeling was present in the piriform cortex (Figure 2A, left), hippocampus (dentate gyrus shown; Figure 2B, left) and thalamus (Figure 2C, left), while CXCL1 labeling was absent in vehicle controls in the same regions (Figure 2A, B, &2C, right). Specific labeling was also absent in secondary only controls at the 12-hour time point (Figure 2D) and in vehicle controls (Figure 2E) as exemplified by the piriform cortex. In the piriform cortex, CXCL1-positive cells were found predominantly in layer II but also in layer III. In the hippocampus, CXCL1-positive cells were found primarily in the granular layer of the dentate gyrus (GrDG) and the CA3 pyramidal layer closest to the dentate gyrus. CXCL1-positive cells were also found in the laterodorsal and lateral posterior nuclei of the thalamus. To identify these cells, sections were co-labeled with antibodies specific for neurons, astrocytes, microglia and endothelial cells and for CXCL1. CXCL1 immunoreactivity was found in

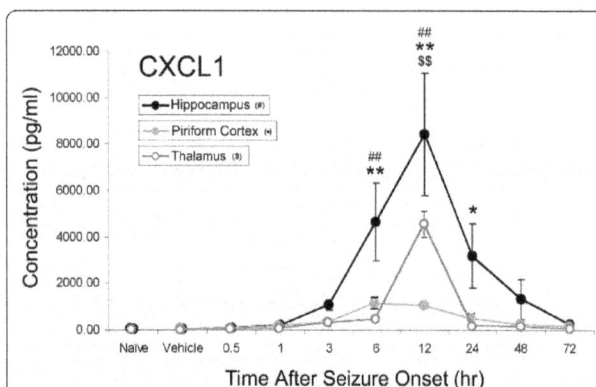

Figure 1 CXCL1 increases in rat brain after GD-induced SE. Concentrations of CXCL1 peak at 6 hours in the piriform cortex (solid gray line) and 12 hours in the hippocampus (solid black line) and thalamus (open gray line). Data are given as pg/ml of tissue lysate and reported as mean ± SEM. Data were analyzed using a one-way ANOVA with a post-hoc Dunnett's analysis comparing to vehicle control. (## $p < 0.01$ hippocampus, * $p < 0.05$, ** $p < 0.01$ piriform cortex, $$ $p < 0.01$ thalamus).

neuronal populations in the regions mentioned above (Figure 2F). CXCL1 diffusely labeled the cytoplasm in these cells with interspersed fine punctate labeling. No co-localization was observed between CXCL1 and astrocytes (Figure 2G) or microglia (Figure 2H) regardless of state of activation. Co-localization was limited in endothelial cells, though a prevalent, but not exclusive, association between CXCL1 and the vasculature was often observed (Figure 2I).

Brain concentrations of MIP-1α significantly increase in response to GD-induced SE
Significant concentration increases were observed for MIP-1α protein in all three brain regions following GD-induced seizure (Figure 3). MIP-1α concentrations significantly increased in the hippocampus at 6 hours (152 ± 42 pg/ml), peaked at 24 hours (247 ± 90 pg/ml) and then rapidly decreased by 48 hours after SE onset compared to vehicle controls (2.06 ± 0.05 pg/ml). In the piriform cortex, MIP-1α concentrations significantly increased at 3 hours (149 ± 14 pg/ml), peaked at 24 hours (200 ± 34 pg/ml) and remained elevated through the 72-hour endpoint (139 ± 22 pg/ml) compared to vehicle controls (<1.94 pg/ml, MinDC). The pattern in the thalamus was different still, where a double peak was observed at 12 hours (245 ± 28 pg/ml) and 48 hours (248 ± 22 pg/ml) compared to controls (18 ± 11 pg/ml).

MIP-1α is expressed by neurons and microglia
Twelve hours following seizure onset, MIP-1α immunolabeling was present in piriform cortex (Figure 4A, left), hippocampus (dentate gyrus shown; Figure 4B, left) and thalamus (Figure 4C, left) but not in vehicle controls (Figure 4A, B &4C, right). Weak to moderate diffuse co-localization with neurons (Figure 4D) was observed in layers II and III of the piriform cortex, the CA1 and CA3 pyramidal layers of the hippocampus and the polymorphic (PoDG) but not the granular layer (GrDG) of the dentate gyrus. Astrocytes were not found to express MIP-1α in any region observed (Figure 4E). Activated microglia strongly expressed MIP-1α in all regions investigated. These cells had a myriad of morphological features including hypertrophy, spheroid shape, blebbing and dystrophy. Specifically, MIP-1α shows a high degree of cellular localization with the dystrophic microglial morphology (Figure 4F). Lastly, MIP-1α-positive cells were closely associated with large blood vessel endothelial cells in the piriform cortex and thalamus but co-localization was not observed (Figure 4G).

Neutrophil influx positively correlates with chemokine expression
To determine whether neutrophil recruitment correlates to increases in CXCL1or MIP-1α, neutrophil counts in

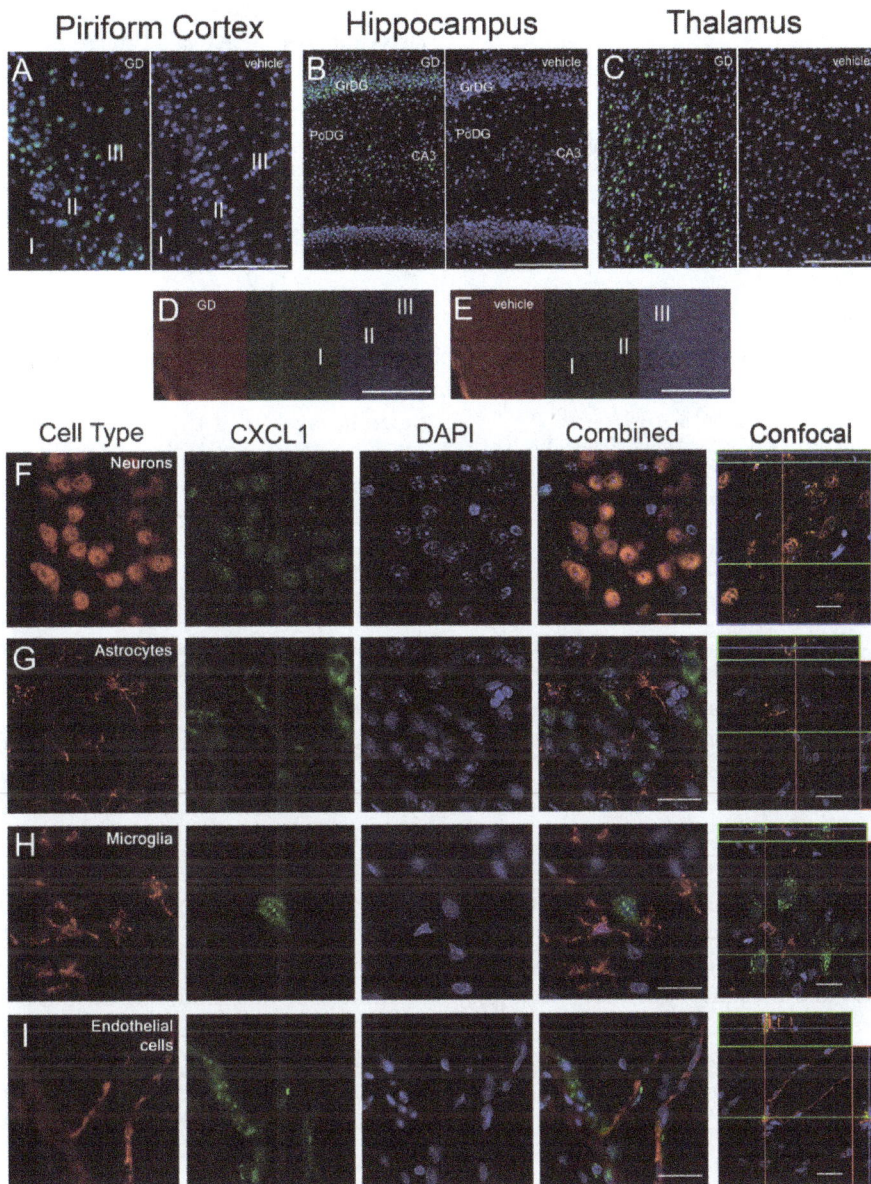

Figure 2 CXCL1 is expressed in neurons and, to a much lesser extent, in endothelial cells after GD-induced SE. Prominent CXCL1 (A-I, green) immunolabeling is present in the piriform cortex, hippocampus and thalamus 12 hours after GD-induced SE (A, B & C; left). CXCL1 is absent in vehicle controls of these same regions (A, B & C; right). In the piriform cortex (A), labeling is observed primarily in layers II and III. In the hippocampus (B), labeling was primarily confined to the CA3 pyramidal layer and granular layer of the dentate gyrus (GrDG) but not evident in the polymorphic layer of the dentate gyrus (PoDG). CXCL1 was located to the laterodorsal and lateral posterior nuclei of the thalamus (C). Labeling was absent in the secondary controls for both 12-hour GD-exposed (D) and vehicle control tissues (E), exemplified by the piriform cortex. Neurons (F, red) and CXCL1 were often found to co-localize (F, yellow). Co-localization was not observed in hypertrophic astrocytes (G, red) or activated microglia (H, red) and was limited in endothelial cells (I, yellow). DAPI (A-I, blue) was used to label the nuclei of each cell. Scale bar: 250 μm (A-E), 50 μm and 20 μm (F-I) for regular and confocal fluorescent microscopy respectively; n = 7 for 12-hour, n = 4 for vehicle controls.

the piriform cortex, hippocampus and thalamus were quantified using stereological techniques and correlated to CXCL1 and MIP-1α concentration data using a one measurement time lag with Pearson's correlation analysis. Neutrophil infiltration significantly increases in all three observed brain regions following GD-induced SE

(Figure 5). No neutrophils were found in vehicle controls in any brain region (0 ± 0 cells/mm^3). In the piriform cortex, neutrophil infiltration significantly increased at 12 (1,117 ± 485 cells/mm^3) and 24 hours (1,565 ± 618 cells/mm^3) but not 6 hours (3 ± 5.8 cells/mm^3) compared to vehicle. Significant, though less

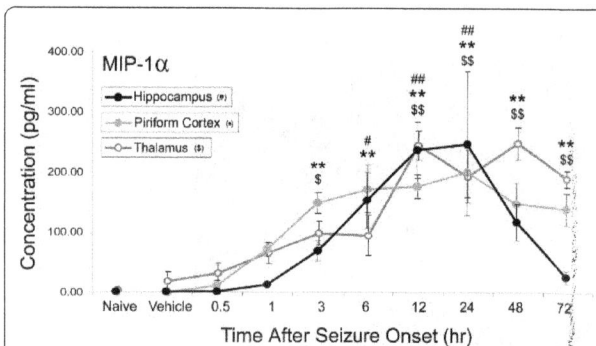

Figure 3 MIP-1α Increases in Rat Brain after GD-induced SE. MIP-1α concentrations significantly increase in the hippocampus, piriform cortex and thalamus following GD-induced SE. MIP-1α concentrations peak at 24 hours after seizure onset in both the hippocampus (solid black line) and piriform cortex (solid gray line). In the thalamus (open gray line), there is a double peak at 12 and 48 hours after seizure onset. Data are given as pg/ml of tissue lysate reported as mean ± SEM. Data were analyzed using a one-way ANOVA with a post-hoc Dunnett's analysis comparing to vehicle control. (# $p < 0.05$, ## $p < 0.01$ hippocampus; ** $p < 0.01$ piriform cortex; $ $p < 0.05$, $$ $p < 0.01$ thalamus).

robust, neutrophil infiltration was also observed in the hippocampus at 12 (128 ± 85 cells/mm^3) and 24 hours (589 ± 10 cells/mm^3) but not 6 hours (0 ± 0 cells/mm^3) compared to vehicle. In contrast, neutrophils in the thalamus significantly increased only at 24 hours ($2,098 \pm 824$ cells/mm^3) and not at 12 hours (158 ± 90 cells/mm^3). Pearson's correlation analysis revealed a positive correlation between CXCL1 concentration and neutrophil infiltration (offset by one time point) in the piriform cortex, hippocampus and thalamus. For MIP-1α, a less robust positive correlation existed in the hippocampus and thalamus compared to CXCL1. No significant correlation was observed in the piriform cortex (Table 1).

Discussion

Neuroinflammation is almost ubiquitous following brain injury, though little is known about this process following damage caused by GD-induced SE. As part of the inflammatory process, resident and systemic inflammatory cells migrate to areas of injury guided by concentration gradients of chemokines and growth factors. This study describes the temporal and regional protein changes of four neutrophil activating and chemotactic factors in the brain, the expression of significantly upregulated factors in resident brain cells, quantification of neutrophil infiltration into the brain, and the correlation between chemokine expression and neutrophil infiltration. Significant expression of two chemokines, CXCL1 and MIP-1α, immediately preceded neutrophil infiltration in brain regions damaged by SE (i.e., the piriform cortex, hippocampus and thalamus). Both chemokines were primarily expressed by neurons; however, CXCL1

was also expressed in endothelial cells, and MIP-1α was also expressed in activated microglia. These data are the first to show the temporal, regional and cellular protein expression of chemokines, consequent neutrophil infiltration and the relationship between these two events following nerve agent exposure and subsequent SE.

Of all the resident brain cell types, neurons appear most susceptible to GD-induced SE damage as shown by substantial neuronal cell death in the piriform cortex, thalamus and portions of the hippocampus [5,27]. Therefore, it is not surprising that neurons become the focal point of the inflammatory response. In fact, the neurons most vulnerable to GD-induced SE, including those in layer II of the piriform cortex [28], strongly expressed both CXCL1 and MIP-1α. Injured neurons have the ability to produce chemokines to recruit and activate inflammatory cells following injury [29-31], and we have now shown expression of CXCL1 and MIP-1α in the GD-induced SE model as well.

Astrocytes did not express CXCL1 or MIP-1α in any brain region despite concurrent neuronal injury. CXCL1 expression by astrocytes does occur following various central nervous system (CNS) insults [32-34], and this expression appears to be dependent on neuronal damage [35]. Similarly, MIP-1α is expressed by astrocytes in SE [36] and experimental autoimmune encephalomyelitis models [37,38]. Though it is unknown exactly why chemokine expression in this model is incongruent with other CNS injury paradigms, it is apparent that chemokine expression is likely insult specific [39], and neutrophil recruitment may not be the main function of astrocytes in this model or at this point in pathology progression. Further, cytokine expression is prominent in both astrocytes (IL-6) and microglia (IL-1) in this model and may function to modulate the neuroinflammatory process rather than to recruit inflammatory cells [11].

Despite a lack of expression in most microglia, MIP-1α was expressed by a number of activated microglia and prominently expressed by those with a dystrophic morphology. MIP-1α expression by active microglia following brain injury has been previously observed [40], though little is known about dystrophic microglia or the expression of inflammatory factors by this morphological type. It is known that dystrophic microglia appear exclusively in progressive neurodegenerative disease states such as Alzheimer's and Huntington's disease and are indicative of concurrent and subsequent neuronal degeneration [41-43], a condition that is accelerated in this model. We have previously shown that another important neutrophil chemoattractant [44] and upregulator of neutrophil infiltration endothelium adhesion molecules [45], IL-1β, was also localized to dystrophic microglia [11]. Therefore, dystrophic microglia appear to have a prominent role in

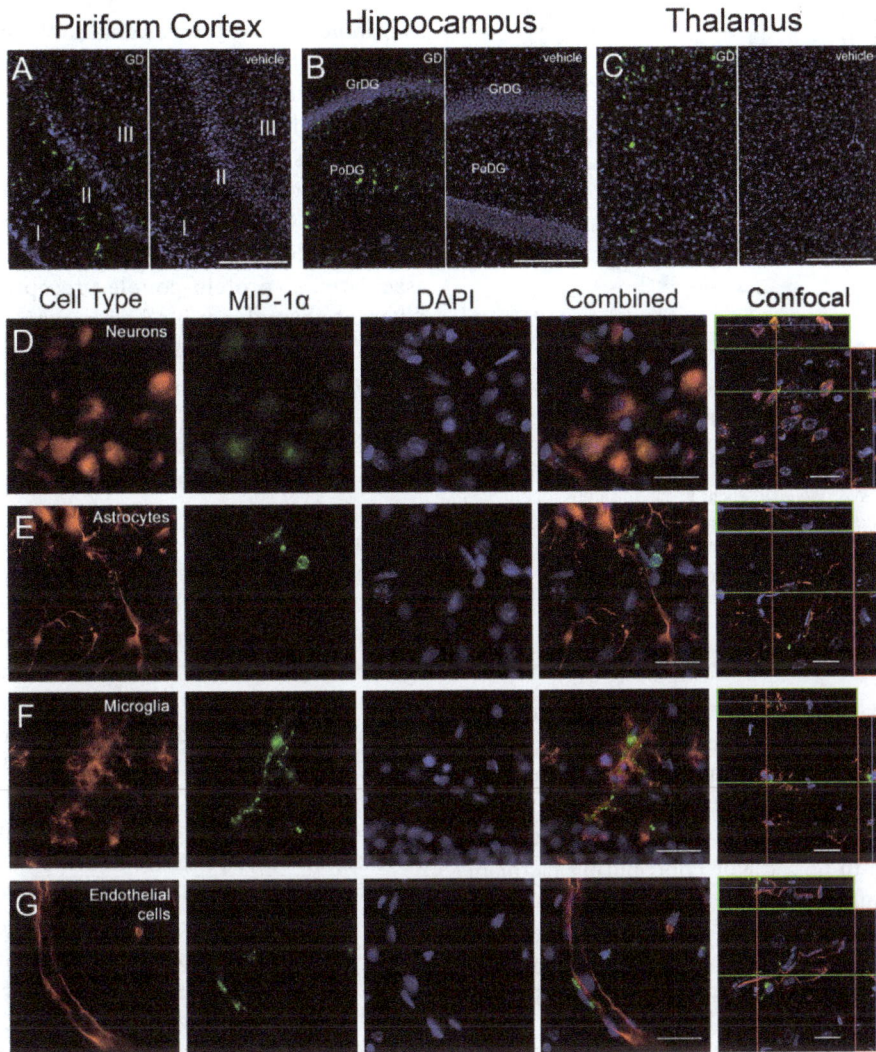

Figure 4 MIP-1α is primarily expressed by neurons and dystrophic microglia after GD-induced SE. MIP-1α immunolabeling (A-G, green) is present in the piriform cortex, hippocampus and thalamus 12 hours after GD-induced SE (A, B & C; left) but absent in vehicle controls of these same regions (A, B & C; right). In the piriform cortex (A), labeling is observed primarily in layers II and III. In the hippocampus (B), labeling was less robust and found primarily in the CA1 and CA3 pyramidal layers as well as in the polymorphic layer of the dentate gyrus (PoDG) but not the granular layer of the dentate gyrus (GrDG). MIP-1α labeling was also less robust in the thalamus (C) and was found primarily in the laterodorsal and lateral posterior nuclei. Neurons (D, red) and MIP-1α frequently co-localized (D, yellow), while no co-localization with astrocytes (E, red) was observed. MIP-1α was primarily expressed by microglia with a dystrophic morphology (F, red). Limited co-localization was observed in endothelial cells (G, red). Scale bar: 250 μm (A-C), 50 μm and 10 μm (D-F) for regular and confocal fluorescent microscopy respectively; n = 9 for 12-hour and n = 4 for vehicle controls.

the recruitment and activation of neutrophils following prolonged SE induced by GD.

Lastly, significant CXCL1 expression precedes a significant influx of neutrophils into vulnerable brain regions (<6 hours in the piriform cortex and hippocampus and <12 hours in the thalamus; Figures 1 &5). A less definitive positive correlation exists for MIP-1α, likely because MIP-1α is highly pleiotropic and also modulates the chemotactic and activation properties of other leukocyte cell types [46,47]. Though there is a strong positive correlation between CXCL1 concentration and consequent neutrophil influx, this relationship does not appear to be proportional. For example, while we observed the highest concentrations of CXCL1 in the hippocampus, this region had the fewest number of infiltrating neutrophils. In contrast, the piriform cortex had the lowest concentration of CXCL1 but had some of the highest numbers of infiltrating neutrophils.

Though little is known about regional differences in brain chemokine expression, there are several variables

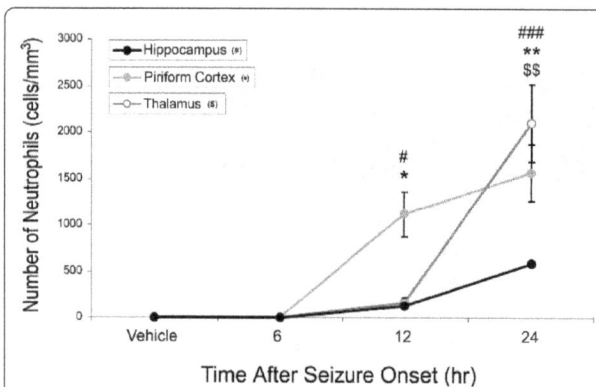

Figure 5 Neutrophil infiltration occurs following significant CXCL1 expression in injured brain regions. Significant increases in neutrophils were observed in the hippocampus (solid black line) and piriform cortex (solid gray line) at 12 and 24 hours following SE onset. Significant increases were observed in the thalamus (open gray line) at 24 hours only. Data are given as cells/mm^3 of tissue reported as mean ± SEM. Data were analyzed using a one-way ANOVA with a post-hoc Newman-Kuel analysis ($^{\#}$ p < 0.05, $^{\#\#\#}$ p < 0.001 in hippocampus; ** p < 0.01 in piriform cortex; $^{\$\$}$ p < 0.01 in thalamus; n = 3 for all brain regions and time points).

that may influence the relationship between chemokine concentration and neutrophil infiltration. First, region specific neutrophil infiltration may rely on other cytokine induced neutrophil chemoattractant (CINC) family members. For example, CXCL1, also known as CINC-2β, was not found to be a major contributing factor in brain neutrophil infiltration following direct IL-1β injection into the brain compared to CINC-1 and CINC-2α [48]. It should be noted, however, that individual chemokine involvement is likely injury specific and these CINCs may not be active in this model. Second, differential IL-1β brain expression may play a role. We have previously documented regional differences in brain IL-1β concentration, an important promoter of neutrophil adhesion, in this model [11]. No significant expression of IL-1β was observed in the hippocampus whereas significant increases in IL-1β were observed in the piriform cortex and thalamus that correspond to neutrophil influx. However, IL-1α, an IL-1 isoform that can

similarly increase CXCL1 expression and cellular adhesion molecules [49], was significantly increased and may serve a similar role as IL-1β in this model. Lastly, differential expression of CXCL1 receptors, CXCR1 and CXCR2, and the associated vascular cell surface glycosaminoglycans (GAGs), may account for the observed discrepancy between CXCL1 expression and neutrophil infiltration. GAGs are essential for forming chemotactic gradients [50] and affect chemokine binding to their associated G-protein-coupled receptors [51]. Because different chemokines bind with varying affinities to different GAGs [50] and GAG and CXCL1 receptor expression are highly dependent on the location, type and subset of the cell [52-56], varying rates of neutrophil infiltration are possibly at different neuroinflammatory foci dictated by these complex interactions.

Conclusion

In conclusion, we have shown that concentrations of CXCL1 and MIP-1α significantly increase in the brain of rats following GD-induced SE. We have also identified specific cell types that express these factors; neurons and endothelial cells primarily express CXCL1, while neurons and dystrophic microglia primarily express MIP-1α. Neutrophil infiltration significantly increases in regions where CXCL1 and MIP-1α expression and neuronal death occur. Lastly, expression of these chemokines precedes neutrophil infiltration, consistent with their chemotactic properties, but infiltration is not necessarily proportional to chemokine concentration. These data suggest a strong activation and recruitment of neutrophils to areas of brain damage modulated, at least partially, by CXCL1 and MIP-1α expression by injured neurons, microglia and endothelial cells following GD-induced SE.

List of abbreviations

CNS: central nervous system; GD: soman; SE: status epilepticus; MIP-1α: macrophage inflammatory protein 1α; CXCL1: chemokine (C-X-C motif) ligand 1; IL: interleukin; G-CSF: granulocyte colony stimulating factor; GM-CSF: granulocyte-macrophage colony stimulating factor; IHC: immunohistochemistry; MinDC: minimum detectable concentration.

Acknowledgements

This work was supported by the U.S. Army Medical Research and Materiel Command and by the Defense Threat Reduction Agency (DTRA) under contract # I10001_04_RC_C and W911NF-07-D-001. The authors would like to thank Ms. Jessica Leuschner, Mr. Colin Smith, Mr. Mayank Patel, Ms. Jennifer Peeling, Ms. Marissa Babnew and Ms. Dominique Scutella for their expert technical support. We would also like to thank Dr. Wolfgang Streit, University of Florida Department of Neuroscience, for his assistance in identifying dystrophic microglia. The findings contained herein are the private views of the author(s) and are not to be construed as official or as reflecting the views of the U.S. Army or Department of Defense.

Authors' contributions

EAJ and RKK both participated in developing the study concept and experimental design. EAJ analyzed data, wrote the manuscript and participated in acquisition of data. TLD, MAG, CEG and AIKC acquired and

Table 1 CXCL1 and MIP-1α expression positively correlates with the infiltration of neutrophils into injured brain.

	Brain Region	Pearson's r	P value	95% CI
CXCL1	Piriform cortex	0.945	0.015	0.377 to 0.996
	Hippocampus	0.946	0.015	0.383 to 0.996
	Thalamus	0.999	<0.001	0.978 to 0.999
MIP-1α	Piriform cortex	0.728	>0.05	-0.431 to 0.980
	Hippocampus	0.943	0.016	0.360 to 0.996
	Thalamus	0.954	0.012	0.452 to 0.997

analyzed data and contributed to the writing of the manuscript. All authors have read, edited and approved the final manuscript.

Competing interests
The authors declare that they have no competing interests.

References
1. Shih TM: **Anticonvulsant effects of diazepam and MK-801 in soman poisoning.** *Epilepsy Res* 1990, 7:105-116.
2. Lallement G, Pernot-Marino I, Baubichon D, Burckhart MF, Carpentier P, Blanchet G: **Modulation of soman-induced neuropathology with an anticonvulsant regimen.** *Neuroreport* 1994, 5:2265-2268.
3. McDonough JH Jr, Dochterman LW, Smith CD, Shih TM: **Protection against nerve agent-induced neuropathology, but not cardiac pathology, is associated with the anticonvulsant action of drug treatment.** *Neurotoxicology* 1995, 16:123-132.
4. Churchill L, Pazdernik TL, Jackson JL, Nelson SR, Samson FE, McDonough JH Jr, McLeod CG Jr: **Soman-induced brain lesions demonstrated by muscarinic receptor autoradiography.** *Neurotoxicology* 1985, 6:81-90.
5. McLeod CG Jr, Singer AW, Harrington DG: **Acute neuropathology in soman poisoned rats.** *Neurotoxicology* 1984, 5:53-57.
6. Ravizza T, Gagliardi B, Noe F, Boer K, Aronica E, Vezzani A: **Innate and adaptive immunity during epileptogenesis and spontaneous seizures: evidence from experimental models and human temporal lobe epilepsy.** *Neurobiol Dis* 2008, 29:142-160.
7. Vezzani A, Granata T: **Brain inflammation in epilepsy: experimental and clinical evidence.** *Epilepsia* 2005, 46:1724-1743.
8. Williams AJ, Berti R, Yao C, Price RA, Velarde LC, Koplovitz I, Schultz SM, Tortella FC, Dave JR: **Central neuro-inflammatory gene response following soman exposure in the rat.** *Neurosci Lett* 2003, 349:147-150.
9. Dillman JF, Phillips CS, Kniffin DM, Tompkins CP, Hamilton TA, Kan RK: **Gene expression profiling of rat hippocampus following exposure to the acetylcholinesterase inhibitor soman.** *Chem Res Toxicol* 2009, 22:633-638.
10. Svensson I, Waara L, Johansson L, Bucht A, Cassel G: **Soman-induced interleukin-1 beta mRNA and protein in rat brain.** *Neurotoxicology* 2001, 22:355-362.
11. Johnson EA, Kan RK: **The acute phase response and soman-induced status epilepticus: temporal, regional and cellular changes in rat brain cytokine concentrations.** *J Neuroinflammation* 2010, 7:40.
12. Manley NC, Bertrand AA, Kinney KS, Hing TC, Sapolsky RM: **Characterization of monocyte chemoattractant protein-1 expression following a kainate model of status epilepticus.** *Brain Res* 2007, 1182:138-143.
13. Emerich DF, Dean RL, Bartus RT: **The role of leukocytes following cerebral ischemia: pathogenic variable or bystander reaction to emerging infarct?** *Exp Neurol* 2002, 173:168-181.
14. Clark RS, Carlos TM, Schiding JK, Bree M, Fireman LA, DeKosky ST, Kochanek PM: **Antibodies against Mac-1 attenuate neutrophil accumulation after traumatic brain injury in rats.** *J Neurotrauma* 1996, 13:333-341.
15. Shaftel SS, Carlson TJ, Olschowka JA, Kyrkanides S, Matousek SB, O'Banion MK: **Chronic interleukin-1beta expression in mouse brain leads to leukocyte infiltration and neutrophil-independent blood brain barrier permeability without overt neurodegeneration.** *J Neurosci* 2007, 27:9301-9309.
16. Wolpe SD, Davatelis G, Sherry B, Beutler B, Hesse DG, Nguyen HT, Moldawer LL, Nathan CF, Lowry SF, Cerami A: **Macrophages secrete a novel heparin-binding protein with inflammatory and neutrophil chemokinetic properties.** *J Exp Med* 1988, 167:570-581.
17. Appelberg R: **Macrophage inflammatory proteins MIP-1 and MIP-2 are involved in T cell-mediated neutrophil recruitment.** *J Leukoc Biol* 1992, 52:303-306.
18. Watanabe K, Konishi K, Fujioka M, Kinoshita S, Nakagawa H: **The neutrophil chemoattractant produced by the rat kidney epithelioid cell line NRK-52E is a protein related to the KC/gro protein.** *J Biol Chem* 1989, 264:19559-19563.
19. Tani M, Fuentes ME, Peterson JW, Trapp BD, Durham SK, Loy JK, Bravo R, Ransohoff RM, Lira SA: **Neutrophil infiltration, glial reaction, and neurological disease in transgenic mice expressing the chemokine N51/KC in oligodendrocytes.** *J Clin Invest* 1996, 98:529-539.
20. Auvin S, Shin D, Mazarati A, Nakagawa J, Miyamoto J, Sankar R: **Inflammation exacerbates seizure-induced injury in the immature brain.** *Epilepsia* 2007, 48(Suppl 5):27-34.
21. De Simoni MG, Perego C, Ravizza T, Moneta D, Conti M, Marchesi F, De Luigi A, Garattini S, Vezzani A: **Inflammatory cytokines and related genes are induced in the rat hippocampus by limbic status epilepticus.** *Eur J Neurosci* 2000, 12:2623-2633.
22. Vezzani A, Moneta D, Richichi C, Aliprandi M, Burrows SJ, Ravizza T, Perego C, De Simoni MG: **Functional role of inflammatory cytokines and antiinflammatory molecules in seizures and epileptogenesis.** *Epilepsia* 2002, 43(Suppl 5):30-35.
23. Dhote F, Peinnequin A, Carpentier P, Baille V, Delacour C, Foquin A, Lallement G, Dorandeu F: **Prolonged inflammatory gene response following soman-induced seizures in mice.** *Toxicology* 2007.
24. Dillman JF, Phillips CS, Fath DM, Tompkins CP, Hamilton TA, Kan RK: **Genomic analysis of rat brain following exposure to soman.** *The Toxicologist CD – An official Journal of the Society of Toxicology* 2007, 96:Abst 1852.
25. Shih TM, McDonough JH Jr: **Neurochemical mechanisms in soman-induced seizures.** *J Appl Toxicol* 1997, 17:255-264.
26. Johnson EA, Svetlov SI, Pike BR, Tolentino PJ, Shaw G, Wang KKW, Hayes RL, Pineda JA: **Cell-specific Upregulation of Survivin After Experimental Traumatic Brain Injury in Rats.** *Journal of Neurotrauma* 2004, 21:1183-1195.
27. Kan RK, Fath DM, Tompkins CP, Hamilton TA: **Systematic characterization of regional and temporal brain injury following status epilepticus induced by chemical warfare nerve agent soman.** *Society for Neuroscience annual meeting; San Diego, CA. Neuroscience Meeting Planner* 2008.
28. Kan RK, Johnson EA, Fath DM, Tompkins CP, Hamilton TA, Hoard-Fruchey H: **Temporal expression of neuroinflammatory markers and brain injury following acute soman poisoning.** *Defence against the Effects of Chemical Hazards: Toxicology, Diagnosis and Medical Countermeasures Meeting Proceedings RTO-MP-HFM-149; Edinburg, Scotland* 2007, 1-1-1-14.
29. Rappert A, Bechmann I, Pivneva T, Mahlo J, Biber K, Nolte C, Kovac AD, Gerard C, Boddeke HW, Nitsch R, Kettenmann H: **CXCR3-dependent microglial recruitment is essential for dendrite loss after brain lesion.** *J Neurosci* 2004, 24:8500-8509.
30. de Jong EK, Dijkstra IM, Hensens M, Brouwer N, van Amerongen M, Liem RS, Boddeke HW, Biber K: **Vesicle-mediated transport and release of CCL21 in endangered neurons: a possible explanation for microglia activation remote from a primary lesion.** *J Neurosci* 2005, 25:7548-7557.
31. Flugel A, Hager G, Horvat A, Spitzer C, Singer GM, Graeber MB, Kreutzberg GW, Schwaiger FW: **Neuronal MCP-1 expression in response to remote nerve injury.** *J Cereb Blood Flow Metab* 2001, 21:69-76.
32. Luo Y, Fischer FR, Hancock WW, Dorf ME: **Macrophage inflammatory protein-2 and KC induce chemokine production by mouse astrocytes.** *J Immunol* 2000, 165:4015-4023.
33. Pineau I, Sun L, Bastien D, Lacroix S: **Astrocytes initiate inflammation in the injured mouse spinal cord by promoting the entry of neutrophils and inflammatory monocytes in an IL-1 receptor/MyD88-dependent fashion.** *Brain Behav Immun* 2010, 24:540-553.
34. Rubio N, Sanz-Rodriguez F: **Induction of the CXCL1 (KC) chemokine in mouse astrocytes by infection with the murine encephalomyelitis virus of Theiler.** *Virology* 2007, 358:98-108.
35. Katayama T, Tanaka H, Yoshida T, Uehara T, Minami M: **Neuronal injury induces cytokine-induced neutrophil chemoattractant-1 (CINC-1) production in astrocytes.** *J Pharmacol Sci* 2009, 109:88-93.
36. Xu JH, Long L, Tang YC, Zhang JT, Hut HT, Tang FR: **CCR3, CCR2A and macrophage inflammatory protein (MIP)-1a, monocyte chemotactic protein-1 (MCP-1) in the mouse hippocampus during and after pilocarpine-induced status epilepticus (PISE).** *Neuropathol Appl Neurobiol* 2009, 35:496-514.
37. Nygardas PT, Maatta JA, Hinkkanen AE: **Chemokine expression by central nervous system resident cells and infiltrating neutrophils during experimental autoimmune encephalomyelitis in the BALB/c mouse.** *Eur J Immunol* 2000, 30:1911-1918.
38. Quinones MP, Kalkonde Y, Estrada CA, Jimenez F, Ramirez R, Mahimainathan L, Mummidi S, Choudhury GG, Martinez H, Adams L, *et al*: **Role of astrocytes and chemokine systems in acute TNFalpha induced demyelinating syndrome: CCR2-dependent signals promote astrocyte activation and survival via NF-kappaB and Akt.** *Mol Cell Neurosci* 2008, 37:96-109.

39. McKimmie CS, Graham GJ: **Astrocytes modulate the chemokine network in a pathogen-specific manner.** *Biochem Biophys Res Commun* 2010, **394**:1006-1011.

40. Cowell RM, Xu H, Galasso JM, Silverstein FS: **Hypoxic-ischemic injury induces macrophage inflammatory protein-1alpha expression in immature rat brain.** *Stroke* 2002, **33**:795-801.

41. Streit WJ, Braak H, Xue QS, Bechmann I: **Dystrophic (senescent) rather than activated microglial cells are associated with tau pathology and likely precede neurodegeneration in Alzheimer's disease.** *Acta Neuropathol* 2009, **118**:475-485.

42. Streit WJ, Sammons NW, Kuhns AJ, Sparks DL: **Dystrophic microglia in the aging human brain.** *Glia* 2004, **45**:208-212.

43. Lopes KO, Sparks DL, Streit WJ: **Microglial dystrophy in the aged and Alzheimer's disease brain is associated with ferritin immunoreactivity.** *Glia* 2008, **56**:1048-1060.

44. Perretti M, Appleton I, Parente L, Flower RJ: **Pharmacology of interleukin-1-induced neutrophil migration.** *Agents Actions* 1993, **38**(Spec No):C64-65.

45. Amantea D, Nappi G, Bernardi G, Bagetta G, Corasaniti MT: **Post-ischemic brain damage: pathophysiology and role of inflammatory mediators.** *FEBS J* 2009, **276**:13-26.

46. Alam R, Forsythe PA, Stafford S, Lett-Brown MA, Grant JA: **Macrophage inflammatory protein-1 alpha activates basophils and mast cells.** *J Exp Med* 1992, **176**:781-786.

47. Rot A, Krieger M, Brunner T, Bischoff SC, Schall TJ, Dahinden CA: **RANTES and macrophage inflammatory protein 1 alpha induce the migration and activation of normal human eosinophil granulocytes.** *J Exp Med* 1992, **176**:1489-1495.

48. Campbell SJ, Wilcockson DC, Butchart AG, Perry VH, Anthony DC: **Altered chemokine expression in the spinal cord and brain contributes to differential interleukin-1beta-induced neutrophil recruitment.** *J Neurochem* 2002, **83**:432-441.

49. Thornton P, McColl BW, Greenhalgh A, Denes A, Allan SM, Rothwell NJ: **Platelet interleukin-1alpha drives cerebrovascular inflammation.** *Blood* 2010, **115**:3632-3639.

50. Kuschert GS, Coulin F, Power CA, Proudfoot AE, Hubbard RE, Hoogewerf AJ, Wells TN: **Glycosaminoglycans interact selectively with chemokines and modulate receptor binding and cellular responses.** *Biochemistry* 1999, **38**:12959-12968.

51. Hoogewerf AJ, Kuschert GS, Proudfoot AE, Borlat F, Clark-Lewis I, Power CA, Wells TN: **Glycosaminoglycans mediate cell surface oligomerization of chemokines.** *Biochemistry* 1997, **36**:13570-13578.

52. Arisaka T, Mitsumata M, Kawasumi M, Tohjima T, Hirose S, Yoshida Y: **Effects of shear stress on glycosaminoglycan synthesis in vascular endothelial cells.** *Ann N Y Acad Sci* 1995, **748**:543-554.

53. Gallagher JT, Turnbull JE, Lyon M: **Patterns of sulphation in heparan sulphate: polymorphism based on a common structural theme.** *Int J Biochem* 1992, **24**:553-560.

54. Danik M, Puma C, Quirion R, Williams S: **Widely expressed transcripts for chemokine receptor CXCR1 in identified glutamatergic, gamma-aminobutyric acidergic, and cholinergic neurons and astrocytes of the rat brain: a single-cell reverse transcription-multiplex polymerase chain reaction study.** *J Neurosci Res* 2003, **74**:286-295.

55. Flynn G, Maru S, Loughlin J, Romero IA, Male D: **Regulation of chemokine receptor expression in human microglia and astrocytes.** *J Neuroimmunol* 2003, **136**:84-93.

56. Horuk R, Martin AW, Wang Z, Schweitzer L, Gerassimides A, Guo H, Lu Z, Hesselgesser J, Perez HD, Kim J, *et al*: **Expression of chemokine receptors by subsets of neurons in the central nervous system.** *J Immunol* 1997, **158**:2882-2890.

12

Metalloprotease Adam10 suppresses epilepsy through repression of hippocampal neuroinflammation

Xinjian Zhu[1*], Xiaolin Li[2], Mengyi Zhu[1], Kangni Xu[1], Li Yang[1], Bing Han[1], Rongrong Huang[1], Aifeng Zhang[3] and Honghong Yao[1]

Abstract

Background: Mice with pilocarpine-induced temporal lobe epilepsy (TLE) are characterized by intense hippocampal neuroinflammation, a prominent pathological hallmark of TLE that is known to contribute to neuronal hyperexcitability. Recent studies indicate that Adam10, a member of a disintegrin and metalloproteinase domain-containing protein (Adam) family, has been involved in the neuroinflammation response. However, it remains unclear whether and how Adam10 modulates neuroinflammation responses in the context of an epileptic brain or whether Adam10 affects epileptogenesis via the neuroinflammation pathway.

Methods: Adult male C57BL/6J mice were subjected to intraperitoneal injection of pilocarpine to induce TLE. Adeno-associated viral (AAV) vectors carrying Adam10 (AAV-Adam10) or lentiviral vectors carrying short hairpin RNA, which is specific to the mouse Adam10 mRNA (shRNA-Adam10), were bilaterally injected into the hippocampus to induce overexpression or knockdown of Adam10, respectively. The specific anti-inflammatory agent minocycline was administered following status epilepticus (SE) to block hippocampal neuroinflammation. Continuous video EEG recording was performed to analyze epileptic behavior. Western blot, immunofluorescence staining, and ELISA were performed to determine Adam10 expression as well as hippocampal neuroinflammation.

Results: In this study, we demonstrate that overexpression of Adam10 in the hippocampus suppresses neuroinflammation and reduces seizure activity in TLE mice, whereas knockdown of Adam10 exacerbates hippocampal neuroinflammation and increases seizure activity. Furthermore, increased seizure activity in Adam10 knockdown TLE mice is dependent on hippocampal neuroinflammation.

Conclusion: These results suggest that Adam10 suppresses epilepsy through repression of hippocampal neuroinflammation. Our findings provide new insights into the Adam10 regulation of development of epilepsy via the neuroinflammation pathway and identify a potential therapeutic target for epilepsy.

Keywords: Metalloprotease, Adam10, Hippocampus, Neuroinflammation, Temporal lobe epilepsy

Background

Adam10 is a member of the ADAM metalloprotease family and is able to cleave the extracellular domains of several membrane-bound proteins in a process called ectodomain shedding [1–3]. One of the major substrates of Adam10 is amyloid precursor protein (APP), for which Adam10 acts as an α-secretase to prevent the excessive production of the pathogenic amyloid β (Aβ) peptide [4, 5], a hallmark of Alzheimer's disease (AD). The processing of APP by Adam10 produces a soluble N-terminal APP fragment (sAPP), which has been shown to exert neurotrophic and neuroprotective effects [6]. Thus, the activation of Adam10 has been suggested as a therapeutic approach for AD patients [4, 7]. Despite the crucial role of Adam10 in AD, recent studies indicate that Adam10 may contribute to other neurological and psychiatric disease. A previous study reported that postnatal disruption of Adam10 in the brain causes

* Correspondence: xinjianzhu@seu.edu.cn
[1]Department of Pharmacology, Medical School of Southeast University, Dingjiaqiao 87th, Nanjing 210009, China

epileptic seizures, learning deficits, altered neuronal spine morphology, and defective synaptic functions [8], suggesting that Adam10 plays a pivotal role in the synaptic and neuronal network activity. This finding is supported by evidence that conditional Adam10$^{-/-}$ mice exhibit mistargeted axons and a dysregulated neuronal network [9]. Additionally, Adam10 expression has been found to be altered in the dentate gyrus of kainic acid-induced epileptic rats [10], indicating an association of Adam10 with epilepsy. It is generally accepted that neuroinflammation is a prominent pathological hallmark of TLE, which is known to contribute to neuronal hyperexcitability in both human patients and animal models [11–14]. These studies indicate that seizure-induced proinflammatory signals may play a pivotal role in recurrent epilepsy. Adam10 has been largely distributed in the astrocytes [15, 16], as well as neurons [17], and it has been found to be responsible for proteolytic processing of CX3CL1, a chemokine primarily expressed in the neurons and astrocytes, which is involved in the neuroinflammation response [16]. However, it remains unclear whether and how Adam10 modulates the neuroinflammatory response in the context of an epileptic brain or whether Adam10 affects epileptogenesis via the neuroinflammation pathway. Thus, in the present study, we sought to explore the role of Adam10 in neuroinflammation of the epileptic brain and to further determine whether Adam10 affects epileptogenesis through neuroinflammation pathways.

Methods
Animals
Male C57BL/6J mice (4–6 weeks old; weighing 19 ± 2 g at the beginning of the experiments) were obtained from Nanjing Biomedical Research Institute of Nanjing University (NBRI) (Nanjing, China). The animals were housed in plastic cages and kept in a regulated environment (22 ± 1 °C) with an artificial 12-h light/dark cycle (lighted from 7:00 A.M. to 7:00 P.M.). Food and tap water were available ad libitum. Procedures for pilocarpine-induced status epilepticus (SE) model and all subsequent experiments were approved by the Animal Care and Use Committee at Medical School of Southeast University. All efforts were made to minimize animal suffering and discomfort and to reduce the number of animals used.

Surgery and virus injection
For adeno-associated viral (AAV) and lentiviral infection, the mice were anesthetized and positioned on a stereotaxic frame (Stoelting, Wood Dale, USA). Vectors (either AAV-Adam10, AAV-Ctrl, or lentiviral shRNA-Adam10, lentiviral shRNA-Ctrl) were bilaterally injected into the hippocampus (coordinates: A/P – 2.2; M/L ± 2.0; D/V 1.9) using 1 µl of viral preparation at a rate of 0.2 µl/min. AAV

constructs used were designed and produced by Han Bio (Shanghai, China, contract number: HH20170303RFF-A AV01). Adam10-shRNA lentiviral particles and control lentiviral particles were purchased from Santa Cruz Biotechnology Inc. (Santa Cruz, TX, USA). For EEG recording, the mice were then subjected to hippocampus depth electrode placement as we previously described [18]. A bipolar twist electrode was placed in the left hippocampus (coordinates: A/P – 2.2; M/L – 2.0; D/V 1.9) for continuous EEG monitoring. In addition to the hippocampal electrodes, four cortical screws with two in front of the bregma for bilateral cortex recording and two behind the lambda for ground and reference. Electrodes are connected with a plastic cap and kept in place with dental cement. Animals were allowed to recover for at least 1 week prior to pilocarpine-induced SE.

Pilocarpine induction of SE and EEG recording
SE model was induced as we previously described [18]. Briefly, the mice were subjected to an intraperitoneal injection of 1 mg/kg methyl-scopolamine (Sigma Aldrich, St. Louis, MO, USA) followed 30 min later by an injection of 300 mg/kg pilocarpine HCL (Sigma Aldrich, St. Louis, MO, USA). Control animals received all drugs and treatments, except they were given saline instead of pilocarpine. After pilocarpine injection, all animals were subjected to continuous video EEG recording with the video EEG monitoring system (Chengyi Inc., Chengdu, China). The seizure intensity was assessed based on Racine scale: stage 1, mouth and facial movements; stage 2, head nodding; stage 3, forelimb clonus; stage 4, seizures characterized by rearing; and stage 5, seizures characterized by rearing and falling [19]. To determine whether neuroinflammation could affect the process of Adam10-regulated epileptogenesis, we treated Adam10 knockdown and control mice with pilocarpine to induce SE, followed by multiple doses of anti-inflammatory agent minocycline (1 mg/kg, Sigma Aldrich, St. Louis, MO, USA) treatment to block neuroinflammation. Animals were then subjected to continuous video EEG recording as described above. Electroencephalographic seizures were differentiated from background noise by the appearance of large-amplitude, high-frequency activity, with the progression of the spike frequency. The behavioral data captured by the synchronized video recording system were used to confirm EEG seizure activity.

Brain tissue processing
For PCR and Western blot experiments, the hippocampus was dissected, snap-frozen and stored at – 80 °C until use. For immunocytochemistry experiment, the mice were euthanized by an intraperitoneal injection of an overdose of urethane and were transcardially perfused with 100 mL of saline (0.9% w/v NaCl), followed by

50 mL of 4% paraformaldehyde in 0.05 M sodium phosphate (pH = 7.4, containing 0.8% NaCl). The mouse brains were removed and post-fixed overnight in 4% paraformaldehyde then were cryoprotected in 30% sucrose in PBS for 72 h. The serial coronal hippocampal sections with a thickness of 25 μm were cut using a cryostat (Leica Microsystems, Wetzlar, Germany), and every sixth section throughout the hippocampus was collected in PBS as free-floating sections and was stored at 4 °C for future immunocytochemistry studies as we previously described [20].

Reverse transcription PCR

The dissected hippocampal tissues were homogenized, and total RNA was extracted with Trizol reagent (Vazyme Biotech, Nanjing, China) according to the manufacturer's instructions. Total mRNA (1 μg) was reverse transcribed using cDNA RT Kits (Vazyme Biotech, Nanjing, China). RNA and cDNA concentrations were measured using a spectrophotometer (OD-1000, Wuyi Technology, Nanjing, China). For reverse transcription PCR, the reaction conditions were 30 cycles of denaturation at 98 °C for 10 s, annealing at 55 °C for 30 s, and extension at 72 °C for 60 s. PCR products were separated by electrophoresis through a 1.5% agarose gel containing 0.5% μg/ml ethidium bromide and imaged using a Gel imaging system (Tanon, Shanghai, China). The endogenous glyceraldehyde 3-phosphate dehydrogenase (GADPH) gene was used to normalize the level of the target mRNA. The primer sequence of Adam10 and GADPH were as follows: Adam10 forward: 5′-CAAC ATCAAGGCAAACTATGCGA-3′, reverse: 5′-CTTAG GTTCACTGTCCAAAGCGA-3′; GADPH forward: 5′-AAGGTCATCCCAGAGCTGAAC-3′, reverse: 5′-TGA AGTCGCAGGAGACAACC-3′.

Western blotting

The dissected hippocampal tissues of the mice were homogenized in tissue lysis buffer (Beyotime Biotech, China). After being lysed for 15 min on ice, the samples were centrifuged at 12,000 rpm for 15 min. The protein content in each supernatant fraction was determined using a BCA protein assay kit (Pierce, Rockford, IL, USA), and samples containing equivalent amounts of protein were applied to 12% acrylamide denaturing gels (SDS-PAGE). After electrophoresis, the proteins were transferred to nitrocellulose membranes (Amersham, Little Chalfont, UK) using a Bio-Rad mini-protein-III wet transfer unit (Hercules, CA, USA) overnight at 4 °C. The membranes were then incubated with 5% non-fat milk in TBST (10 mmol/l Tris pH = 7.6, 150 mmol/L NaCl, 0.01%Tween-20) for 1 h at room temperature followed by three washes then were incubated with mouse anti-Adam10 (1:2000; Santa Cruz, TX, USA), rabbit

anti-iNOS (1:5000; Abcam, Temecula, CA, USA), rabbit anti-COX-2 (1:2500; Abcam, Temecula, CA, USA), mouse anti-NF-κB (1:2500; Santa Cruz, TX, USA), and rabbit anti-β-actin (1:5000; Sigma-Aldrich, St. Louis, USA) in TBST overnight at 4 °C. After several washes with TBST buffer, the membranes were incubated for 1 h with HRP-linked secondary antibody (Boster Bioengineering, Wuhan, China) diluted 1:5,000, followed by four washes. The membranes were then processed with enhanced chemiluminescence (ECL) Western blot detection reagents (Millipore, Billerica, MA, USA). Signals were digitally captured using a MicroChemi chemiluminescent image analysis system (DNR Bio-imaging Systems, Jerusalem, Israel). Blots were quantified using the ImageJ software (NIH, Bethesda, MD, USA).

Immunocytochemistry

The immunocytochemistry studies were performed on free-floating sections as described previously [20]. Briefly, the sections were heated (65 °C for 50 min) in antigen unmasking solution (2xSSC/formamide), incubated in 2 M HCl (30 °C for 30 min), rinsed in 0.1 M boric acid (pH 8.5) for 10 min, incubated in 1% H_2O_2 in PBS for 30 min, and blocked in PBS containing 3% normal goat serum, 0.3% (w/v) Triton X-100, and 0.1% BSA (room temperature for 1 h), followed by incubation with mouse anti-Adam10 (1:200; Santa Cruz, TX, USA), rabbit anti-Iba-1 (1:200; Wako, Osaka, Japan), and mouse anti-GFAP (1:100, Boster, Bioengineering, Wuhan, China) antibody at 4 °C overnight. For DAB staining, the sections were developed with super ABC kit (Boster, Wuhan, China). For immunofluorescence assay, the sections were incubated with a TRITC-conjugated goat anti-rabbit antibody (1:200; Cwbiotech, Beijing, China) for Iba-1 staining and a TRITC-conjugated goat anti-mouse antibody (1:200; Cwbiotech, Beijing, China) for Adam10 and GFAP staining, respectively. The sections were then rinsed and mounted on gelatin-coated slides in DAPI antifade mounting medium (SouthernBiotech, Birmingham, AL, USA). The images of Adam10, Iba-1, and GFAP staining were captured with a confocal laser scanning microscope (Olympus LSM-GB200, Japan). The quantitative analyses of the Adam10, Iba-1, and GFAP immunostaining were performed using the ImageJ software (NIH, Bethesda, MD, USA) as described in our previous study [21, 22].

Enzyme-linked immunosorbent assay

The mouse IL-1β and TNF-α ELISA was performed according to the manufacturer's protocol. Briefly, hippocampal lysates were incubated with reaction buffer. The mixture was incubated for 2.5 h at room temperature before protease activity was detected using a microplate reader (BioTek, USA). The samples for each ELISA were run in duplicate, and each ELISA was repeated at least three times, using the mouse IL-1β and TNF-α ELISA kits (ExCell Bio, Shanghai, China).

Statistical analysis

All data are presented as the means ± SEM. Statistical significance was determined by using unpaired two-tailed Student's t test for the two groups' comparison and by using one-way or two-way ANOVA for multi-group comparisons. Tukey's test was used for post hoc comparisons. Differences were considered to be significant for values of $p < 0.05$.

Results

Adam10 expression is decreased in the hippocampus of pilocarpine-induced SE mice

A growing body of evidence suggests a possible link between Adam10 and epilepsy [8, 10, 23, 24]. To test this hypothesis, we first assessed Adam10 expression in different brain regions of mice. Our immunohistochemistry results show clear nuclear staining of Adam10 in the hippocampal CA1 region, DG, striatum, and cortex, with strong Adam10 expression in the hippocampal CA1 region and DG (Fig. 1a), suggesting that Adam10 may have important functions in the hippocampus. A

great number of clinical and experimental studies have consistently reported that the hippocampus is involved in the generation and propagation of seizures in the brain [25–30]. Based on these facts, we speculate that Adam10 plays an important role in the development of epilepsy through regulation of neural activities in the hippocampus.

To investigate the expression pattern of Adam10 in the hippocampus of TLE mice, we examined the hippocampal Adam10 protein levels following pilocarpine-induced SE, which serves as a model of TLE. Our Western blotting data show that Adam10 protein levels in the hippocampus start to progressively decrease from day 14 to day 28 post-SE (Fig. 1b, c). Immunofluorescence data reveal that Adam10-positive cells in the hippocampal CA1 region are significantly decreased at day 28 post-SE compared to those of the control animals (Fig. 1d, e), which further confirmed the decrease of Adam10 expression in the hippocampus of pilocarpine-induced SE mice. Taken together, these results indicate that pilocarpine-induced SE results in a progressive decrease of Adam10 expression in a time-dependent manner.

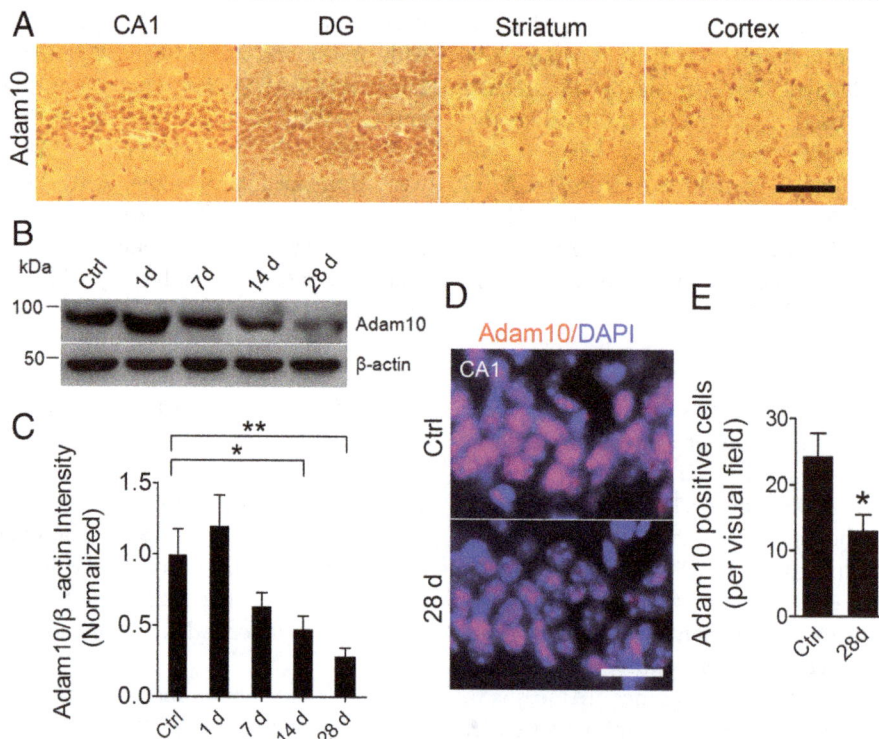

Fig. 1 Adam10 expression is decreased in the hippocampus of TLE mice. **a** Representative images showing the expression of Adam10 protein in the CA1, DG, striatum, and cortex area of the mouse brain by DAB staining ($n = 4$). **b, c** Western blots and quantification of Adam10 protein level in Ctrl and days 1, 7, 14, and 28 post-SE mice ($F_{4,20} = 7.40$, $p = 0.020$, 14 days vs Ctrl; $p = 0.006$, 28 days vs Ctrl) ($n = 5$). **d** Representative images of the immunostaining of Adam10 in the hippocampal CA1 region of the Ctrl and day 28 post-SE mice, respectively. **e** Bar graphs showing the quantification of Adam10-positive cells in Ctrl and day 28 post-SE mice ($p = 0.02$) ($n = 4$). *$p < 0.05$ and **$p < 0.01$ compared with Ctrl mice, unpaired two-tailed Student's t test, and one-way ANOVA. Scale bar = 100 μm in **a** and 20 μm in **d**

Neuroinflammation is triggered in the hippocampus after pilocarpine-induced SE

Neuroinflammation is implicated as a pathogenic mechanism in a variety of neurological disorders including epilepsy. To determine whether neuroinflammation is present in the hippocampus of pilocarpine-induced SE mice, we first examined the inflammatory mediators iNOS and COX-2 and the transcription factor NF-κB, which is responsible for the induction of inflammatory mediators in the hippocampus of pilocarpine-induced SE mice. Our Western blotting results reveal that the hippocampal protein levels of the inflammatory mediators iNOS and COX-2 and the transcription factor NF-κB are significantly increased at days 14 and 28 post-SE compared to those of the control animals (Fig. 2a–d). To further confirm the neuroinflammation in the hippocampus of SE mice, we detected the levels of the cytokines IL-1β and TNF-α by ELISA. Notably, we find that, similar to the changing trend of the above inflammatory mediators and the transcription factor in the hippocampus of SE mice, the production of IL-1β and TNF-α is significantly increased at days 14 and 28 post-SE compared to those of the control mice (Fig. 2e, f). Taken together, these results suggest that SE triggers neuroinflammation in the hippocampus.

Overexpression of Adam10 decreases spontaneous seizures in TLE mice

The AAV vector carrying Adam10 and an empty construct or a ZsGreen gene, which is a green fluorescent protein to be used as an indicator (Fig. 3a). Single-clone PCR identification of Adam10 expression is shown in Fig. 3b. Each AAV vector was bilaterally injected into the hippocampal CA1 region (Fig. 3c). As expected, in the AAV-ZsGreen-treated mice, hippocampal CA1 neurons show robust expression of ZsGreen 2 weeks after the virus injection (Fig. 3d), suggesting high AAV infection efficiency. Quantification of mRNA (Fig. 3e, f) and protein (Fig. 3g, h) levels by RT-PCR and Western blotting 2 weeks after the virus injection validated the overexpression of Adam10 in the mouse hippocampus. Further analysis of Adam10 expression in the hippocampal CA1 region by immunofluorescence reveals that Adam10-overexpressing mice show a higher percentage of Adam10-positive cells than those of the control mice

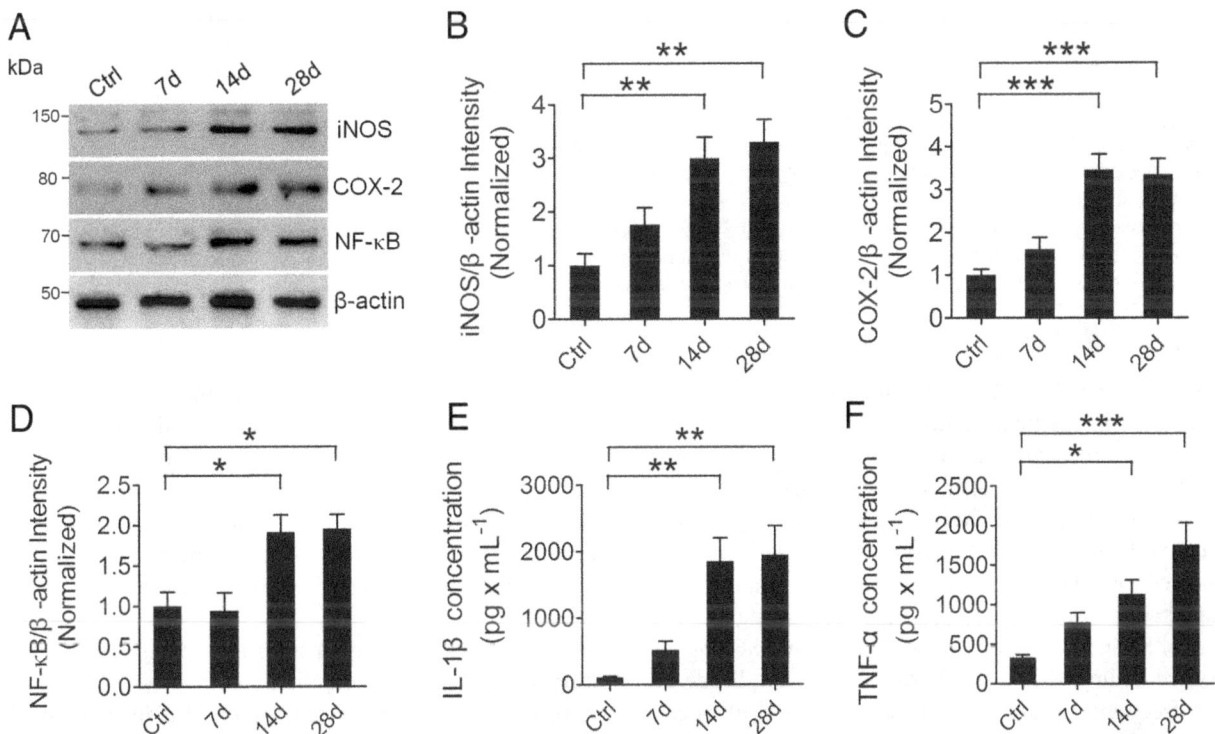

Fig. 2 Inflammation-related proteins and cytokines are increased in the hippocampus of TLE mice. **a** Western blotting showing the protein levels of the inflammation-related proteins iNOS and COX-2 and NF-κB in the hippocampus of Ctrl and 7, 14, and 28 days post-SE mice. **b–d** Bar graphs showing the quantification of iNOS ($F_{3,16} = 9.60$, $p = 0.004$, 14 days vs Ctrl; $p = 0.001$, 28 days vs Ctrl), COX-2 ($F_{3,16} = 17.02$, $p < 0.001$, 14 days vs Ctrl; $p < 0.001$, 28 days vs Ctrl), and NF-κB ($F_{3,16} = 7.76$, $p = 0.025$, 14 days vs Ctrl; $p = 0.018$, 28 days vs Ctrl), which are represented as the intensity ratios of these proteins to β-actin ($n = 5$). **e, f** Bar graphs showing the concentration of IL-1β ($F_{3,16} = 10.32$, $p = 0.004$, 14 days vs Ctrl; $p = 0.002$, 28 days vs Ctrl) and TNF-α ($F_{3,16} = 11.41$, $p = 0.027$, 14 days vs Ctrl; $p < 0.001$, 28 days vs Ctrl) in the hippocampus of Ctrl and 7, 14, and 28 day post-SE mice, which were detected by ELISA ($n = 5$). *$p < 0.05$, **$p < 0.01$, ***$p < 0.001$, and one-way ANOVA

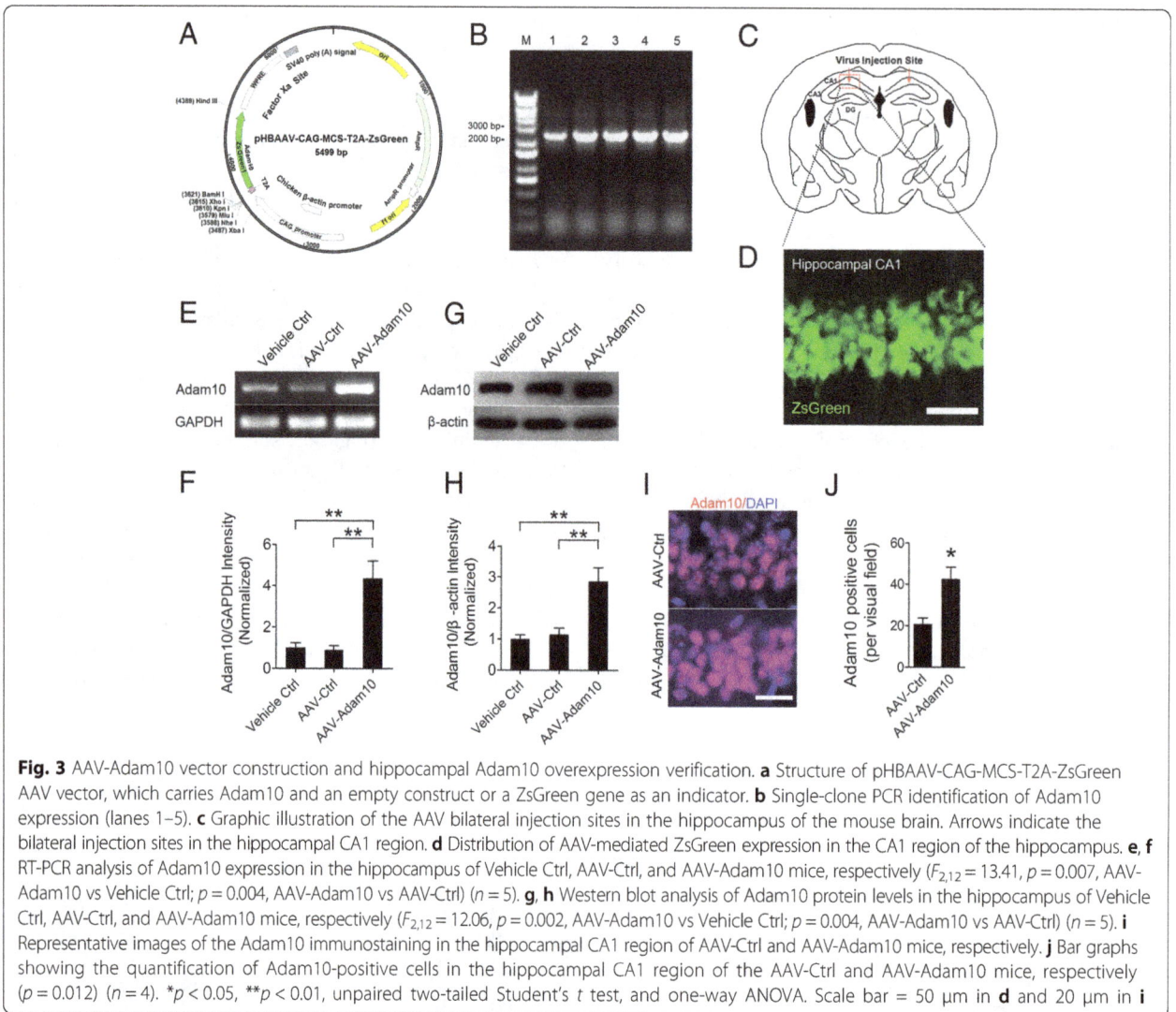

Fig. 3 AAV-Adam10 vector construction and hippocampal Adam10 overexpression verification. **a** Structure of pHBAAV-CAG-MCS-T2A-ZsGreen AAV vector, which carries Adam10 and an empty construct or a ZsGreen gene as an indicator. **b** Single-clone PCR identification of Adam10 expression (lanes 1–5). **c** Graphic illustration of the AAV bilateral injection sites in the hippocampus of the mouse brain. Arrows indicate the bilateral injection sites in the hippocampal CA1 region. **d** Distribution of AAV-mediated ZsGreen expression in the CA1 region of the hippocampus. **e**, **f** RT-PCR analysis of Adam10 expression in the hippocampus of Vehicle Ctrl, AAV-Ctrl, and AAV-Adam10 mice, respectively ($F_{2,12} = 13.41$, $p = 0.007$, AAV-Adam10 vs Vehicle Ctrl; $p = 0.004$, AAV-Adam10 vs AAV-Ctrl) ($n = 5$). **g**, **h** Western blot analysis of Adam10 protein levels in the hippocampus of Vehicle Ctrl, AAV-Ctrl, and AAV-Adam10 mice, respectively ($F_{2,12} = 12.06$, $p = 0.002$, AAV-Adam10 vs Vehicle Ctrl; $p = 0.004$, AAV-Adam10 vs AAV-Ctrl) ($n = 5$). **i** Representative images of the Adam10 immunostaining in the hippocampal CA1 region of AAV-Ctrl and AAV-Adam10 mice, respectively. **j** Bar graphs showing the quantification of Adam10-positive cells in the hippocampal CA1 region of the AAV-Ctrl and AAV-Adam10 mice, respectively ($p = 0.012$) ($n = 4$). *$p < 0.05$, **$p < 0.01$, unpaired two-tailed Student's t test, and one-way ANOVA. Scale bar = 50 μm in **d** and 20 μm in **i**

(Fig. 3i, j), which further confirmed the overexpression of Adam10 in the hippocampus.

To determine whether the overexpression of Adam10 affects the epileptogenesis in the pilocarpine-induced TLE mice, we bilaterally treated the hippocampus of the mice with Vehicle Ctrl, AAV-Ctrl, or AAV-Adam10, followed by pilocarpine-induced SE. All animals were subjected to continuous video EEG monitoring from the start of SE induction until 4 weeks following SE (Fig. 4a). EEG recording shows the burst of large amplitude and high-frequency spikes in both the cortex and hippocampus of SE mice (Fig. 4b). SE analysis shows that AAV-Adam10 treatment did not alter the onset of SE (Fig. 4c) as well as SE duration (Fig. 4d). AAV-Adam10 treatment reduced seizure severity at 15–30 and 30–45 min after SE (Fig. 4e). Following the episode of SE, we monitored the spontaneous recurrent seizures (SRS) by video EEG recording continuously for 4 weeks. Our

data reveal that the latency to the onset of SRS and the electrographic SRS duration remain similar between the AAV-Adam10-treated and the control mice (Fig. 4f, h). However, AAV-Adam10 treatment significantly decreased SRS frequency (Fig. 4g). Taken together, these results suggest that overexpression of Adam10 in the hippocampus decreases spontaneous seizures in TLE mice.

Overexpression of Adam10 suppresses SE-induced hippocampal neuroinflammation

A recent study indicates that Adam10 is involved in the process of neuroinflammation [16]. To investigate whether Adam10 regulates the neuroinflammation in the hippocampus of TLE mice, we treated mice with AAV-Adam10 in order to overexpress Adam10 in the hippocampus, followed by pilocarpine-induced SE. Four weeks after SE, we examined the hippocampal neuroinflammation (Fig. 4a). Our Western blotting results reveal

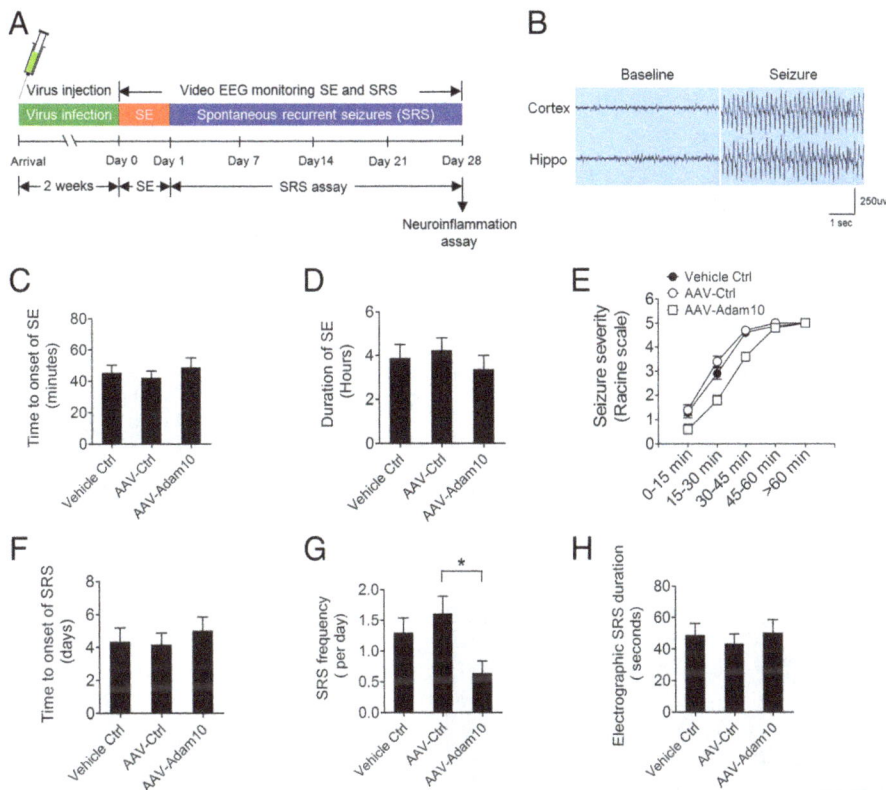

Fig. 4 Adam10 overexpression decreases spontaneous seizures in TLE mice. **a** Schematic diagram of the experimental design. Mice were bilaterally injected with the virus into the hippocampus, and after 2 weeks of recovery, these mice were induced for SE and continuously video EEG monitored for 4 weeks for SE and SRS analysis. These mice were then sacrificed after the EEG recording was completed at day 28 post-SE to detect hippocampal neuroinflammation. **b** A typical EEG recording of the baseline and seizure in the cortex and hippocampus. **c** Bar graph showing the average time to onset of SE in the Vehicle Ctrl, AAV-Ctrl, and AAV-Adam10 mice ($n = 12$). **d** Bar graph showing the quantification of SE duration in the Vehicle Ctrl, AAV-Ctrl, and AAV-Adam10 mice ($n = 10$). **e** Line graphs showing the seizure severity during SE development in the Vehicle Ctrl, AAV-Ctrl, and AAV-Adam10 mice (at 15–30 min, $F_{2,27} = 14.02$, $p = 0.004$, AAV-Adam10 vs Vehicle Ctrl; $p < 0.001$, AAV-Adam10 vs AAV-Ctrl; at 30–45 min, $F_{2,27} = 7.41$, $p = 0.032$, AAV-Adam10 vs Vehicle Ctrl; $p = 0.026$, AAV-Adam10 vs AAV-Ctrl) ($n = 10$). **f** Bar graph showing the average time to onset of first spontaneous seizure in the Vehicle Ctrl, AAV-Ctrl, and AAV-Adam10 mice ($n = 6$). **g** Bar graph showing the SRS frequency in the Vehicle Ctrl, AAV-Ctrl, and AAV-Adam10 mice ($F_{2,15} = 4.23$, $p = 0.031$, AAV-Adam10 vs AAV-Ctrl) ($n = 6$). **h** Bar graph showing the quantification of electrographic SRS duration in the Vehicle Ctrl, AAV-Ctrl, and AAV-Adam10 mice ($n = 6$). *$p < 0.05$ and one-way ANOVA

that the inflammatory mediators iNOS and COX-2 and the inflammatory transcription factor NF-κB are significantly suppressed by hippocampal Adam10 overexpression (Fig. 5a–d). ELISA reveals that after hippocampal Adam10 overexpression, IL-β production is slightly reduced (Fig. 5e), while TNF-α production is significantly decreased compared to those levels in the control animals (Fig. 5f). We next investigated the effects of Adam10 overexpression on glial activation in the hippocampus of TLE mice. Our immunofluorescence data reveal that 4 weeks after SE, the fluorescence intensities of both Iba-1 and GFAP are decreased in the hippocampus of Adam10-overexpressing mice compared to those levels in the control mice (Fig. 5g–i). Notably, the image analysis shows that, in comparison with the control mice, the numbers of GFAP and Iba-1 immunopositive cells in the CA1 region of AAV-Adam10-treated mice

are dramatically reduced, and the cells are forming fewer ramifications (Fig. 5g). Taken together, these data suggest that the overexpression of Adam10 suppresses SE-induced hippocampal neuroinflammation.

Knockdown of Adam10 increases spontaneous seizures in TLE mice

To investigate whether reducing Adam10 expression could play a role in the epileptogenesis in TLE mice, we bilaterally injected lentivirus carrying control or Adam10-shRNA (Fig. 6a) into the hippocampal CA1 regions of mice. A cop-GFP control lentiviral particle, which contains the full-length cop-GFP gene for high-level expression of the fluorescent protein, was used to test the lentiviral infection efficiency. Our results show a robust cop-GFP expression in the hippocampal CA1 region (Fig. 6b), suggesting high lentiviral infection efficiency. Furthermore, the efficiency of

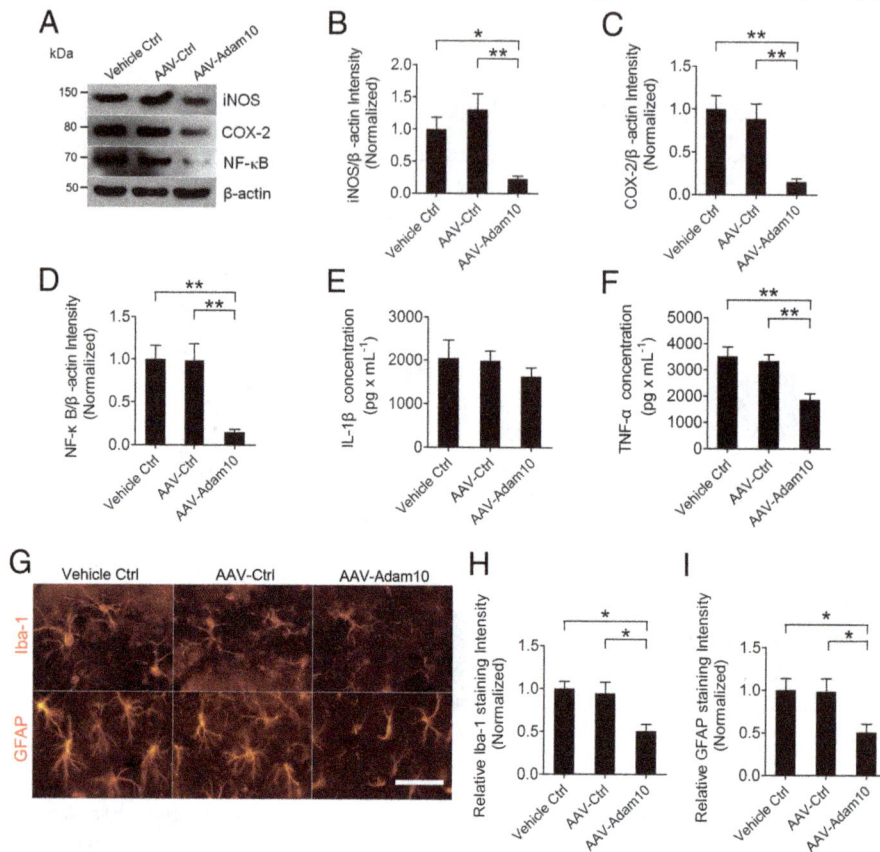

Fig. 5 Adam10 overexpression suppresses hippocampal neuroinflammation in TLE mice. **a** Western blotting showing the protein levels of inflammation-related proteins iNOS and COX-2 and NF-κB in the hippocampus of Vehicle Ctrl, AAV-Ctrl, and AAV-Adam10-treated TLE mice. **b–d** Bar graphs showing the quantification of iNOS ($F_{2,12} = 9.86$, $p = 0.024$, AAV-Adam10 vs Vehicle Ctrl; $p = 0.003$, AAV-Adam10 vs AAV-Ctrl), COX-2 ($F_{2,12} = 11.27$, $p = 0.003$, AAV-Adam10 vs Vehicle Ctrl; $p = 0.007$, AAV-Adam10 vs AAV-Ctrl), and NF-κB ($F_{2,12} = 11.05$, $p = 0.004$, AAV-Adam10 vs Vehicle Ctrl; $p = 0.005$, AAV-Adam10 vs AAV-Ctrl), which were represented as the intensity ratios of these proteins to β-actin ($n = 5$). **e, f** Bar graphs showing the concentration of IL-1β ($F_{2,12} = 0.59$, $p = 0.572$) and TNF-α ($F_{2,12} = 10.11$, $p = 0.004$, AAV-Adam10 vs Vehicle Ctrl; $p = 0.009$, AAV-Adam10 vs AAV-Ctrl) in the hippocampus of Ctrl, AAV-Ctrl, and AAV-Adam10-treated TLE mice as detected by ELISA ($n = 5$). **g** Representative images of the immunostaining of Iba-1 and GFAP in the hippocampal CA1 region of the Ctrl, AAV-Ctrl, and AAV-Adam10 mice, respectively. **h, i** Bar graphs showing the quantification of Iba-1- ($F_{2,12} = 7.31$, $p = 0.012$, AAV-Adam10 vs Vehicle Ctrl; $p = 0.024$, AAV-Adam10 vs AAV-Ctrl) and GFAP ($F_{2,12} = 4.61$, $p = 0.039$, AAV-Adam10 vs Vehicle Ctrl; $p = 0.042$, AAV-Adam10 vs AAV-Ctrl)-positive cells in the hippocampal CA1 region of the Ctrl, AAV-Ctrl, and AAV-Adam10 mice, respectively ($n = 4$). *$p < 0.05$, **$p < 0.01$, and one-way ANOVA. Scale bar = 50 μm in **g**

Adam10 silencing was confirmed by RT-PCR and Western blotting analysis 2 weeks after the lentivirus injection, which respectively show a significant reduction of mRNA (Fig. 6c, d) and protein (Fig. 6e, f) levels of Adam10. Immunofluorescence reveals that shRNA-Adam10-treated mice showed fewer Adam10-positive cells than those of the shRNA-control mice (Fig. 6g, h), which confirmed the knockdown of Adam10 in the hippocampus.

To further determine whether Adam10 affects epileptogenesis in the pilocarpine-induced SE mice, we treated mice with Vehicle Ctrl, lentivirus carrying shRNA-Ctrl, and shRNA-Adam10 in the hippocampus, followed by pilocarpine-induced SE. All animals were subjected to continuous video EEG monitoring as described in Fig. 4a. We then analyzed the SE episode and SRS of Vehicle

Ctrl and shRNA-Ctrl- and shRNA-Adam10-treated mice. SE analysis shows that shRNA-Adam10 treatment did not alter the onset of SE (Fig. 7a) as well as SE duration (Fig. 7b). Furthermore, shRNA-Adam10 treatment increased the seizure severity at 15–30 min after SE (Fig. 7c). Following the episode of SE, we monitored the SRS continuously for 4 weeks. Our data show that the latency to the onset of SRS and the electrographic SRS duration remain similar between the shRNA-Adam10-treated and the control mice (Fig. 7d, f). However, shRNA-Adam10 treatment significantly increased the SRS frequency (Fig. 7e). Taken together, these results suggest that knockdown of Adam10 increases spontaneous seizures in pilocarpine-induced TLE mice.

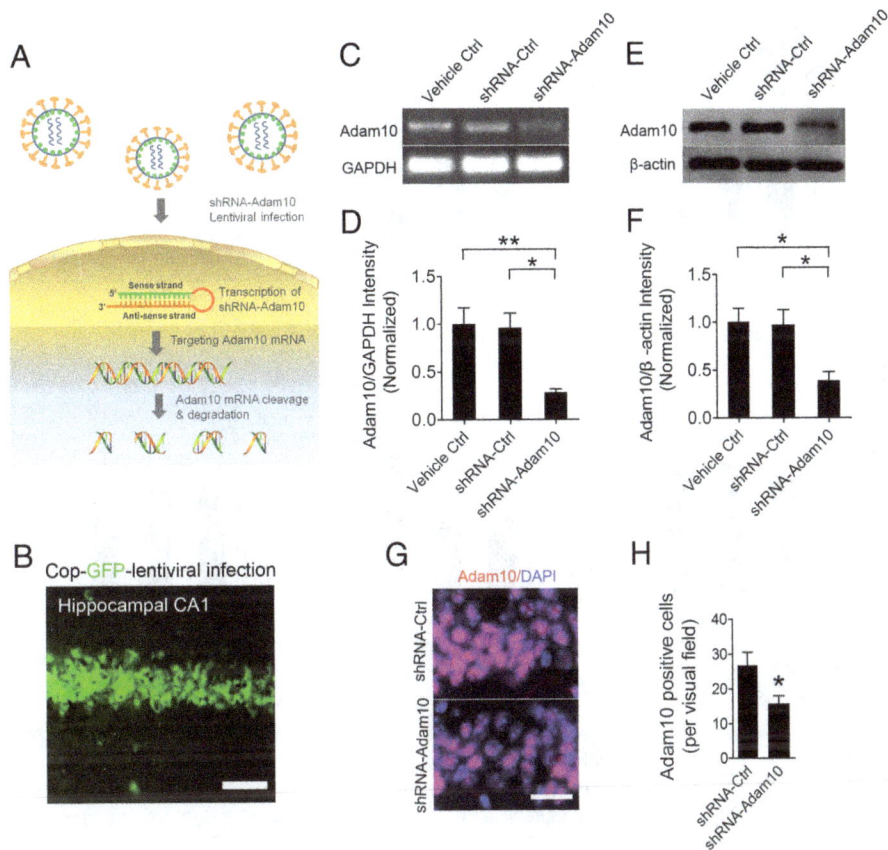

Fig. 6 shRNA-mediated Adam10 knockdown in the hippocampus. **a** Action mode of shRNA-mediated Adam10 knockdown via lentiviral vector infection. **b** Distribution of lentivirus-mediated cop-GFP expression in the CA1 region of the hippocampus. **c, d** RT-PCR analysis of Adam10 expression in the hippocampus of Vehicle Ctrl, shRNA-Ctrl, and shRNA-Adam10 mice, respectively ($F_{2,12} = 8.84$, $p = 0.008$, shRNA-Adam10 vs Vehicle Ctrl; $p = 0.032$, shRNA-Adam10 vs shRNA-Ctrl) ($n = 5$). **e, f** Western blot analysis of Adam10 protein levels in the hippocampus of Vehicle Ctrl, shRNA-Ctrl, and shRNA-Adam10 mice, respectively ($F_{2,12} = 6.38$, $p = 0.021$, shRNA-Adam10 vs Vehicle Ctrl; $p = 0.027$, shRNA-Adam10 vs shRNA-Ctrl) ($n = 5$). **g** Representative images of the immunostaining of Adam10 in the hippocampal CA1 region of the shRNA-Ctrl and shRNA-Adam10 mice, respectively. **h** Bar graph showing the quantification of Adam10-positive cells in the hippocampal CA1 region of shRNA-Ctrl and shRNA-Adam10 mice, respectively ($p = 0.014$) ($n = 4$). *$p < 0.05$, **$p < 0.01$, unpaired two-tailed Student's t test, and one-way ANOVA. Scale bar = 50 μm in **b** and 20 μm in **g**

Knockdown of Adam10 exacerbates hippocampal neuroinflammation in TLE mice

We next determined whether the knockdown of Adam10 had any effect on hippocampal neuroinflammation in pilocarpine-induced SE mice. For this purpose, we first examined the inflammatory mediators iNOS and COX-2 and the inflammatory transcription factor NF-κB by Western blotting. Our results reveal that both the inflammatory mediators iNOS and COX-2 and the inflammatory transcription factor NF-κB are significantly increased in shRNA-Adam10-treated mice compared to the levels in Vehicle Ctrl- and shRNA-Ctrl-treated mice 4 weeks after SE (Fig. 8a–d). Consistently, ELISA reveals that after the hippocampal Adam10 knockdown, both IL-β and TNF-α productions are significantly increased (Fig. 8e, f). We next investigated the effects of Adam10 knockdown on glial activation in the hippocampus. Our immunofluorescence data reveal that 4 weeks after SE,

the fluorescence intensities of both Iba-1 and GFAP are significantly increased in the hippocampus of Adam10 knockdown mice compared to those of the control mice (Fig. 8g–i). Notably, the image analysis shows that the numbers of GFAP and Iba-1 immunopositive cells in the CA1 region of shRNA-Adam10-treated mice are dramatically increased in comparison with those of Vehicle Ctrl and shRNA-Ctrl mice, and the cells form more ramifications (Fig. 8g). Taken together, these data suggest that knockdown of Adam10 exacerbates hippocampal neuroinflammation in pilocarpine-induced TLE mice.

Increased seizure activity by Adam10 knockdown is dependent on hippocampal neuroinflammation

Beyond its role as a pathological hallmark of epilepsy, we hypothesized that neuroinflammation could affect the process of Adam10-regulated epileptogenesis. To test this hypothesis, we treated Adam10 knockdown and

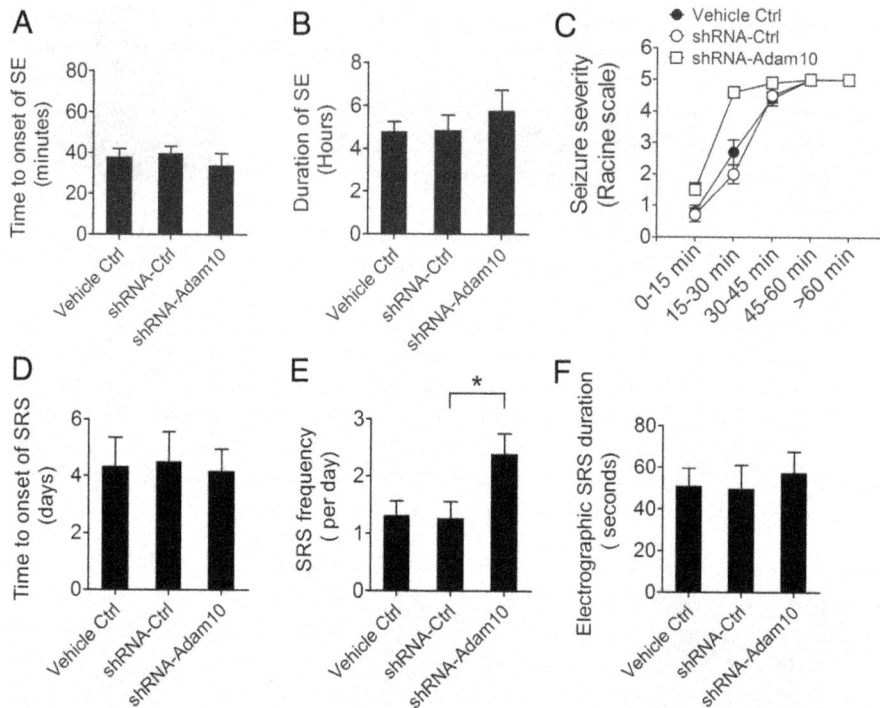

Fig. 7 Adam10 knockdown increases spontaneous seizures in TLE mice. **a** Bar graph showing the average time to onset of SE in the Vehicle Ctrl, shRNA-Ctrl, and shRNA-Adam10 mice ($n = 12$). **b** Bar graph showing the quantification of SE duration in the Vehicle Ctrl, shRNA-Ctrl, and shRNA-Adam10 mice ($n = 10$). **c** Line graphs showing the seizure severity during SE development in the Vehicle Ctrl, shRNA-Ctrl, and shRNA-Adam10 mice (at 15–30 min, $F_{2,27} = 19.95$, $p < 0.001$, shRNA-Adam10 vs Vehicle Ctrl; $p < 0.001$, shRNA-Adam10 vs shRNA-Ctrl) ($n = 10$). **d** Bar graph showing the average time to onset of the first spontaneous seizure in the Vehicle Ctrl, shRNA-Ctrl, and shRNA-Adam10 mice ($n = 6$). **e** Bar graph showing the SRS frequency in the Vehicle Ctrl, shRNA-Ctrl, and shRNA-Adam10 mice ($F_{2,15} = 4.55$, $p = 0.043$, shRNA-Adam10 vs shRNA-Ctrl) ($n = 6$). **f** Bar graph showing the quantification of electrographic SRS duration in the Vehicle Ctrl, shRNA-Ctrl, and shRNA-Adam10 mice ($n = 6$). *$p < 0.05$ and one-way ANOVA

control mice with pilocarpine to induce SE, followed by multiple doses of the anti-inflammatory agent minocycline to block neuroinflammation. All animals were subjected to continuous video EEG monitoring from the start of SE induction until 4 weeks post-SE (Fig. 9a). We then analyzed the SRS in these mice. Our results show that minocycline treatment significantly suppressed the Adam10 knockdown-induced increase of SRS (Fig. 9b).

To confirm the anti-inflammatory effect of minocycline, we used Western blotting to examine the hippocampal protein levels of the inflammatory mediators iNOS and COX-2 and the inflammatory transcription factor NF-κB after minocycline treatment. Our results reveal that minocycline treatment suppresses the Adam10 knockdown-induced increase in expression of the inflammatory mediators iNOS and COX-2 and the inflammatory transcription factor NF-κB (Fig. 9c–f). Furthermore, we have observed a remarkable reduction of iNOS (Fig. 9d) and NF-κB (Fig. 9f) expression after minocycline treatment in shRNA-Ctrl-treated mice. Consistent with the Western blotting results, ELISA reveals that minocycline suppressed the Adam10 knock

down-induced increase in the production of IL-1β and TNF-α (Fig. 9g, h). Moreover, minocycline treatment decreased TNF-α levels in ShRNA-Ctrl mice (Fig. 9h).

Taken together, these results suggest that increased seizure activity in the Adam10 knockdown TLE mice is dependent on hippocampal neuroinflammation.

Discussion

Adam10 was initially identified as an alpha-secretase in the processing of the amyloid precursor protein, which is involved in Alzheimer's disease. Recent studies shed light on the link between Adam10 and another neurological disease, such as epilepsy. Our findings that Adam10 is abundantly expressed in the hippocampal region highlight the importance of Adam10 for the regulation of neural activities in the hippocampus. The hippocampus is a region of the forebrain, which is highly vulnerable to excitotoxic injury and is largely involved in epileptic seizures. Therefore, it is plausible that the Adam10 gene regulates the development of epilepsy via modulation of hippocampal neural circuit activities. We have shown that Adam10 expression in the hippocampus

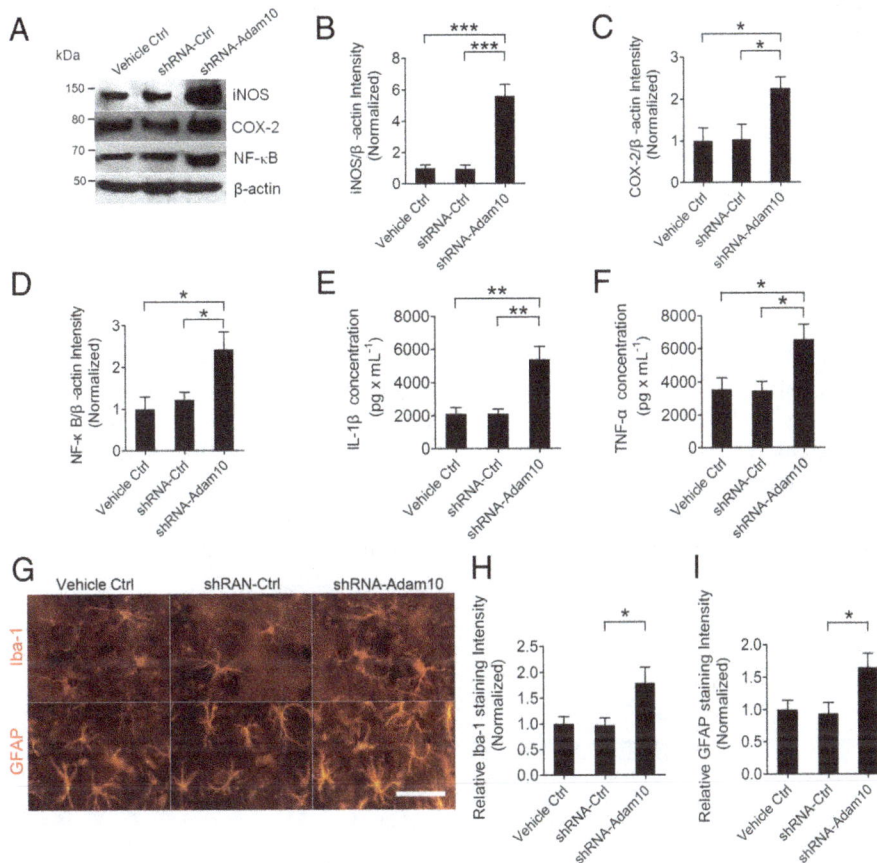

Fig. 8 Adam10 knockdown exacerbates hippocampal neuroinflammation in TLE mice. **a** Western blotting showing the protein levels of the inflammation-related proteins iNOS and COX-2 and NF-κB in the hippocampus of Vehicle Ctrl, shRNA-Ctrl, and shRNA-Adam10-treated TLE mice. **b–d** Bar graphs showing the quantification of iNOS ($F_{2,12} = 32.09$, $p < 0.001$, shRNA-Adam10 vs Vehicle Ctrl; $p < 0.001$, shRNA-Adam10 vs shRNA-Ctrl), COX-2 ($F_{2,12} = 5.32$, $p = 0.035$, shRNA-Adam10 vs Vehicle Ctrl; $p = 0.041$, shRNA-Adam10 vs shRNA-Ctrl), and NF-κB ($F_{2,12} = 5.82$, $p = 0.020$, shRNA-Adam10 vs Vehicle Ctrl; $p = 0.049$, shRNA-Adam10 vs shRNA-Ctrl), which were represented as the intensity ratios of these proteins to β-actin ($n = 5$). **e, f** Bar graphs showing the concentration of IL-1β ($F_{2,12} = 12.78$, $p = 0.003$, shRNA-Adam10 vs Vehicle Ctrl; $p = 0.003$, shRNA-Adam10 vs shRNA-Ctrl) and TNF-α ($F_{2,12} = 5.66$, $p = 0.035$, shRNA-Adam10 vs Vehicle Ctrl; $p = 0.030$, shRNA-Adam10 vs shRNA-Ctrl) in the hippocampus of Vehicle Ctrl, shRNA-Ctrl, and shRNA-Adam10-treated TLE mice, as detected by ELISA ($n = 5$). **g** Representative images of the immunostaining of Iba-1 and GFAP in the hippocampal CA1 region of the Vehicle Ctrl, shRNA-Ctrl, and shRNA-Adam10 mice, respectively. **h, i** Bar graphs showing the quantification of Iba-1- ($F_{2,12} = 4.70$, $p = 0.047$, shRNA-Adam10 vs shRNA-Ctrl) and GFAP ($F_{2,12} = 4.88$, $p = 0.039$, shRNA-Adam10 vs shRNA-Ctrl)-positive cells in the hippocampal CA1 region of the Vehicle Ctrl, shRNA-Ctrl, and shRNA-Adam10 mice, respectively ($n = 4$). *$p < 0.05$, **$p < 0.01$, ***$p < 0.001$, and one-way ANOVA. Scale bar = 50 μm in **g**

progressively decreases from day 14 to day 28 post-SE. Consistent with our findings, a previous study reported that Adam10 mRNA levels were significantly downregulated in the CA1 and CA3 pyramidal cell layers of the hippocampus at 24 h after a kainic acid-induced generalized seizure [10].

Recent studies implicate neuroinflammation as playing a crucial role in the pathophysiological processes of both animal and human TLE [31–33]. It has been reported that neuroinflammation occurs following SE in rodent brains and is associated with the process of chronic recurrence of spontaneous seizures [34]. Here, we demonstrate that the inflammatory mediators iNOS and COX-2 and the transcription factor NF-κB in the

hippocampus of pilocarpine-induced TLE mice are significantly increased, which is consistent with previous reports [35, 36]. Additionally, the proinflammatory cytokines IL-1β and TNF-α are increased as well.

Neuroinflammation in TLE mice is characterized by the production of inflammatory mediators and cytokines as well as glial activation [32, 37]. It has been reported that glia activation occurs following prolonged seizures and is considered to be involved in the subsequent proinflammatory cytokine production [34, 38]. Consistently, in this study, we found that both microglia and astrocytes are significantly activated in the hippocampus of TLE mice. It has been suggested that seizure activities lead to the production of proinflammatory mediators, such as IL-1β and TNF, which in turn affect seizure severity and recurrence [34]. Furthermore, systemic injection of lipopolysaccharide, an inducer of inflammation in the brain, increases the seizure susceptibility [39, 40]. In agreement with these studies, we find here that neuroinflammation in the hippocampus of TLE mice is accompanied by increased spontaneous seizure recurrence after SE. Combined with previous data, our findings imply that prolonged SE activates microglia and astrocytes and induces inflammatory mediators and cytokines, which may contribute to the increased spontaneous seizure recurrence in TLE mice.

Adam10 has been suggested to be involved in the neuroinflammation process under the conditions of epilepsy. Herein, we demonstrate that overexpression of Adam10 in the hippocampus suppresses neuroinflammation and reduces seizure activities, while inhibition of Adam10 exacerbates hippocampal neuroinflammation and

increases seizure activity in TLE mice. Consistent with our findings, a previous study by Clement et al. reported that overexpression of Adam10 decreased seizure activity and suppressed neuroinflammation by reducing glia activation in a kainate-induced seizure model [41]. Interestingly, Clement et al. also demonstrated that when there is a lack of APP expression, overexpression of Adam10 leads to increased neuroinflammation and seizure activity [41]. These findings suggest that the action of Adam10 may be dependent on its substrates. To further investigate whether the effect of Adam10 on seizure activity is dependent on hippocampal neuroinflammation in TLE mice, we induced SE in Adam10 knockdown mice, followed by the treatment with the anti-inflammatory agent minocycline. We demonstrated that minocycline treatment suppressed the Adam10 knockdown-induced increase of spontaneous recurrent seizures. Minocycline is known as an inhibitor of microglial activation which

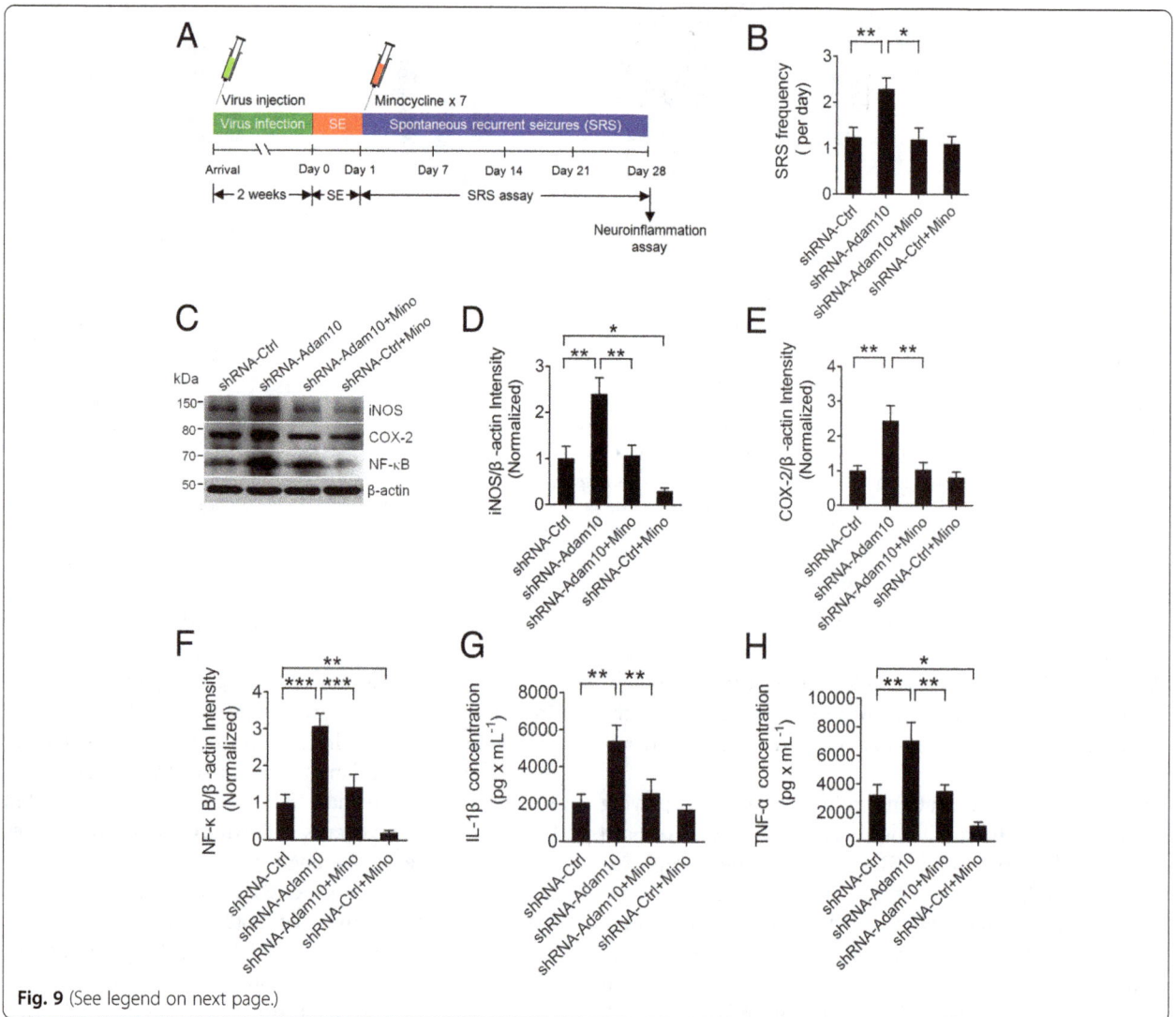

Fig. 9 (See legend on next page.)

(See figure on previous page.)

Fig. 9 Increased seizure activity by Adam10 knockdown is dependent on hippocampal neuroinflammation. **a** Schematic diagram of the experimental design. Mice were bilaterally injected into the hippocampus with either Vehicle Ctrl or lentivirus carrying the shRNA-Ctrl or shRNA-Adam10. Following 2 weeks of recovery, the mice were induced to SE, and 24 hours after the SE induction, they were treated with minocycline (50 mg/kg, i.p.) seven times at 24-hour intervals. The mice were continuously video EEG monitored for 4 weeks for SRS analysis. The mice were then sacrificed after the EEG recording was completed at day 28 post-SE for analysis of hippocampal neuroinflammation. **b** Bar graph showing the SRS frequency in the shRNA-Ctrl, shRNA-Adam10, and shRNA-Adam10 + Minocycline- and shRNA-Ctrl + Minocycline-treated TLE mice. A two-way ANOVA revealed a significant main effect of Adam10 knockdown ($F_{1,20} = 6.60$, $p = 0.02$), minocycline treatment ($F_{1,20} = 7.90$, $p = 0.011$), and Adam10 knockdown × minocycline interaction ($F_{1,20} = 4.69$, $p = 0.043$) on SRS frequency. A Tukey post hoc test revealed that SRS frequency was significantly increased in shRNA-Adam10 mice compared to that in shRNA-Ctrl mice ($p = 0.003$). Minocycline treatment suppressed the shRNA-Adam10-induced increase of SRS frequency ($p = 0.02$), while the minocycline-treated shRNA-Ctrl mice did not show any significant difference of SRS frequency compared to the shRNA-Ctrl mice ($p = 0.087$) ($n = 6$). **c** Western blotting showing the protein levels of the inflammation-related proteins iNOS, COX-2, and NF-κB in the hippocampus of shRNA-Ctrl, shRNA-Adam10, and shRNA-Adam10 + Minocycline- and shRNA-Ctrl + Minocycline-treated TLE mice. **d–f** Bar graphs showing the quantification of iNOS, COX-2, and NF-κB as measured by the intensity ratios of these proteins to β-actin. For iNOS, a two-way ANOVA revealed a significant main effect of both Adam10 knockdown ($F_{1,16} = 19.13$, $p < 0.001$) and minocycline treatment ($F_{1,16} = 16.67$, $p < 0.001$) on iNOS protein level, but there was no significant interaction between Adam10 knockdown and minocycline treatment ($F_{1,16} = 1.60$, $p = 0.224$). A Tukey post hoc test revealed that the iNOS protein content was significantly increased in shRNA-Adam10 mice compared to that in shRNA-Ctrl mice ($p = 0.001$). Minocycline treatment suppressed the shRNA-Adam10-induced increase in iNOS protein level ($p = 0.002$), Moreover, the iNOS protein level in minocycline-treated shRNA-Ctrl mice was significantly decreased compared to that in shRNA-Ctrl mice ($p = 0.044$). For COX-2, a two-way ANOVA revealed a significant main effect of Adam10 knockdown ($F_{1,16} = 9.98$, $p = 0.006$), minocycline treatment ($F_{1,16} = 9.05$, $p = 0.008$), and Adam10 knockdown × minocycline interaction ($F_{1,16} = 5.37$, $p = 0.034$) on the COX-2 protein level. A Tukey post hoc test revealed that COX-2 protein content was significantly increased in shRNA-Adam10 mice compared to that in shRNA-Ctrl mice ($p = 0.001$). Minocycline treatment suppressed the shRNA-Adam10-induced increase in COX-2 protein level ($p = 0.002$), while the minocycline-treated shRNA-Ctrl mice did not show any significant difference in the COX-2 protein content compared to that in shRNA-Ctrl mice ($p = 0.631$). For NF-κB, a two-way ANOVA revealed a significant main effect of both Adam10 knockdown ($F_{1,16} = 37.88$, $p < 0.001$) and minocycline treatment ($F_{1,16} = 20.67$, $p < 0.001$) on the NF-κB protein level, but there was no significant interaction between Adam10 knockdown and minocycline treatment ($F_{1,16} = 2.46$, $p = 0.136$). A Tukey post hoc test revealed that the NF-κB protein content was significantly increased in shRNA-Adam10 mice compared to that in shRNA-Ctrl mice ($p < 0.001$). Minocycline treatment suppressed the shRNA-Adam10-induced increase in NF-κB protein level ($p < 0.001$). Moreover, the NF-κB protein level in minocycline-treated shRNA-Ctrl mice was significantly decreased compared to the levels in the shRNA-Ctrl mice ($p = 0.008$) ($n = 5$). **g, h** Bar graphs showing the concentration of IL-1β and TNF-α in the hippocampus of shRNA-Ctrl, shRNA-Adam10, and shRNA-Adam10 + Minocycline- and shRNA-Ctrl + Minocycline-treated TLE mice as detected by ELISA. For IL-1β, a two-way ANOVA revealed a significant main effect of both Adam10 knockdown ($F_{1,16} = 11.14$, $p = 0.004$) and minocycline treatment ($F_{1,16} = 6.31$, $p = 0.023$) on IL-1β concentration, but there was no significant interaction between Adam10 knockdown and minocycline treatment ($F_{1,16} = 3.781$, $p = 0.070$). A Tukey post hoc test revealed that the IL-1β concentration was significantly increased in shRNA-Adam10 mice compared to that in shRNA-Ctrl mice ($p = 0.002$). Minocycline treatment suppressed the shRNA-Adam10-induced increase in IL-1β concentration ($p = 0.006$), while the minocycline-treated shRNA-Ctrl mice did not show any significant difference in IL-1β concentration compared to that in shRNA-Ctrl mice ($p = 0.693$). For TNF-α, a two-way ANOVA revealed a significant main effect of both Adam10 knockdown ($F_{1,16} = 16.09$, $p = 0.001$) and minocycline treatment ($F_{1,16} = 13.32$, $p = 0.002$) on TNF-α concentration, but there was no significant interaction between Adam10 knockdown and minocycline treatment ($F_{1,16} = 0.83$, $p = 0.375$). A Tukey post hoc test revealed that the TNF-α concentration was significantly increased in shRNA-Adam10 mice compared to that in shRNA-Ctrl mice ($p = 0.003$). Minocycline treatment suppressed the shRNA-Adam10-induced increase in TNF-α concentration ($p = 0.005$). Moreover, the TNF-α concentration in minocycline-treated shRNA-Ctrl mice was significantly decreased compared to that in shRNA-Ctrl mice ($p = 0.041$) ($n = 5$). *$p < 0.05$, **$p < 0.01$, ***$p < 0.001$, and two-way ANOVA

selectively inhibits microglia-related gene expression [42]. Therefore, it is possible that minocycline suppresses seizure activity in Adam10 knockdown mice through repression of microglia-mediated neuroinflammation.

Conclusions

Our data identify Adam10 as a key regulator of hippocampal neuroinflammation-dependent seizure activity in pilocarpine-induced TLE mice. Our results suggest that the modulation of hippocampal neuroinflammation via Adam10 could play a pivotal role in the development of epilepsy.

Abbreviations
AAV: Adeno-associated virus; AD: Alzheimer's disease; Adam: A disintegrin and metalloproteinase domain-containing protein; Aβ: Amyloid β; ELISA: Enzyme-linked immunosorbent assay; sAPP: Soluble N-terminal APP fragment; SE: Status epilepticus; TLE: Temporal lobe epilepsy

Funding
This work was supported by grants from the National Natural Science Foundation of China (81673413 to Xinjian Zhu), Natural Science Foundation of Jiangsu Province (BK20141335 to Xinjian Zhu), the Fundamental Research Funds for the Central Universities (2242017K3DN33 and 2242017K40095 to Xinjian Zhu), the Specialized Research Fund for the Doctoral Program of Higher Education (20130092120043 to Xinjian Zhu), and the Scientific Research Foundation of State Education Ministry for the Returned Overseas Chinese Scholars (No. 311, 2015 to Xinjian Zhu).

Authors' contributions
XZ and XL designed the research. XZ, MZ, KX, LY, BH, and RH performed the research. AZ and HY provided technical help. XZ analyzed the data and wrote the paper. All authors read and approved the final manuscript.

Consent for publication
Not applicable.

Competing interests

The authors declare that they have no competing interests.

Author details

[1]Department of Pharmacology, Medical School of Southeast University, Dingjiaqiao 87th, Nanjing 210009, China. [2]Department of Geriatrics, The First Affiliated Hospital of Nanjing Medical University, Nanjing, China. [3]Department of Pathology, Medical School of Southeast University, Nanjing, China.

References

1. Reiss K, Saftig P. The "a disintegrin and metalloprotease" (ADAM) family of sheddases: physiological and cellular functions. Semin Cell Dev Biol. 2009;20:126–37.
2. Reiss K, Maretzky T, Ludwig A, Tousseyn T, de Strooper B, Hartmann D, Saftig P. ADAM10 cleavage of N-cadherin and regulation of cell-cell adhesion and beta-catenin nuclear signalling. EMBO J. 2005;24:742–52.
3. Weber S, Saftig P. Ectodomain shedding and ADAMs in development. Development. 2012;139:3693–709.
4. Postina R, Schroeder A, Dewachter I, Bohl J, Schmitt U, Kojro E, Prinzen C, Endres K, Hiemke C, Blessing M, et al. A disintegrin-metalloproteinase prevents amyloid plaque formation and hippocampal defects in an Alzheimer disease mouse model. J Clin Invest. 2004;113:1456–64.
5. Kuhn PH, Wang H, Dislich B, Colombo A, Zeitschel U, Ellwart JW, Kremmer E, Rossner S, Lichtenthaler SF. ADAM10 is the physiologically relevant, constitutive alpha-secretase of the amyloid precursor protein in primary neurons. EMBO J. 2010;29:3020–32.
6. Chasseigneaux S, Allinquant B. Functions of Abeta, sAPPalpha and sAPPbeta : similarities and differences. J Neurochem. 2012;120(Suppl 1):99–108.
7. Endres K, Fahrenholz F, Lotz J, Hiemke C, Teipel S, Lieb K, Tuscher O, Fellgiebel A. Increased CSF APPs-alpha levels in patients with Alzheimer disease treated with acitretin. Neurology. 2014;83:1930–5.
8. Prox J, Bernreuther C, Altmeppen H, Grendel J, Glatzel M, D'Hooge R, Stroobants S, Ahmed T, Balschun D, Willem M, et al. Postnatal disruption of the disintegrin/metalloproteinase ADAM10 in brain causes epileptic seizures, learning deficits, altered spine morphology, and defective synaptic functions. J Neurosci. 2013;33:12915–28. 12928a.
9. Kuhn PH, Colombo AV, Schusser B, Dreymueller D, Wetzel S, Schepers U, Herber J, Ludwig A, Kremmer E, Montag D, et al. Systematic substrate identification indicates a central role for the metalloprotease ADAM10 in axon targeting and synapse function. Elife. 2016;5:1–29.
10. Ortiz RM, Karkkainen I, Huovila AP, Honkaniemi J. ADAM9, ADAM10, and ADAM15 mRNA levels in the rat brain after kainic acid-induced status epilepticus. Brain Res Mol Brain Res. 2005;137:272–5.
11. Pernot F, Heinrich C, Barbier L, Peinnequin A, Carpentier P, Dhote F, Baille V, Beaup C, Depaulis A, Dorandeu F. Inflammatory changes during epileptogenesis and spontaneous seizures in a mouse model of mesiotemporal lobe epilepsy. Epilepsia. 2011;52:2315–25.
12. Maroso M, Balosso S, Ravizza T, Iori V, Wright CI, French J, Vezzani A. Interleukin-1beta biosynthesis inhibition reduces acute seizures and drug resistant chronic epileptic activity in mice. Neurotherapeutics. 2011;8:304–15.
13. Crespel A, Coubes P, Rousset MC, Brana C, Rougier A, Rondouin G, Bockaert J, Baldy-Moulinier M, Lerner-Natoli M. Inflammatory reactions in human medial temporal lobe epilepsy with hippocampal sclerosis. Brain Res. 2002;952:159–69.
14. Lehtimaki KA, Keranen T, Palmio J, Peltola J. Levels of IL-1beta and IL-1ra in cerebrospinal fluid of human patients after single and prolonged seizures. Neuroimmunomodulation. 2010;17:19–22.
15. Karkkainen I, Rybnikova E, Pelto-Huikko M, Huovila AP. Metalloprotease-disintegrin (ADAM) genes are widely and differentially expressed in the adult CNS. Mol Cell Neurosci. 2000;15:547–60.
16. O'Sullivan SA, Gasparini F, Mir AK, Dev KK. Fractalkine shedding is mediated by p38 and the ADAM10 protease under pro-inflammatory conditions in human astrocytes. J Neuroinflammation. 2016;13:189.
17. Wang JY, Darbinyan A, White MK, Darbinian N, Reiss K, Amini S. Involvement of IRS-1 interaction with ADAM10 in the regulation of neurite extension. J Cell Physiol. 2014;229:1039–46.
18. Zhu X, Han X, Blendy JA, Porter BE. Decreased CREB levels suppress epilepsy. Neurobiol Dis. 2012;45:253–63.
19. Racine RJ. Modification of seizure activity by electrical stimulation. II Motor seizure. Electroencephalogr Clin Neurophysiol. 1972;32:281–94.
20. Zhu X, Shen K, Bai Y, Zhang A, Xia Z, Chao J, Yao H. NADPH oxidase activation is required for pentylenetetrazole kindling-induced hippocampal autophagy. Free Radic Biol Med. 2016;94:230–42.
21. Zhu X, Dong J, Shen K, Bai Y, Zhang Y, Lv X, Chao J, Yao H. NMDA receptor NR2B subunits contribute to PTZ-kindling-induced hippocampal astrocytosis and oxidative stress. Brain Res Bull. 2015;114:70–8.
22. Zhu X, Dong J, Han B, Huang R, Zhang A, Xia Z, Chang H, Chao J, Yao H. Neuronal nitric oxide synthase contributes to PTZ kindling epilepsy-induced hippocampal endoplasmic reticulum stress and oxidative damage. Front Cell Neurosci. 2017;11:377.
23. Tao H, Zhao J, Zhou X, Ma Z, Chen Y, Sun F, Cui L, Zhou H, Cai Y, Chen Y, et al. Promoter variants of the ADAM10 gene and their roles in temporal lobe epilepsy. Front Neurol. 2016;7:108.
24. Saftig P, Lichtenthaler SF. The alpha secretase ADAM10: a metalloprotease with multiple functions in the brain. Prog Neurobiol. 2015;135:1–20.
25. Cendes F, Sakamoto AC, Spreafico R, Bingaman W, Becker AJ. Epilepsies associated with hippocampal sclerosis. Acta Neuropathol. 2014;128:21–37.
26. Cho KO, Lybrand ZR, Ito N, Brulet R, Tafacory F, Zhang L, Good L, Ure K, Kernie SG, Birnbaum SG, et al. Aberrant hippocampal neurogenesis contributes to epilepsy and associated cognitive decline. Nat Commun. 2015;6:6606.
27. Buckmaster PS, Wen X, Toyoda I, Gulland FM, Van Bonn W. Hippocampal neuropathology of domoic acid-induced epilepsy in California sea lions (Zalophus californianus). J Comp Neurol. 2014;522:1691–706.
28. Buckmaster PS, Lew FH. Rapamycin suppresses mossy fiber sprouting but not seizure frequency in a mouse model of temporal lobe epilepsy. J Neurosci. 2011;31:2337–47.
29. Pallud J, Haussler U, Langlois M, Hamelin S, Devaux B, Deransart C, Depaulis A. Dentate gyrus and hilus transection blocks seizure propagation and granule cell dispersion in a mouse model for mesial temporal lobe epilepsy. Hippocampus. 2011;21:334–43.
30. Chatzikonstantinou A. Epilepsy and the hippocampus. Front Neurol Neurosci. 2014;34:121–42.
31. Strauss KI, Elisevich KV. Brain region and epilepsy-associated differences in inflammatory mediator levels in medically refractory mesial temporal lobe epilepsy. J Neuroinflammation. 2016;13:270.
32. Jimenez-Pacheco A, Diaz-Hernandez M, Arribas-Blazquez M, Sanz-Rodriguez A, Olivos-Ore LA, Artalejo AR, Alves M, Letavic M, Miras-Portugal MT, Conroy RM, et al. Transient P2X7 receptor antagonism produces lasting reductions in spontaneous seizures and gliosis in experimental temporal lobe epilepsy. J Neurosci. 2016;36:5920–32.
33. Leal B, Chaves J, Carvalho C, Rangel R, Santos A, Bettencourt A, Lopes J, Ramalheira J, Silva BM, da Silva AM, Costa PP. Brain expression of inflammatory mediators in mesial temporal lobe epilepsy patients. J Neuroimmunol. 2017;313:82–8.
34. Vezzani A, French J, Bartfai T, Baram TZ. The role of inflammation in epilepsy. Nat Rev Neurol. 2011;7:31–40.
35. Miller JA, Kirkley KA, Padmanabhan R, Liang LP, Raol YH, Patel M, Bialecki RA, Tjalkens RB. Repeated exposure to low doses of kainic acid activates nuclear factor kappa B (NF-kappaB) prior to seizure in transgenic NF-kappaB/EGFP reporter mice. Neurotoxicology. 2014;44:39–47.
36. Teocchi MA, Ferreira AE, da Luz de Oliveira EP, Tedeschi H, D'Souza-Li L. Hippocampal gene expression dysregulation of Klotho, nuclear factor kappa B and tumor necrosis factor in temporal lobe epilepsy patients. J Neuroinflammation. 2013;10:53.
37. Das A, Wallace GC, Holmes C, McDowell ML, Smith JA, Marshall JD, Bonilha L, Edwards JC, Glazier SS, Ray SK, Banik NL. Hippocampal tissue of patients with refractory temporal lobe epilepsy is associated with astrocyte activation, inflammation, and altered expression of channels and receptors. Neuroscience. 2012;220:237–46.
38. Vezzani A, Friedman A, Dingledine RJ. The role of inflammation in epileptogenesis. Neuropharmacology. 2013;69:16–24.
39. Galic MA, Riazi K, Heida JG, Mouihate A, Fournier NM, Spencer SJ, Kalynchuk LE, Teskey GC, Pittman QJ. Postnatal inflammation increases seizure susceptibility in adult rats. J Neurosci. 2008;28:6904–13.
40. Auvin S, Mazarati A, Shin D, Sankar R. Inflammation enhances epileptogenesis in the developing rat brain. Neurobiol Dis. 2010;40:303–10.
41. Clement AB, Hanstein R, Schroder A, Nagel H, Endres K, Fahrenholz F, Behl C. Effects of neuron-specific ADAM10 modulation in an in vivo model of acute excitotoxic stress. Neuroscience. 2008;152:459–68.

13

NLRP1 inflammasome is activated in patients with medial temporal lobe epilepsy and contributes to neuronal pyroptosis in amygdala kindling-induced rat model

Chen-Chen Tan[1†], Jian-Guo Zhang[2,3†], Meng-Shan Tan[4†], Hua Chen[5], Da-Wei Meng[2,3], Teng Jiang[6], Xiang-Fei Meng[1], Ying Li[5], Zhen Sun[1], Meng-Meng Li[1], Jin-Tai Yu[1,4,6,7*] and Lan Tan[1,4,6*]

Abstract

Background: Temporal lobe epilepsy (TLE) is often characterized pathologically by severe neuronal loss in the hippocampus. Understanding the mechanisms of neuron death is key to preventing the neurodegeneration associated with TLE. However, the involvement of neuronal loss to the epileptogenic process has yet to be fully determined. Recent studies have shown that the activation of NLRP1 can generate a functional caspase-1-containing inflammasome *in vivo* to drive the proinflammatory programmed cell death termed 'pyroptosis', which has a key role in the pathogenesis of neurological disorders. To the best of our knowledge, there are no reported studies that performed detailed identification and validation of NLRP1 inflammasome during the epileptogenic process.

Methods: We first compared expression of NLRP1 and caspase-1 in resected hippocampus from patients with intractable mesial temporal lobe epilepsy (mTLE) with that of matched control samples. To further examine whether the activation of NLRP1 inflammasome contributes to neuronal pyroptosis, we employed a nonviral strategy to knock down the expression of NLRP1 and caspase-1 in the amygdala kindling-induced rat model. Proinflammatory cytokines levels and hippocampal neuronal loss were evaluated after 6 weeks of treatment in these NLRP1 or caspase-1 deficiency TLE rats.

Results: Western blotting detected upregulated NLRP1 levels and active caspase-1 in mTLE patients in comparison to those levels seen in the controls, suggesting a role for this inflammasome in mTLE. Moreover, we employed direct *in vivo* infusion of nonviral small interfering RNA to knockdown NLRP1 or caspase-1 in the amygdala kindling-induced rat model, and discovered that these NLRP1 or caspase-1 silencing rats resulted in significantly reduced neuronal pyroptosis.

Conclusions: Our data suggest that NLRP1/caspase-1 signaling participates in the seizure-induced degenerative process in humans and in the animal model of TLE and points to the silencing of NLRP1 inflammasome as a promising strategy for TLE therapy.

Keywords: NLRP1, pyroptosis, inflammasome, Caspase-1, temporal lobe epilepsy

* Correspondence: yu-jintai@163.com; dr.tanlan@163.com
†Equal contributors
[1]Department of Neurology, Qingdao Municipal Hospital, School of Medicine, Qingdao University, No.5 Donghai Middle Road, Qingdao 266071, China
[4]College of Medicine and Pharmaceutics, Ocean University of China, No.5 Yushan Road, Qingdao 266003, China
Full list of author information is available at the end of the article

Background

Temporal lobe epilepsy (TLE), a serious, chronic neuro-logical syndrome in patients presenting refractory seizures, is characterized pathologically by selective neuronal cell loss and mossy fiber sprouting in hippocampus and limbic system. Hippocampal sclerosis (HS) is the most common lesion found in patients with mTLE. Experimental studies in animal models of epilepsy and human brain tissue have revealed a role of progressive damage and consider-able neuronal death in vulnerable areas such as the hippocampus of TLE [1,2]. However, the exact molecular pathogenic mechanisms of neuronal loss are not com-pletely understood.

Recently, a novel inflammasome signaling pathway has been uncovered, and a wealth of information link-ing the activation of inflammasome to neurological dis-orders pathogenesis has emerged [3]. The NLRP1 inflammasome was first characterized as a member of the NLRP family, whose activation can generate a func-tional caspase-1-containing inflammasome *in vivo* to drive the proinflammatory programmed cell death termed 'pyroptotic death' [4]. Like apoptosis, pyroptosis requires the proteolytic activation of specific caspases: caspase 3 and 7 for apoptosis and caspase-1 for pyroptosis. In contrast to apoptosis, which is often anti-inflammatory, pyroptosis is predicted to be proinflammatory due to the rapid loss of cell membrane integrity and release of cytosolic contents [5]. In addition, inhibition of the NLRP1 inflammasome could reduce the innate im-mune response and ameliorate detrimental conse-quences inflammation [6,7]. As a critical component of the inflammasome, NLRP1 appears to be expressed ra-ther ubiquitously, and high NLRP1 levels were also found in the brain, in particular in pyramidal neurons and oligodendrocytes [8]. Although current data re-garding NLRP1 functions are far scarcer than those that described for other inflammasome, various studies have proposed its crucial role in neurological diseases such as neurodegenerative pathologies, in which in-flammatory events and neuronal death have a clear causal role [9]. Thus, we hypothesized that the activa-tion of NLRP1-inflammasome may have key roles in the pathogenesis of TLE, in which inflammatory events and neuronal death contribute powerful pathogenetic forces [10,11]. To test this hypothesis, we first investigated whether the expression profiles of the NLRP1 inflamma-some components, including NLRP1 and caspase-1, are altered in resected hippocampus from patients with in-tractable mTLE when compared to matched control sam-ples. Next, we applied small interfering RNAs (siRNAs) to knock down NLRP1 and caspase-1 in the brain of amyg-dala kindling-induced TLE rat model and measured the NLRP1 component alterations as well as the functional outcomes.

Methods

Temporal lobe epilepsy patients and control group

We collected the hippocampus samples of mTLE pa-tients. Patients recruited in this study have a diagnosis of refractory epilepsy according to the definition of phar-macoresistant epilepsy [12]. The 24-h EEG monitoring indicated that widespread sharp or spike or slow-waves originated from unilateral temporal lobe. In addition, there was ipsilateral hippocampal sclerosis identified by MRI or low metabolism in ipsilateral mesial temporal lobe identified by 18F-FDG PET, without other patho-logical changes. Surgery was determined by a neurologist and a neurosurgery specialist in consultation. During the operation, cortical electrode monitoring confirmed that epilepsy-like waves originated from the inferior temporal lobe. All patients showed HS, with appreciable neuronal loss and reactive gliosis in CA1, CA3 and CA4. It was infeasible to obtain brain tissues of normal hippocampus cortex, so that normal temporal cortex tissues were used as negative control. Considering the difficulty in finding 'real' controls in human studies, in our experiments we used 'healthy' surgical samples from patients with other pathologies. Seizure absence was determined by the pa-tient's report to the neurologist during the scheduled visits. Therefore, for comparative purposes, we used six specimens of nonepileptic tissues from Histologically normal specimens (control samples) in accordance with all legal requirements. None of the patients in the con-trol group had a history of systematic diseases. We also used autopsy hippocampal tissue as a second control tis-sue for these studies to avoid problems due to the localization of specific expression. Autopsy hippocampal tissues from six patients with no known history of epi-lepsy and other systematic diseases were used as con-trols. The average postmortem interval was within 12 h after death. Routine neuropathological examination of tissue sections of these control hippocampal samples showed no pathologic changes. The brain tissues were separated as needed and immediately preserved in liquid nitrogen. Clinicopathological data are presented in Table 1, Additional file 1: Figure S1, and Additional file 2: Figure S2. The study was approved by the Ethics Committee of Qingdao Municipal Hospital. Informed consent was ob-tained from the patients and their legal guardians on the use of their brain tissues in this research.

Animals

To avoid the interference of estrogen on neuroinflam-mation [13], only male rats were used in this study. Adult male Sprague-Dawley rats weighing 260 to 300 g were obtained from the Experimental Animal Center of Qingdao University. They were housed in a standard animal room on a 12 h light/dark cycle with a controlled temperature and humidity, and given free access to food

Table 1 Clinical data of temporal lobe epilepsy patient group and control groups

(a) Clinical data of temporal lobe epilepsy patient group

Case	Sex	Age, y	Seizure type	Duration, y	EEG, sp ori	MRI/PET	HS
1	M	27	CPS, SGS	24	R-T	R-HS/R-T[a]	Wyler III
2	F	24	CPS	22	L-T	L-HS/L-T[a]	Wyler IV
3	F	23	CPS	10	L-T	L-HS/ -	Wyler III
4	F	33	CPS	26	L-T	L-HS/ -	Wyler III
5	M	26	CPS	20	R-T	R-HS/R-T[a]	Wyler IV
6	F	26	CPS	10	L-T	L-HDA/L-T[a]	Wyler III

(b) Clinical data of normal temporal cortex tissues control group

Case	Sex	Age, y	Tissue sources
1	M	29	Operative route of benign neoplasm in deep area of brain
2	M	38	Adjacent normal cortex in surgical evacuation of meningioma
3	M	23	Operative route of benign neoplasm in deep area of brain
4	F	37	Adjacent normal cortex in surgical evacuation of BGH
5	F	31	Adjacent normal cortex in surgical evacuation of IH
6	M	33	Operative route of benign neoplasm in deep area of brain

(c) Clinical data of postmortem hippocampal tissue control group

Case	Sex	Age, y	Cause of death
1	M	45	Sudden cardiac death
2	M	24	Car accident
3	F	19	Car accident
4	M	32	Pulmonary artery embolism
5	F	25	Amniotic fluid embolism
6	F	23	Amniotic fluid embolism

BGH, basal ganglia hemorrhage; CPS, complex partial seizure; F, female; HAD, hippocampal degenerative atrophy; HS, hippocampal sclerosis, IH, intracerebral hematoma; L, left; M, male; R, right; SGS, secondarily generalized seizure; sp ori, spikes origin; T, temporal lobe; y, year.
[a]Indicates that the positron emission tomography (PET) shows low metabolism.

and water. All experiments were performed in strict accordance with the National Institute of Health Guide for the Care and Use of Laboratory Animals. Animal care and sacrifice were conducted according to methods approved by the Qingdao University Animal Experimentation Committee. All efforts were made to minimize the number of animals used and their suffering.

Electrode implantation and temporal lobe epilepsy induction

Rats were positioned in a stereotaxic apparatus (Stoelting, USA, www.stoeltingco.com) under deep anesthesia (10% chloral hydrate, 3.5 mL/kg, i.p.). An electrode was implanted into the right basolateral amygdala (AP: -3.0 mm; L: -4.8 mm; V: -8.8 mm) [14,15]. The electrode was connected to a miniature receptacle, which were fixed to the skull using dental cement anchored with stainless steel screws. All rats underwent an identical surgical procedure, which were performed with the use of antiseptic technique.

After electrode implantation, the rats were allowed to recover for 2 weeks. Seizures were induced by a 20-minute amygdala stimulation (100 ms train of 1 ms, 60 Hz bipolar pulses, 400 µA, every 0.5 s) using a ML1101 electronic stimulator. Electroencephalograms of the right amygdala were recorded with a digital amplifier (AD Instrument, Racine, WI, USA). Following electrical stimulation, rats were video-monitored for 8 weeks. The rats with chronic TLE were identified by occurrence of frequent seizures (at least 2 times IV/V spontaneous seizures per week) from 1 week after electrical stimulation. Control rats were handled in the same manner but did not receive any electrical stimulation. Moreover, our preliminary experiments showed that this amygdala stimulation model is effective.

siRNA administration in rat brain

We prepared the Entranster in vivo- siRNA mixture according to the manufacturer's instructions. Briefly, 50 µg NLRP1 siRNA (Santa Cruz Biotechnology, Inc., Dallas, Texas, USA) or caspase-1 siRNA (Santa Cruz Biotechnology, Inc., Dallas, Texas, USA) or control siRNA (Santa Cruz Biotechnology, Inc., Dallas, Texas, USA) was resuspended in 50 µL RNAse-free water to make a siRNA solution. Then, 50 µL NLRP1 siRNA or control siRNA solution was mixed with 50 µL Entranster *in vivo* transfection reagent (Engreen, Inc., Beijing, China) and 100 µL artificial cerebrospinal fluid (aCSF, composition in mmol/L: NaCl 130, KCl 2.99, $CaCl_2$ 0.98, $MgCl_2 \cdot 6H_2O$ 0.80, $NaHCO_3$ 25, $Na_2HPO_4 \cdot 12H_2O$ 0.039, $NaH_2PO_4 \cdot 2H_2O$ 0.46) to get a 200-µL *in vivo* transfection mixture. NLRP1 siRNA or caspase-1 siRNA at this dose was well tolerated, and no signs of neurotoxicity including hind-limb paralysis, vocalization, food intake, or neuroanatomic damage were observed in the preliminary study.

We filled an osmotic pump (Model 2006; ALZET Inc., Cupertino, CA, USA) with the *in vivo* transfection mixture or aCSF alone. Meanwhile, rats were anesthetized with 10% chloral hydrate (0.3 mL/100 g, intraperitoneal) and were fixed in a stereotactic frame (Stoelting, USA, www.stoeltingco.com). A brain-infusion cannula (ALZET Inc., Cupertino, CA, USA) coupled via vinyl tubing to the osmotic pump was implanted into the dorsal third ventricle (AP: -1.8 mm; L: -0 mm; V: -5 mm) of rats with chronic TLE 8 weeks after electrical stimulation. Meanwhile, the osmotic pump was placed subcutaneously between the scapulae of rat, and the siRNAs were continuously infused into the brain at a flow rate of 0.15 µL/hour for 6 weeks by the osmotic pumps. All surgical procedures were ere performed with the use of antiseptic technique.

Behavioral assessment of seizure

All animals were assessed for amygdala stimulation induced seizures during the first 24 h postsurgery. At the 8th week postsurgery, all animals were re-evaluated for behavioral progression of seizures 4 h/day for 5 consecutive days to record the spontaneous seizures and scored according to Racine's classification [16]: 0, no reaction; 1, stereotypic mounting, eye blinking, and/or mild facial clonus; 2, head nodding and/or multiple facial clonus; 3, myoclonic jerks in the forelimbs; 4, clonic convulsions in the forelimbs with rearing; and 5, generalized clonic convulsions and loss of balance. Numbers and rates of animals with seizures (at least 2 times IV/V spontaneous seizures) during the first 24 h post-surgery and on the 6th week post-treatment were recorded.

Brain tissue preparation

Rats were sacrificed under deep anesthesia for the following biochemical assays:

1. For western blot analysis, quantitative real-time polymerase chain reaction (PCR), and enzyme-linked immunosorbent assay (ELISA), the rats were perfused transcardially with 0.9% saline (pH7.4). Then, the samples were rapidly isolated and placed in liquid nitrogen until use.

2. For cresyl violet staining and TUNEL analysis, rats were perfused transcardially with 0.9% saline (pH 7.4), followed by a fixative solution containing 4% paraformaldehyde in PBS (pH 7.4). Then, the brains were removed and fixed in the same fixative at 4°C until use.

3. For double immunofluorescence staining, rat brain was removed without perfusion, embedded in tissue freezing medium, and immediately frozen at -40°C. Frozen tissue was stored at -80°C until sectioning.

Western blotting

Tissues samples were digested with RIPA lysis buffer (50 mmol/L Tris-HCl, 150 mmol/L NaCl, 1% Nonidet-40, 0.5% sodium deoxycholate, 1 mmol/L EDTA, 1 mmol/L PMSF) with protease inhibitors (pepstatin 1 µg/mL, aprotinin 1 µg/mL, leupeptin 1 µg/mL) for 30 min and the protein concentration was determined using the Bradford assay kit (Bio-Rad Laboratories, Hercules, CA, USA). Different samples with an equal amount of protein were separated using 8-12% SDS-polyacrylamide gels and transferred to PVDF membranes. After blocking with 10% non-fat milk at room temperature, the membranes were incubated with primary antibodies against NALP1 (1:1000; Novus Biologicals, Inc., Littleton, CO, USA), NeuN (1:500; Chemicon, www.chemicon.com.br), cleaved caspase-1 (1:200; Cambridge, UK), cleaved IL-1β (1:500; Santa Cruz Biotechnology, Inc., Dallas, Texas, USA), and β-actin (1:1000; Santa Cruz Biotechnology, Inc., Dallas, Texas, USA) at 4°C overnight. After rinsing, the membranes were appropriately incubated with horseradish peroxidase (HRP)-conjugated suitable secondary antibodies (1:5000; Zhongshan Inc., Beijing, China) for 2 h at room temperature. Cross-reactivity was visualized using ECL western blotting detection reagents and analyzed by scanning densitometry using a BioSpectrum Imaging System (UVP, Upland, CA, USA).

Real-time PCR

Total RNA was extracted using TRIzol reagent (Invitrogen Life Technologies, Carlsbad, CA, USA), using the protocol supplied by the manufacturer. Total RNA was reverse transcribed to cDNA by the Reverse Transcription System (Bio-Rad, Hercules, CA, USA). The reaction was performed at 42°C for 50 min, 95°C for 5 min, and 5°C for 5 min, then the cDNA was stored in -20°C. Amplification was carried out with the Stratagene Mx3000P real-time PCR system (Stratagene, LaJolla, CA, USA) with a SYBR Green PCR technology (Takara Bio, Inc., Shiga, Japan). Reverse transcription was performed in a final volume of 20 µL containing 2 µL cDNA, 10 µL SYBR Green, 0.4 µL ROX Reference Dye, 0.4 µL forward and reverse primer (1 mol/L), and 6.8 µL nuclease-free water. The optimal conditions were 40 cycles of 95°C for 30 s, 60°C for 32 s, and 72°C for 30 s. Relative quantification was given by the CT values, determined for triplicate reactions of SE samples and sham samples for each gene. Total RNA concentrations from each sample were normalized by quantity of β-actin mRNA, and the target genes' expression was evaluated by ratio of the number of target mRNA to β-actin mRNA. Relative expression of genes was obtained by the $2^{-\triangle\triangle CT}$ method. Primers were purchased from Invitrogen as follows (name: forward primer, reverse primer): *nlrp1*: 5'-gccctggagacaaagaatcc-3', 5'-agtgggcatcgtcatgtgt-3'; *caspase-1*: 5'-aaggtcctgagggcaaa gag-3', 5'-gtgttgcagataatgagggc-3'; *β-actin*: 5'-agggaaatcg tgcgtgac-3', 5'-cgctcattgccgatagtg-3'.

ELISA

Levels of secreted IL-1β were measured using commercially available ELISA kit (R&D Systems, Minneapolis, MN, USA) according to the manufacturer's instructions. ELISA was conducted by technicians who were blinded to the experimental groups. The results are expressed in pg/mL.

Nissl staining and TUNEL assay

Nissl staining was employed to detect surviving neurons. The brains were embedded in paraffin and cut into 7-μm sections. Next, the paraffin-embedded sections were dewaxed and rehydrated according to the standard protocols. Then, the sections were stained in 1% cresyl violet at 50°C for 5 minutes. After being rinsed with water, the sections were dehydrated in increasing concentrations of ethanol, mounted on the slides, and examined with a light microscope. Only the neurons with violet nucleus and the intact morphology were counted as surviving neurons. Besides, we used a cell death detection kit (In Situ Cell Death Detection Kit, POD; Roche, www.roche.com) for TUNEL assay to detect neuronal apoptosis. We employed TUNEL assay via a commercial kit according to the manufacturer instructions. Briefly, the paraffin-embedded sections of samples received deparaffinization and rehydration treatments, and then were incubated with proteinase-K for 15 min at room temperature followed by three washes in PBS. The TUNEL reaction mixture was added and incubated for 60 min at 37°C. Next, sections were washed with PBS and two drops of peroxidase-streptavidin conjugate solution in blocking buffer was applied. Then, the sections were incubated for 30 min at room temperature, washed again with PBS and exposed to 0.03% diaminobenzidine in 0.01% H_2O_2. Lastly, sections were counterstained with Mayer's hematoxylin, dehydrated, mounted on the slides and examined with a microscope equipped with a charge-coupled device camera. We identified the neurons with deep black nuclei as TUNEL-positive neurons. Cell counting was performed on five randomly selected non-

overlapping fields of per slide. The densities of surviving neurons or TUNEL-positive neurons in the hippocampus of the scanned digital images were calculated using Image-Pro Express software (Media Cybernetics, Silver Spring, MD, USA). The total cell counts were averaged from five sections per animal. The survival index was defined as follows: surviving index (%) = 100× (number of surviving neurons/total number of neurons). Furthermore, the TUNEL-positive neurons index was defined as follows: TUNEL-positive neurons index (%) = 100× (TUNEL-positive neurons/total neurons).

Immunofluorescence staining

For immunofluorescence studies, 20-μm-thick sections were obtained by cryosectioning at -20°C, mounted on a glass slide, and incubated at room temperature for 1 hour. Next, the sections were fixed in ice-cold acetone for 10 minutes and then dried on a heater for 10 minutes at 40°C. Then, sections were blocked with 5% BSA and 0.1% TritonX-100 for 2 hours. After a single wash with PBS, sections were incubated overnight at 4°C with a rabbit polyclonal antibody against NALP1 (1:1000; Novus Biologicals, Inc., Littleton, CO, USA) combined with a mouse monoclonal antibody against NeuN (1:200; Chemicon, www.chemicon.com.br). Afterward, sections were washed in PBS and incubated respectively with FITC conjugated anti-rabbit IgG (1:200; Santa Cruz Biotechnology, Inc., Dallas, Texas, USA) and TRITC conjugated anti-mouse IgG (1:200; Zhongshan Inc., Beijing, China) in a dark and humidified container for 1 h at 37°C. After that, the sections were washed with PBS and sealed with a cover slip. The slides were analyzed with a fluorescence microscopy (Olympus, Inc, Tokyo, Japan). To ensure the specificity of the immunoblotting procedure, control experiments were performed in which the corresponding primary antibody was omitted. Under these conditions, no signal was observed.

Statistical analysis

Statistical analysis was conducted by SPSS software 17.0 (IBM, Inc., Armonk, NY, USA). After confirming normal distribution with the skewness and kurtosis statistic test, an independent sample t-test or one-way ANOVA followed by a least significant difference (LSD) post hoc test was used to analyze differences among groups. All data are expressed as mean ± standard deviation. $P < 0.05$ was considered statistically significant.

Results

NLRP1 inflammasome components were upregulated in human mesial temporal lobe epilepsy

We first investigated whether the expression of NLRP1 was altered in the brains of individuals with pharmacoresistant mTLE. Total proteins were extracted from the surgically obtained hippocampus samples and control samples and subjected to western blot analysis. We found that the NLRP1 levels of TLE patients were significantly elevated, while the levels of NeuN were slightly reduced compared to control samples (Figure 1a, b). Using double immunofluorescence staining to colocalize NLRP1 with neuronal marker NeuN, our results further demonstrated the increased neuronal expression of NLRP1 in the NeuN-positive neurons of mTLE patients (Figure 1c). After that, we further investigated the expression profiles of caspase-1. We found that the expression of caspase-1, an indicator of pyroptosis, showed a robust increase in hippocampus of chronic mTLE than that of controls (Figure 1d). Moreover, we have confirmed that the difference between the two control groups was not statistically significant (see Additional file 3: Figure S3).

Inhibition of NLRP1-attenuated neuron pyroptosis in temporal lobe epilepsy rats

Next, we investigate the possible mechanism involved in the neuron pyroptosis with increased NLRP1 level. Toward this end, we knocked down brain NLRP1 expression of TLE rats by using *in vivo* nonviral RNA interference methodology [17]. To evaluate the silencing efficiency of siRNA infusion, the gene expression and protein level of NLRP1 protein were detected by quantitative real-time PCR and western blotting, respectively. Compared with control siRNA, NLRP1 siRNA significantly reduced the gene expression of NLRP1 in brain

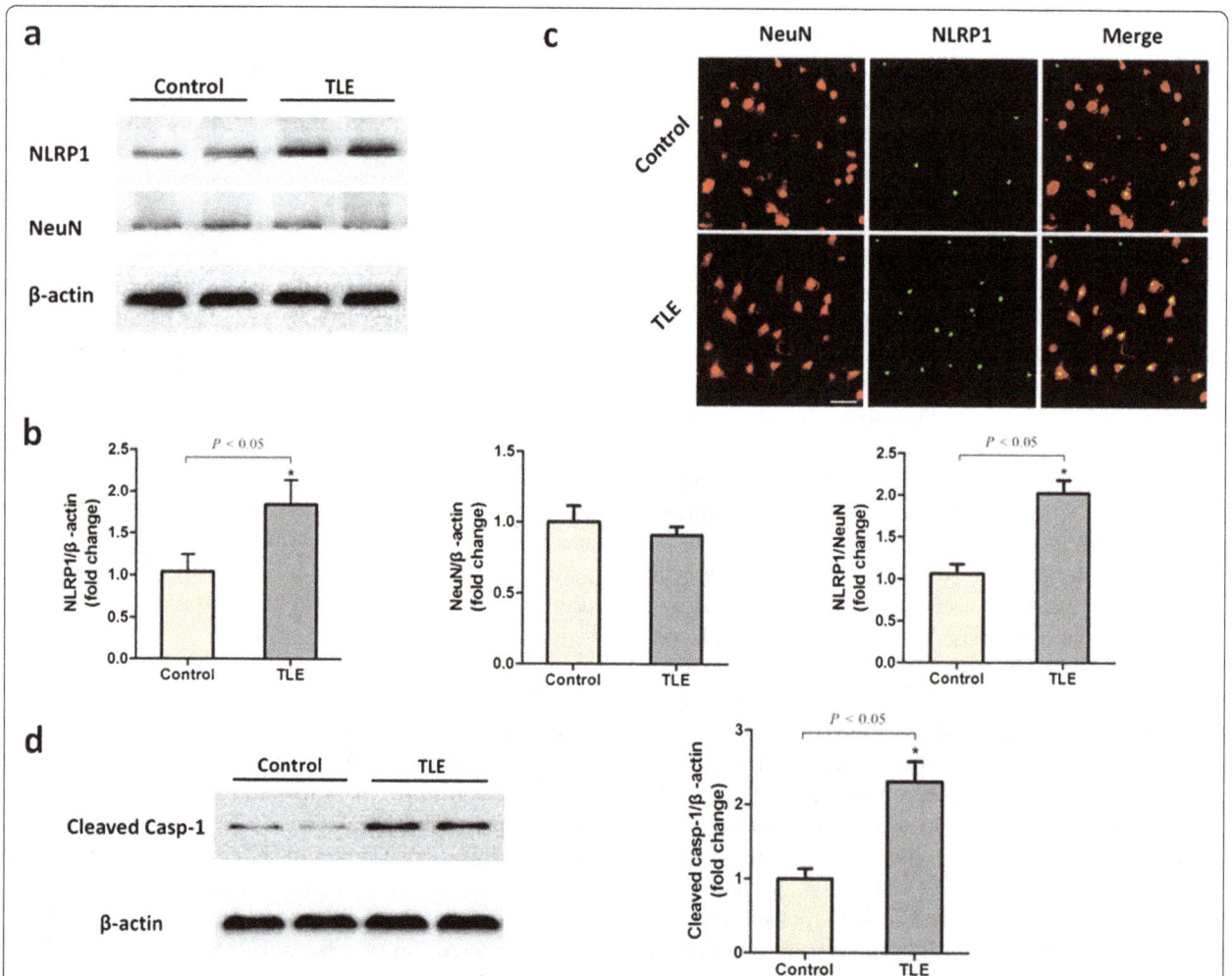

Figure 1 Increased expression of NLRP1 and caspase-1 in the neurons of temporal lobe epilepsy (TLE) patient brains. (a) Cerebral NLRP1 and NeuN levels from Case 1 TLE patient and Case 1 'healthy control' individual were detected by western blot analysis. β -actin was used as loading control. **(b)** Levels of NLRP1, NeuN and NLRP1/NeuN were quantified by densitometric measurement. Values are the mean ± standard deviation. **(c)** Double immunofluorescent detection of NLRP1 in the NeuN-positive neurons of Case 6 TLE patient and Case 6 'healthy control' individual. **(d)** The expression level of active caspase-1 (20KD) in Case 3 TLE patient and Case 3 'healthy control' individual was analyzed using the western blot assay. Tissue samples from hippocampus of the TLE group and control group were immunostained using anti-NLRP1 and anti-NeuN antibodies and examined under a fluorescence microscope. Scale bars: 20 μm. n = 6 individuals per group.

(see Additional file 4: Figure S4a). Consistent with the changes in gene expression, TLE rats infused with NLRP1 siRNA showed a dramatic reduction in hippocampus NLRP1 protein levels. Incidentally, the NLRP1 levels and gene expression between control-siRNA treated and No siRNA treated cells do not differ (see Additional file 4: Figure S4b), excluding an effect of siRNA transfection on gene expression or the protein level of NLRP1.

Then, we investigate the effects of NLRP1 inhibition on neuron pyroptosis in TLE rats. The TUNEL staining assay was firstly used to characterize the pyroptotic effects of NLRP1. Compared to the control-siRNA group, the increased number of TUNEL-positive cells in the hippocampus of TLE rats could be inhibited by NLRP1 siRNA treatment (Figure 2a, b). In addition, cresyl violet staining showed that NLRP1 siRNA led to less obvious neuronal loss in hippocampus of TLE rat brain (Figure 2c, d). We

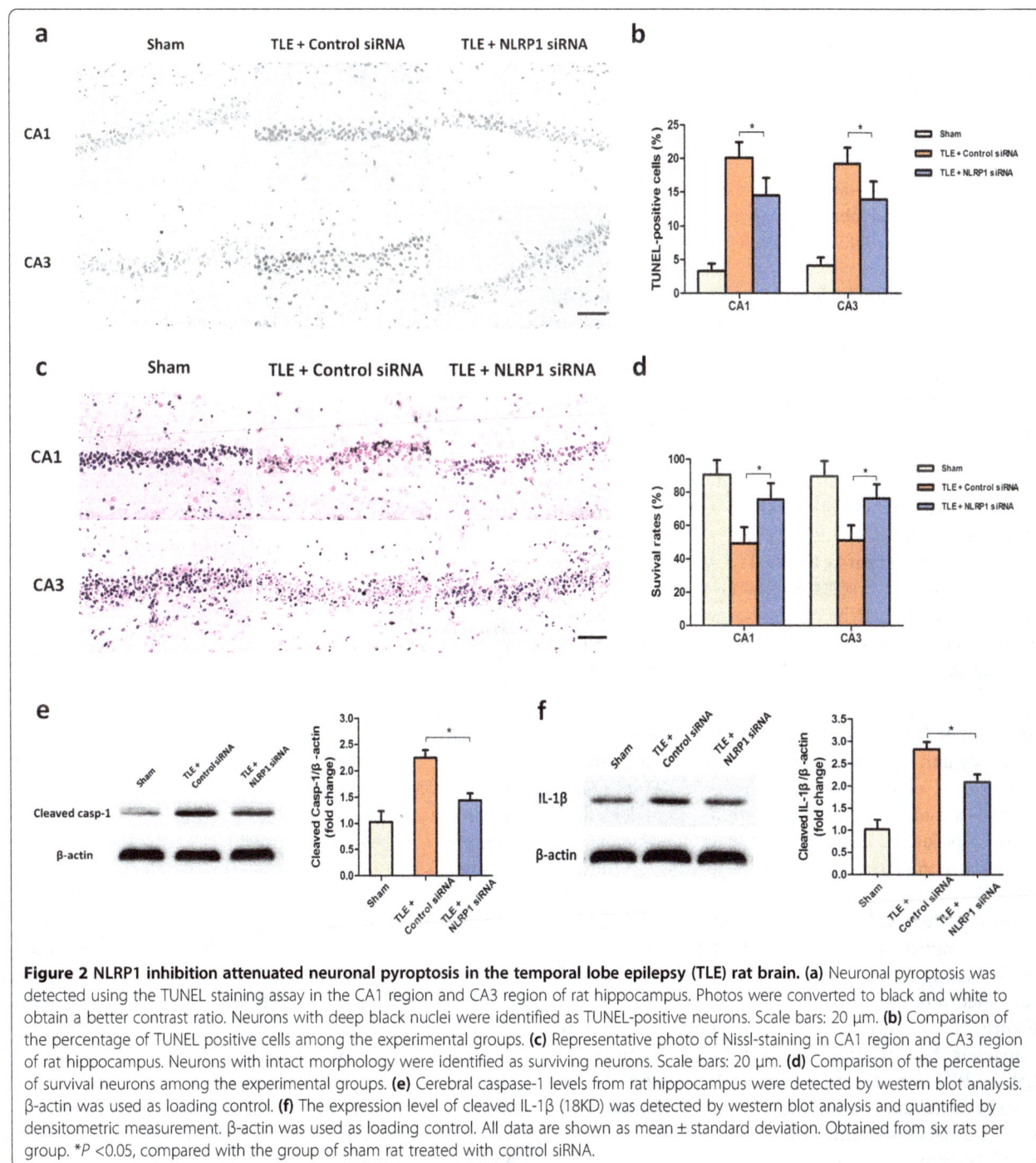

Figure 2 NLRP1 inhibition attenuated neuronal pyroptosis in the temporal lobe epilepsy (TLE) rat brain. (a) Neuronal pyroptosis was detected using the TUNEL staining assay in the CA1 region and CA3 region of rat hippocampus. Photos were converted to black and white to obtain a better contrast ratio. Neurons with deep black nuclei were identified as TUNEL-positive neurons. Scale bars: 20 μm. **(b)** Comparison of the percentage of TUNEL positive cells among the experimental groups. **(c)** Representative photo of Nissl-staining in CA1 region and CA3 region of rat hippocampus. Neurons with intact morphology were identified as surviving neurons. Scale bars: 20 μm. **(d)** Comparison of the percentage of survival neurons among the experimental groups. **(e)** Cerebral caspase-1 levels from rat hippocampus were detected by western blot analysis. β-actin was used as loading control. **(f)** The expression level of cleaved IL-1β (18KD) was detected by western blot analysis and quantified by densitometric measurement. β-actin was used as loading control. All data are shown as mean ± standard deviation. Obtained from six rats per group. *P <0.05, compared with the group of sham rat treated with control siRNA.

further examined the changes in caspase-1, which has been known to play a central role in the execution of pyroptosis. Western blot analysis was performed to measure the caspase-1 expression. As indicated in the Figure 2e, the NLRP1 siRNA treatment could reduce the active caspase-1 levels in TLE rats. In addition to pyroptosis, NLRP1 inflammasome is also responsible for caspase-1-dependent processing of the key pro-inflammatory cytokine IL-1β to an active secreted form [18,19]. In particular, the activation of IL-1β, which is involved in inflammatory cycle, is demonstrated to play a key role in TLE pathology [20]. Therefore, we also inspected the cerebral IL-1β levels by western blot. Similarly, NLRP1 siRNA treatment also changes the expression of active IL-1β (Figure 2f) in the brain of TLE rats.

Inhibition of NLRP1 reduced seizure frequency and severity in temporal lobe epilepsy rats

To investigate the effects of NLRP1 siRNA on seizure frequency and severity in TLE rats, we assessed seizures of TLE rats during the first 24 h post-surgery and 6th week post-treatment. Our study demonstrated that sham rats after 6 weeks of treatment with NLRP1 siRNA or control siRNA showed no signs of seizure activity during the first 24 h post-surgery and/or 6th week post-treatment. In contrast, all rats (100%) in the TLE rats with control siRNA exhibited high scores of seizures within the first 24 h post-surgery and 77.8% of them had seizure activity on the 6th week post-treatment. Meanwhile, TLE rats with NLRP1 siRNA showed lower seizure activity as compared to the TLE group with control siRNA within the first 24 h (100%) and only 44.4% of them had seizure activity on the 6th week post-treatment and this difference versus TLE rats with control siRNA was significant for the 6th week post-treatment (Table 2a).

Inhibition of Caspase-1 alleviated pyroptosis and seizure frequency and severity in temporal lobe epilepsy rats

As caspase-1 play a central role in the process of neuron pyroptosis and IL-1β secretion, we also knocked down brain caspase-1 in TLE rats by *in vivo* nonviral RNA interference methodology for 6 weeks (see Additional file 1: Figure S1c,d). We found a marked reduction of TUNEL-positive cell densities in the CA1 and CA3 of TLE rat hippocampus (Figure 3a, b). Furthermore, cresyl violet staining showed that NLRP1 siRNA led to less obvious neuronal loss in hippocampus of TLE rat brain (Figure 3c, d). These results are consistent with the changes in NLRP1 siRNA-treated TLE rats, supporting that NLRP1 acts through caspase-1 to exert the observed effects. In addition, the expression of active IL-1β showed a decrease trend in the TLE rats with caspase-1 siRNA (Figure 3e, f).

Table 2 Numbers and rates of animals with seizures during the first 24 h postsurgery and on the 6th week post-treatment in experimental groups

(a) Results from sham and temporal lobe epilepsy rats after 6 weeks of treatment with NLRP1 siRNA or control siRNA

	Within 24 h post-stimulation		On the 6th week post-treatment	
	Number	Rate (%)	Number	Rate (%)
Sham + Control siRNA	0/18	0	0/18	0
Sham + NLRP1 siRNA	0/18	0	0/18	0
TLE + Control siRNA	18/18	100	14/18	77.8
TLE + NLRP1 siRNA	18/18	100	8/18	44.4[a]

(b) Results from sham and TLE rats after 6 weeks of treatment with Caspase-1 siRNA or control siRNA

Sham + Control siRNA	0/18	0	0/18	0
Sham + Caspase-1 siRNA	0/18	0	0/18	0
TLE + Control siRNA	18/18	100	14/18	77.8
TLE + Caspase-1 siRNA	18/18	100[b]	7/18	38.9[b]

[a]P <0.01 (versus TLE + Control siRNA).
[b]P <0.01 (versus TLE + Control siRNA).

As indicated from the Table 2b, sham rats after 6 weeks of treatment with caspase-1 siRNA or control siRNA showed no signs of seizure activity during the first 24 h post-surgery and/or 6th week post-treatment. While control siRNA-treated TLE rats showed high seizure frequency and severity. In contrast, caspase-1 siRNA treatment could largely reduce seizure frequency and severity in TLE rats. Only 38.9% of them had seizure activity on the 6th week post-treatment and this difference versus TLE rats with control siRNA was significant.

Discussion

Temporal lobe epilepsy (TLE) is often characterized pathologically by severe neuronal loss in the hippocampus. Understanding the mechanisms of cell death is a key for preventing the neurodegeneration associated with TLE. However, the involvement of neuronal death to the epileptogenic process has yet to be fully determined. Recent studies shown that the activation of NLRP1 inflammasome can generate a functional caspase-1-containing inflammasome *in vivo* to drive the proinflammatory programmed cell death termed 'pyroptotic death' [5], which have key roles in the pathogenesis of neurological disorders [4,21,22]. NLRP1 is also highly expressed in pyramidal neurons of the brain [8]. In addition, inflammasome activation especially the NLRP1 is under current investigation across a broad spectrum of neurological diseases, including infections, acute sterile brain injury and chronic neurodegenerative diseases [23]. However, to the best of our knowledge, there are no reported studies that performed a detailed identification and validation of NLRP1 inflammasome during the epileptogenic process.

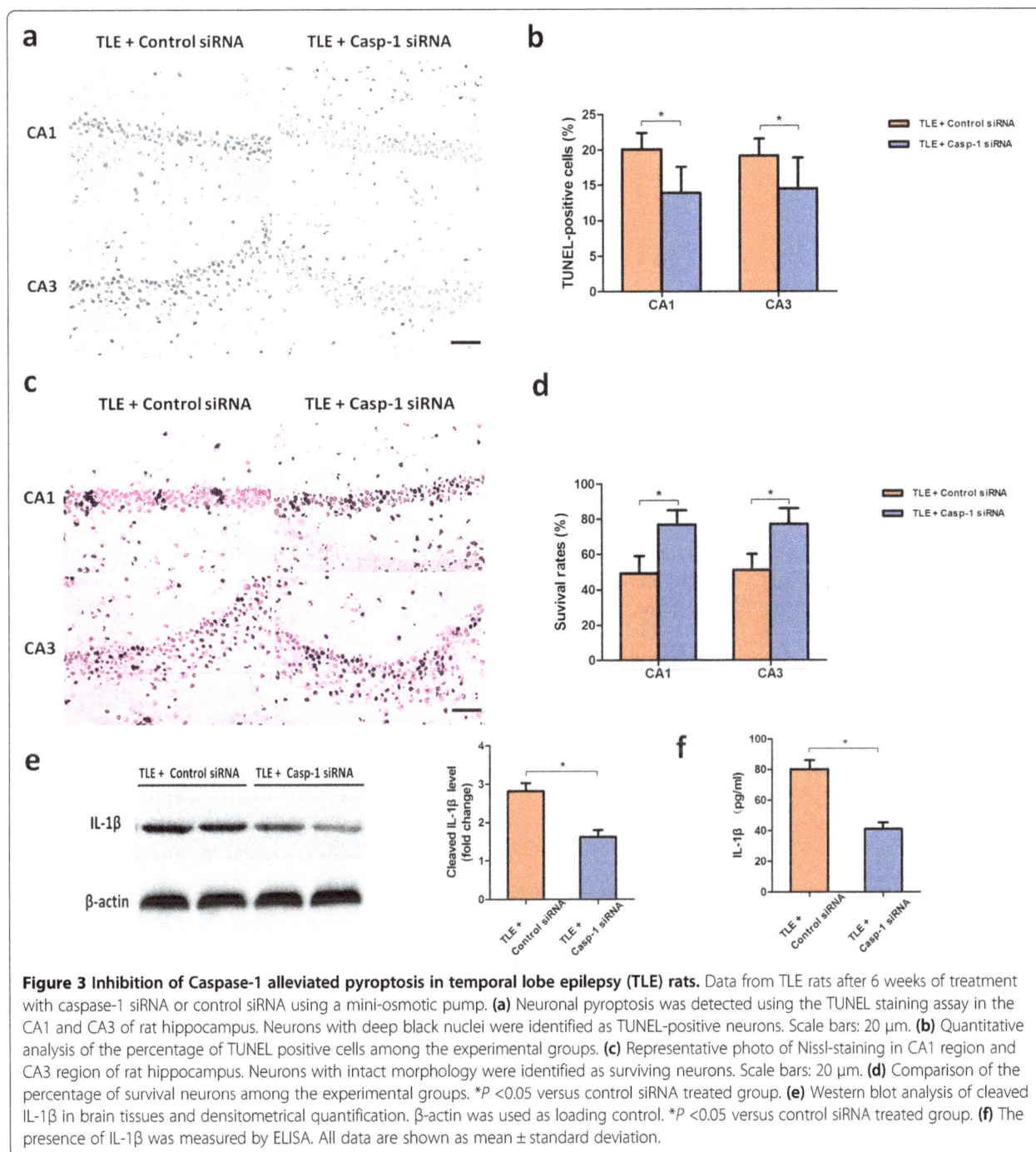

Figure 3 Inhibition of Caspase-1 alleviated pyroptosis in temporal lobe epilepsy (TLE) rats. Data from TLE rats after 6 weeks of treatment with caspase-1 siRNA or control siRNA using a mini-osmotic pump. **(a)** Neuronal pyroptosis was detected using the TUNEL staining assay in the CA1 and CA3 of rat hippocampus. Neurons with deep black nuclei were identified as TUNEL-positive neurons. Scale bars: 20 μm. **(b)** Quantitative analysis of the percentage of TUNEL positive cells among the experimental groups. **(c)** Representative photo of Nissl-staining in CA1 region and CA3 region of rat hippocampus. Neurons with intact morphology were identified as surviving neurons. Scale bars: 20 μm. **(d)** Comparison of the percentage of survival neurons among the experimental groups. *P <0.05 versus control siRNA treated group. **(e)** Western blot analysis of cleaved IL-1β in brain tissues and densitometrical quantification. β-actin was used as loading control. *P <0.05 versus control siRNA treated group. **(f)** The presence of IL-1β was measured by ELISA. All data are shown as mean ± standard deviation.

Hence, we hypothesized that the activation of NLRP1-inflammasome may have key roles in the pathogenesis of mTLE, in which neuronal death combined with inflammation contributes powerful pathogenetic forces [24].

Our study was for first time to examine whether the NLRP1-dependent pyroptosis is a potential mechanism in TLE pathogenesis in refractory medial temporal lobe epilepsy patients. We compared expression of NLRP1 and caspase-1 in resected hippocampus from patients with intractable mTLE to matched control samples. The present study detected upregulated NLRP1 and caspase-1 levels within mTLE samples than controls. Meanwhile, the cellular localization of NLRP1 on the neuron in the mTLE patient brains was demonstrated by the double immunofluorescence staining, consistent with the findings from the other studies [9]. These elevated NLRP1 inflammasome levels may be induced by potassium (K$^+$) efflux, which is causative of the generation or spread of seizure activity in TLE [25,26].

Moreover, we knocked down brain NLRP1 expression by implanting mini-osmotic pumps for direct infusion of siRNA to investigate its role on neuronal pyroptosis in the TLE rat model evoked by amygdala stimulation. This amygdala stimulation model of chronic TLE in rats provides a useful tool for studies aimed at understanding the mechanisms of TLE and exploring the new therapeutic strategy for this disease [27,28]. RNA interference technology has emerged as a potentially superior alternative to the traditional approaches for assessing gene function in adult animals to understand the genes implicated in neuropsychiatric disorders [17,29]. Moreover, application of the nonviral infusion of siRNA into the ventricular system could achieve a widespread sequence-specific gene knockdown in the brain [30]. For the characteristics of rapid, inexpensive, and specific knockdown of target genes in the whole brain, this method could provide a useful tool to accelerate the functional investigation of broadly expressed target genes implicated in neurological disorders. In our study, we found that this approach effectively downregulates the levels of NLRP1 mRNA and protein in TLE rat brain. Meanwhile, compared to no siRNA treated TLE rat, the treatment with control siRNA did not alter cerebral NLRP1 mRNA and protein levels, thus excluding an effect of pump-mediated infusion on NLRP1 expression levels. For the first time, we revealed that NLRP1 siRNA treatment

could significantly reduce TUNEL-positive cell densities and the active caspase-1 expression levels in TLE rats, supporting a fundamental role for NLRP1-mediated pyroptosis in TLE-induced neuronal losses in the hippocampus.

Meanwhile, we should notice that NLRP1 inflammasome is also responsible for caspase-1-dependent processing of the key pro-inflammatory cytokine IL-1β to an active secreted form [18,19]. Pro-inflammatory cytokines, including IL-1β, are known to modulate effects of neurotoxic neurotransmitters discharged during excitation or inflammation in the central nervous system (CNS) [31]. Moreover, current studies pointed out that the inflammatory mechanism contributes powerful pathogenetic forces in the process of TLE [10]. And recent studies found that IL-1β was proconvulsant in animal models of TLE, increasing the time spent in seizures and reducing the onset time of the first seizure [32]. Hence, the elevated levels of IL-1β in TLE are believed to serve as a part of inflammatory cycle that regulates TLE pathology. Our current research has found that NLRP1 siRNA treatment could change the expression of active IL-1β in the brain of TLE rat. However, we should notice that there may be another pathway involved in caspase-1-dependent processing of the key pro-inflammatory cytokine IL-1β. Previous studies have pointed out that NLRP3 inflammasome also can activate caspase-1 to induce IL-1β secretion [28]. In contrast to the activation of NLRP3, inflammasome mainly expressed in microglia, which is essential for the secretion of pro-inflammatory cytokines

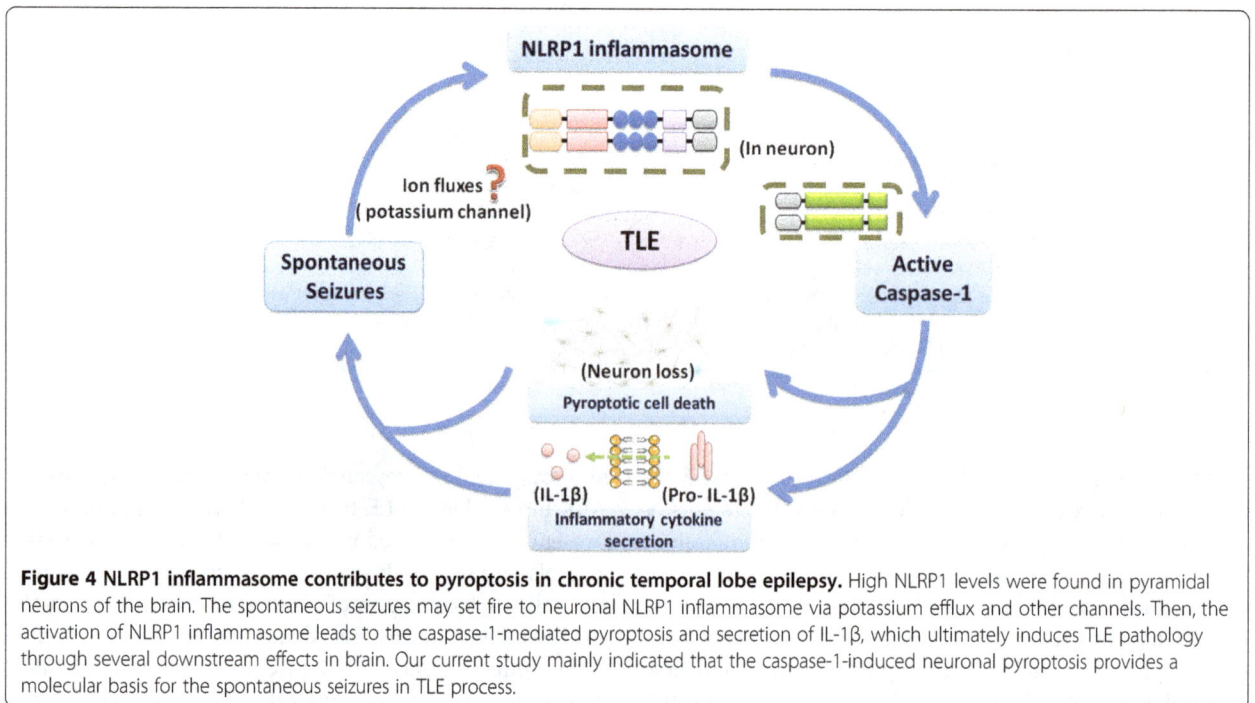

Figure 4 NLRP1 inflammasome contributes to pyroptosis in chronic temporal lobe epilepsy. High NLRP1 levels were found in pyramidal neurons of the brain. The spontaneous seizures may set fire to neuronal NLRP1 inflammasome via potassium efflux and other channels. Then, the activation of NLRP1 inflammasome leads to the caspase-1-mediated pyroptosis and secretion of IL-1β, which ultimately induces TLE pathology through several downstream effects in brain. Our current study mainly indicated that the caspase-1-induced neuronal pyroptosis provides a molecular basis for the spontaneous seizures in TLE process.

and subsequent inflammatory events, the NLRP1 mainly expressed in neuron, which is essential for the pyroptotic cell death in TLE pathogenesis.

To further investigate whether the NLRP1 acts through caspase-1 to exert the observed effects of pyroptosis, we also knocked down brain caspase-1 by this *in vivo* nonviral RNA interference methodology in TLE rats. Consistent biochemical results were found between caspase-1 siRNA and NLRP1 siRNA-treated TLE rats, supporting that NLRP1 acts through caspase-1 signaling to exert the effects of pyroptosis. The only difference was that silencing caspase-1 could markedly reduce active IL-1β expression in the TLE rats. As we all know, caspase-1 is a critical pathway by which inflammasomes contribute to the downstream effects. Beside the NLRP1, other inflammasome such as NLRP3 also can activate caspase-1 to induce IL-1β secretion.

This study also has some limitations. For example, we cannot rule out the possibility that the 6-week infusion of NLRP1 siRNA is not enough to cause obvious changes in TLE-like neuropathology. However, the limited duration (maximum 6 weeks) of osmotic pumps suitable for rat prevented us from observing long-term effects of NLRP1 knockdown. Second, there are limited ways to stimulate or stably overexpress NLRP1 in brain. Hence, we cannot provide more direct evidence on the role of NLRP1 in neuroinflammation and pyroptotic cell death here. However, it is still worth mentioning that our findings have important clinical implications. Although current available interventions can provide benefits for TLE, none prevents or cures the disease. Thus, the inhibition of neuronal pyroptosis is a neuroprotective response and pyroptosis could be restrained to open exciting new therapeutic perspectives for TLE. Thus, because inhibition of NLRP1 inflammasome had several potentially beneficial effects on neuronal pyroptosis and inflammation response in the TLE process, modulation of NLRP1 inflammasome may be explored as a promising strategy for the development of TLE therapy.

Conclusions

Our present study first demonstrates that cerebral expression of NLRP1 was upregulated in refractory medial temporal lobe epilepsy patients. The increase in NLRP1 levels can activate caspase-1 signaling responsible for neuronal pyroptosis and inflammation cytokine release (Figure 4). Using the pump-mediated *in vivo* infusion of nonviral siRNA to knock down NLRP1 in the brain of TLE rats, our study further indicated that inhibition of NLRP1 inflammasome represents a potential clinical benefit of therapeutic interventions that target inflammasome assembly and activity.

Additional files

Additional file 1: Figure S1. Magnetic resonance imaging (MRI) manifestations of all cases in the temporal lobe epilepsy (TLE) patient group. (a) Case 1 showed right hippocampal sclerosis. (b) Case 2 showed left hippocampal sclerosis. (c) Case 5 showed right hippocampal sclerosis. (d) Case 6 showed left hippocampal degenerative atrophy.

Additional file 2: Figure S2. Positron emission tomography (PET) manifestations of cases in the temporal lobe epilepsy (TLE) patient group. (a) Case 1 showed low metabolism in the right temporal lobe. (b) Case 2 showed low metabolism in the left temporal lobe. (c) Case 5 showed low metabolism in the right temporal lobe. (d) Case 6 showed low metabolism in the left temporal lobe. Case 3 and Case 4 did not receive PET test.

Additional file 3: Figure S3. Expression of NLRP1 and caspase-1 in the neurons of two control groups. (a) Cerebral NLRP1 and NeuN levels from two controls were detected by western blot analysis. β -actin was used as loading control. Levels of NLRP1, NeuN and NLRP1/NeuN were quantified by densitometric measurement. Values are the mean ± standard deviation. (b) The expression level of active caspase-1 (20KD) was analyzed using the western blot assay. n = 6 individuals per group. Control 1 indicates the normal temporal cortex tissues; Control 2 indicates postmortem control hippocampal tissue.

Additional file 4: Figure S4. Short interfering RNA (siRNA) targeting NLRP1 or caspase-1 effectively downregulated NLRP1 or caspase-1 in brain of TLE rat model. (a) Messenger RNA levels of NLRP1 in brain of temporal lobe epilepsy (TLE) rats after a 6-week infusion of artificial cerebrospinal fluid (aCSF), control siRNA, or NLRP1 siRNA. (b) Protein levels of NLRP1 in the brain of the TLE rats after a 6-week infusion of artificial cerebrospinal fluid (aCSF), control siRNA, or NLRP1 siRNA. Data are expressed as a fold change relative to sham group. (c) Messenger RNA levels of caspase-1 in brain of TLE rats in sham, 6-week infusion of control siRNA, or caspase-1 siRNA groups. (d) Protein levels of caspase-1 in brain of TLE rats in sham, 6-week infusion of control siRNA or caspase-1 siRNA groups. Data are expressed as a fold change relative to TLE rats infused with control siRNA. Columns represent mean ± standard deviation. n = 6 rats per group.

Abbreviations

ELISA: enzyme-linked immunosorbent assay; HS: hippocampal sclerosis; IL: interleukin; NLRP1: nucleotide binding and domain-like receptor family pyrin domain-containing 1; siRNA: small interfering RNA; PCR: polymerase chain reaction; TLE: temporal lobe epilepsy; TUNEL: terminal deoxynucleotidyl transferase-mediated dUTP end-labeling.

Competing interests

The authors declare that they have no competing interests.

Authors' contributions

CCT, MST and JTY designed and performed experiments, analyzed data, and drafted the first draft. CCT, JGZ, HC, DWM, YL and LT collected the brain specimens and clinical data. XFM, SZ and MML performed experiments. TJ analyzed data and drafted the first draft. LT and JTY designed and supervised experiments. All authors have read and approved the final version of the manuscript.

Acknowledgements

This work was supported by grants from the National Natural Science Foundation of China (81000544, 81171209, 81371406), the Shandong Provincial Natural Science Foundation, China (ZR2010HQ004, ZR2011HZ001), the Medicine and Health Science Technology Development Project of Shandong Province (2011WSA02018, 2011WSA02020), and the Shandong Provincial Outstanding Medical Academic Professional Program.

Author details

[1]Department of Neurology, Qingdao Municipal Hospital, School of Medicine, Qingdao University, No.5 Donghai Middle Road, Qingdao 266071, China. [2]Department of Functional Neurosurgery, Beijing Neurosurgical Institute, Capital Medical University, No.6, Tiantan Xili, Beijing 100050, China. [3]Department of Neurosurgery, Beijing Tiantan Hospital, Capital Medical

University, No.6, Tiantan Xili, Beijing 100050, China. [4]College of Medicine and Pharmaceutics, Ocean University of China, No.5 Yushan Road, Qingdao 266003, China. [5]Department of Pathology, Qingdao Municipal Hospital, School of Medicine, Qingdao University, No.5 Donghai Middle Road, Qingdao 266071, China. [6]Department of Neurology, Qingdao Municipal Hospital, Nanjing Medical University, No.5 Donghai Middle Road, Qingdao 266071, China. [7]Memory and Aging Center, Department of Neurology, University of California, San Francisco, CA 94158, USA.

References

1. Dericioglu N, Soylemezoglu F, Gursoy-Ozdemir Y, Akalan N, Saygi S, Dalkara T. Cell death and survival mechanisms are concomitantly active in the hippocampus of patients with mesial temporal sclerosis. Neuroscience. 2013;237:56–65.

2. Yamamoto A, Murphy N, Schindler CK, So NK, Stohr S, Taki W, et al. Endoplasmic reticulum stress and apoptosis signaling in human temporal lobe epilepsy. J Neuropathol Exp Neurol. 2006;65:217–25.

3. Tan MS, Yu JT, Jiang T, Zhu XC, Tan L. The NLRP3 Inflammasome in Alzheimer's Disease. Mol Neurobiol. 2013;48:875–82.

4. Masters SL, Gerlic M, Metcalf D, Preston S, Pellegrini M, O'Donnell JA, et al. NLRP1 inflammasome activation induces pyroptosis of hematopoietic progenitor cells. Immunity. 2012;37:1009–23.

5. Bergsbaken T, Fink SL, Cookson BT. Pyroptosis: host cell death and inflammation. Nat Rev Microbiol. 2009;7:99–109.

6. de Rivero Vaccari JP, Lotocki G, Alonso OF, Bramlett HM, Dietrich WD, Keane RW. Therapeutic neutralization of the NLRP1 inflammasome reduces the innate immune response and improves histopathology after traumatic brain injury. J Cereb Blood Flow Metab. 2009;29:1251–61.

7. Abulafia DP, de Rivero Vaccari JP, Lozano JD, Lotocki G, Keane RW, Dietrich WD. Inhibition of the inflammasome complex reduces the inflammatory response after thromboembolic stroke in mice. J Cereb Blood Flow Metab. 2009;29:534–44.

8. Kummer JA, Broekhuizen R, Everett H, Agostini L, Kuijk L, Martinon F, et al. Inflammasome components NALP 1 and 3 show distinct but separate expression profiles in human tissues suggesting a site-specific role in the inflammatory response. J Histochem Cytochem. 2007;55:443–52.

9. Fann DY, Lee SY, Manzanero S, Tang SC, Gelderblom M, Chunduri P, et al. Intravenous immunoglobulin suppresses NLRP1 and NLRP3 inflammasome-mediated neuronal death in ischemic stroke. Cell Death Dis. 2013;4:e790.

10. Vezzani A, French J, Bartfai T, Baram TZ. The role of inflammation in epilepsy. Nat Rev Neurol. 2011;7:31–40.

11. Kumar G, Mittal S, Moudgil SS, Kupsky WJ, Shah AK. Histopathological evidence that hippocampal atrophy following status epilepticus is a result of neuronal necrosis. J Neurol Sci. 2013;334:186–91.

12. Kwan P, Arzimanoglou A, Berg AT, Brodie MJ, Allen Hauser W, Mathern G, et al. Definition of drug resistant epilepsy: consensus proposal by the ad hoc Task Force of the ILAE Commission on Therapeutic Strategies. Epilepsia. 2010;51:1069–77.

13. Bjorling DE, Wang ZY. Estrogen and neuroinflammation. Urology. 2001;57:40–6.

14. Sun Z, Yu JT, Jiang T, Li MM, Tan L, Zhang Q. Genome-wide microRNA profiling of rat hippocampus after status epilepticus induced by amygdala stimulation identifies modulators of neuronal apoptosis. PLoS ONE. 2013;8:e78375.

15. Li MM, Jiang T, Sun Z, Zhang Q, Tan CC, Yu JT, et al. Genome-wide microRNA expression profiles in hippocampus of rats with chronic temporal lobe epilepsy. Sci Rep. 2014;4:4734.

16. Racine RJ. Modification of seizure activity by electrical stimulation. II. Motor seizure. Electroencephalogr Clin Neurophysiol. 1972;32:281–94.

17. Thakker DR, Hoyer D, Cryan JF. Interfering with the brain: use of RNA interference for understanding the pathophysiology of psychiatric and neurological disorders. Pharmacol Ther. 2006;109:413–38.

18. Denes A, Lopez-Castejon G, Brough D. Caspase-1: is IL-1 just the tip of the ICEberg? Cell Death Dis. 2012;3:e338.

19. Levandowski CB, Mailloux CM, Ferrara TM, Gowan K, Ben S, Jin Y, et al. NLRP1 haplotypes associated with vitiligo and autoimmunity increase interleukin-1beta processing via the NLRP1 inflammasome. Proc Natl Acad Sci U S A. 2013;110:2952–6.

20. Noe FM, Polascheck N, Frigerio F, Bankstahl M, Ravizza T, Marchini S, et al. Pharmacological blockade of IL-1beta/IL-1 receptor type 1 axis during epileptogenesis provides neuroprotection in two rat models of temporal lobe epilepsy. Neurobiol Dis. 2013;59:183–93.

21. Kovarova M, Hesker PR, Jania L, Nguyen M, Snouwaert JN, Xiang Z, et al. NLRP1-dependent pyroptosis leads to acute lung injury and morbidity in mice. J Immunol. 2012;189:2006–16.

22. Tan MS, Tan L, Jiang T, Zhu XC, Wang HF, Jia CD, et al. Amyloid-beta induces NLRP1-dependent neuronal pyroptosis in models of Alzheimer's disease. Cell Death Dis. 2014;5:e1382.

23. Walsh JG, Muruve DA, Power C. Inflammasomes in the CNS. Nat Rev Neurosci. 2014;15:84–97.

24. Wasterlain CG, Niquet J, Thompson KW, Baldwin R, Liu H, Sankar R, et al. Seizure-induced neuronal death in the immature brain. Prog Brain Res. 2002;135:335–53.

25. Steinhauser C, Seifert G, Bedner P. Astrocyte dysfunction in temporal lobe epilepsy: K+ channels and gap junction coupling. Glia. 2012;60:1192–202.

26. Arlehamn CS, Petrilli V, Gross O, Tschopp J, Evans TJ. The role of potassium in inflammasome activation by bacteria. J Biol Chem. 2010;285:10508–18.

27. Nissinen J, Halonen T, Koivisto E, Pitkanen A. A new model of chronic temporal lobe epilepsy induced by electrical stimulation of the amygdala in rat. Epilepsy Res. 2000;38:177–205.

28. Ghiringhelli F, Apetoh L, Tesniere A, Aymeric L, Ma Y, Ortiz C, et al. Activation of the NLRP3 inflammasome in dendritic cells induces IL-1beta-dependent adaptive immunity against tumors. Nat Med. 2009;15:1170–8.

29. Cryan JF, Thakker DR, Hoyer D. Emerging use of non-viral RNA interference in the brain. Biochem Soc Trans. 2007;35:411–5.

30. Thakker DR, Natt F, Husken D, Maier R, Muller M, van der Putten H, et al. Neurochemical and behavioral consequences of widespread gene knockdown in the adult mouse brain by using nonviral RNA interference. Proc Natl Acad Sci U S A. 2004;101:17270–5.

31. Kanemoto K, Kawasaki J, Miyamoto T, Obayashi H, Nishimura M. Interleukin (IL)1beta, IL-1alpha, and IL-1 receptor antagonist gene polymorphisms in patients with temporal lobe epilepsy. Ann Neurol. 2000;47:571–4.

32. Maroso M, Balosso S, Ravizza T, Liu J, Bianchi M, Vezzani A. Interleukin-1 type 1 receptor/Toll-like receptor signalling in epilepsy: the importance of IL-1beta and high-mobility group box 1. J Intern Med. 2011;270:319.

14

Tumor necrosis factor-α-mediated threonine 435 phosphorylation of p65 nuclear factor-κB subunit in endothelial cells induces vasogenic edema and neutrophil infiltration in the rat piriform cortex following status epilepticus

Ji-Eun Kim[1,2,4†], Hea Jin Ryu[1,2†], Soo Young Choi[2,3*] and Tae-Cheon Kang[1,2*]

Abstract

Background: Status epilepticus (SE) induces severe vasogenic edema in the piriform cortex (PC) accompanied by neuronal and astroglial damages. To elucidate the mechanism of SE-induced vasogenic edema, we investigated the roles of tumor necrosis factor (TNF)-α in blood-brain barrier (BBB) disruption during vasogenic edema and its related events in rat epilepsy models provoked by pilocarpine-induced SE.

Methods: SE was induced by pilocarpine in rats that were intracerebroventricularly infused with saline-, and soluble TNF p55 receptor (sTNFp55R) prior to SE induction. Thereafter, we performed Fluoro-Jade B staining and immunohistochemical studies for TNF-α and NF-κB subunits.

Results: Following SE, most activated microglia showed strong TNF-α immunoreactivity. In addition, TNF p75 receptor expression was detected in endothelial cells as well as astrocytes. In addition, only p65-Thr435 phosphorylation was increased in endothelial cells accompanied by SMI-71 expression (an endothelial barrier antigen). Neutralization of TNF-α by soluble TNF p55 receptor (sTNFp55R) infusion attenuated SE-induced vasogenic edema and neuronal damages via inhibition of p65-Thr435 phosphorylation in endothelial cells. Furthermore, sTNFp55R infusion reduced SE-induced neutrophil infiltration in the PC.

Conclusion: These findings suggest that impairments of endothelial cell functions via TNF-α-mediated p65-Thr 485 NF-κB phosphorylation may be involved in SE-induced vasogenic edema. Subsequently, vasogenic edema results in extensive neutrophil infiltration and neuronal-astroglial loss.

Keywords: Astrocyte, Blood brain barrier, Endothelium, Epilepsy, Immunohistochemistry

Background

Status epilepticus (SE) is a medical emergency with significant mortality [1]. SE has been defined as continuous seizure activity, which causes neuronal cell death, epileptogenesis and learning impairment [2,3]. Some brain regions vulnerable to SE play a role in the generation and propagation of paroxysmal activity in experimental epilepsy models. The piriform cortex (PC) is one of the most susceptible brain regions to seizure-induced damage in the kainate, pilocarpine and other models of temporal lobe epilepsy (TLE) [4-6]. Pilocarpine, a cholinergic agonist, induces SE in rodents. This pilocarpine-induced SE, similar to human TLE, shows massive neuronal loss in the hippocampus followed by glial proliferation. This neuronal damage in the pilocarpine model is not restricted to the hippocampus, but often extends to extrahippocampal limbic structures. Indeed,

* Correspondence: sychoi@hallym.ac.kr; tckang@hallym.ac.kr
† Contributed equally
[1]Department of Anatomy and Neurobiology, College of Medicine, Hallym University, Chunchon, Kangwon-Do 200-702, South Korea
[2]Institute of Epilepsy Research, College of Medicine, Hallym University, Chunchon, Kangwon-Do 200-702, South Korea

pilocarpine-induced SE results in acute neuronal damages within layers II and III of the PC [5,6].

SE also induces severe vasogenic edema in the PC accompanied by neuronal and astroglial damages [5-8]. Brain edema proceeds in two phases, early cytotoxic edema phase and late vasogenic edema phase. Early cytotoxic osmotic edema is due to excess stimulation of glutamatergic pathways during SE, which increases intracellular Na^+ and Ca^{2+} concentrations. The vasogenic edema results from dysfunction of endothelial cells and the blood-brain barrier (BBB). Many studies have reported increased permeability of the BBB during epileptic activity [9-13]. A fast and significant increase in systemic blood pressure, particularly shown during tonic epileptic seizures, induces a marked vasodilation of the large cerebral arteries and an increase in blood pressure in capillaries, small arteries, and veins leading to leakage of the BBB [9]. Loss of BBB integrity is not only due to an abrupt increase in the intraluminal pressure but also influenced by the properties of cerebral tissue. Indeed, an acute increase in blood pressure or epileptic activity causes an increase in pinocytosis at the level of the cerebral endothelium [11-13].

Recently, reports have also emphasized that seizure or epilepsy is a prolonged inflammatory condition, and that seizure activity rapidly increases the synthesis and release of various interleukins in rodent brain areas involved in seizure onset and their generalization. Cytokines act on endothelial cells and change the permeability of the BBB, which exerts significant effects on neuronal viability and excitability [14,15]. Indeed, Sztriha [16] reported that dexamethasone pretreatment reduces vasogenic edema in thalamus following kainic acid-induced seizure. Among cytokines, tumor necrosis factor-α (TNF-α) is a 17 kDa protein that is produced mainly by activated macrophages and T cells in the immune system. TNF-α is expressed at low levels in normal brain and is rapidly upregulated in glia, neurons and endothelial cells in various pathophysiological conditions, including SE [17,18]. TNF-α shows various effects on brain function depending on its local tissue concentration, the type of target cells, and especially the specific receptor subtype: TNF receptor I, or p55 receptor (TNFp55R); and TNF receptor II, or p75 receptor (TNFp75R) [19]. Furthermore, TNF-α induces macrophage inflammatory protein-2 (MIP-2) that recruits neutrophils under pathological conditions, including SE [14,20]. Neurons, microglia, and astrocytes produce MIP-2 when incubated with pro-inflammatory cytokines such as TNF-α and/or interleukin-1β (IL-1β) or after injury [21-23]. Indeed, we have recently reported that SE-mediated MIP-2 expression is relevant to leukocyte infiltrations following SE in an IL-1β-independent manner [20]. However, the relationship between the TNF-α system and BBB disruption/neutrophil infiltration during

vasogenic edema formation induced by epileptogenic insults has not been fully clarified. Therefore, in the present study, we investigated the roles of TNF-α in vasogenic edema and its related events in rat epilepsy models provoked by pilocarpine-induced SE.

Methods
Experimental animals
This study utilized progeny of Sprague-Dawley (SD) rats (male, 9 - 11 weeks old) obtained from Experimental Animal Center, Hallym University, Chunchon, South Korea. The animals were provided with a commercial diet and water *ad libitum* under controlled temperature, humidity and lighting conditions (22 ± 2°C, 55 ± 5% and a 12:12 light/dark cycle with lights). Animal protocols were approved by the Institutional Animal Care and Use Committee of Hallym University. Procedures involving animals and their care were conducted in accord with our institutional guidelines that comply with NIH Guide for the Care and Use of Laboratory Animals (NIH Publications No. 80-23, 1996). In addition, we have made all efforts to minimize the number of animals used and their suffering.

Intracerebroventricular drug infusion
Rats were divided into two groups: vehicle (saline)-treated and soluble TNFp55 receptor (sTNFp55R, 50 µg/ml; Sigma-Aldrich Co., St. Louis, MO)-treated groups. The dosage of sTNFp55R was determined as the highest dose that induced SE of comparable severity in 100% of animals with 5% mortality in the preliminary study. Animals were anesthetized (Zolretil, 50 mg/kg, i.m.; Virbac Laboratories, France) and placed in a stereotaxic frames. For the osmotic pump implantation, holes were drilled through the skull to introduce a brain infusion kit 1 (Alzet, Cupertino, CA) into the right lateral ventricle (1 mm posterior; 1.5 mm lateral; -3.5 mm depth; flat skull position with bregma as reference), according to the atlas of Paxinos and Watson [24]. The infusion kit was sealed with dental cement and connected to an osmotic pump (1007D, Alzet, Cupertino, CA). The pump was placed in a subcutaneous pocket in the dorsal region. Animals received 0.5 µl/hr of vehicle or compound for 1 week. Therefore, the dose of sTNFp55R was 0.6 µg/day per each animal. The compounds began to be immediately infused after surgery. Since the volume of vasogenic edema peaked at 2-3 days after SE in our previous studies [5-8,20], we chose this time point. Thus, our experimental schedules at least inhibit the function of TNF-α from 3 days prior to SE to 4 days after SE when the volume of vasogenic edema peaked.

Seizure induction
Three days after surgery, rats were treated with pilocarpine (380 mg/kg, i.p.; Sigma-Aldrich Co., St. Louis, MO)

at 20 min after methylscopolamine (5 mg/kg, i.p.; Sigma-Aldrich Co., St. Louis, MO). Using this treatment paradigm, behavioral seizures typically began within 20-40 min. Approximately 80% of pilocarpine treated rats showed acute behavioral features of SE (including akinesia, facial automatisms, limbic seizures consisting of forelimb clonus with rearing, salivation, masticatory jaw movements, and falling). We applied the 2 hr-SE rat model, because > 90% of the rats that we monitored in our previous studies [25] displayed spontaneous, recurrent seizures within 1-3 months after pilocarpine-induced status epilepticus. Diazepam (10 mg/kg, i.p.; Hoffman Ia Roche, Neuilly sur-Seine) was administered 2 hours after onset of SE and repeated, as needed. The rats were then observed 3 - 4 hours a day in the vivarium for general behavior and occurrence of spontaneous seizures. Non-experienced SE (non-SE) rats (showing only acute seizure behaviors during 10 - 30 min, n = 8) and age-matched normal rats were used as controls (n = 7).

Tissue processing

At designated time points (non-SE: 12 hr, 1 day, 2 days, 3 days, 4 days and 1 week after SE; n = 5, for each time point), animals were perfused transcardially with phosphate-buffered saline (PBS) followed by 4% paraformaldehyde in 0.1 M phosphate buffer (PB, pH 7.4) under urethane anesthesia (1.5 g/kg, i.p.; Sigma-Aldrich Co., St. Louis, MO). The brains were removed, and postfixed in the same fixative for 4 hr. The brain tissues were cryoprotected by infiltration with 30% sucrose overnight. Thereafter, the entire hippocampus was frozen and sectioned with a cryostat at 30 μm and consecutive sections were contained in six-well plates containing PBS. For stereological study, every sixth section in the series throughout the entire hippocampus was used in some animals.

Immunohistochemistry

Free-floating sections were first incubated with 10% normal goat serum for 30 min at room temperature. They were then incubated in rabbit anti-MPO IgG (1:100, Thermo fisher scientific) or rabbit anti-MIP-2 IgG (1:200, Invitrogen, Carlsbad, CA) in PBS containing 0.3% Triton X-100 (Sigma-Aldrich Co., St. Louis, MO) and 2% normal goat serum(Sigma-Aldrich Co., St. Louis, MO) overnight at room temperature. After washing three times for 10 min with PBS, the sections were incubated sequentially, in goat anti-rabbit or horse anti-mouse IgG (Vector, Burlingame, CA) and ABC complex (Vector, Burlingame, CA), diluted 1:200 in the same solution as the primary antiserum. Between the incubations, the tissues were washed with PBS three times for 10 min each. To confirm vasogenic edema, some tissue

sections were reacted for serum-proteins using horse anti-rat IgG (Vector, Burlingame, CA) as a primary antibody. The sections were visualized with 3,3'-diaminobenzidine (DAB, Sigma-Aldrich Co., St. Louis, MO) in 0.1 M Tris buffer and mounted on the gelatin-coated slides. The immunoreactions were observed under the Axioscope microscope (Carl Zeiss, Munchen-Hallbergmoos). For negative controls, rat hippocampal tissues were incubated with 1 μg of the antibody that was pre-incubated with 1 μg of purified peptide for 1 hr at room temperature or incubated with pre-immune serum instead of the primary antibody. For negative controls, tissues were incubated with pre-immune serum instead of primary antibody.

Double immunofluorescence study

Sections were incubated with 3% bovine serum albumin in PBS for 30 min at room temperature. Sections were then incubated in a mixture of goat anti-TNF-α IgG (1:1000, R&D systems, Minneapolis, MN)/mouse anti-OX-42 IgG (1:100, Serotec, Cambridge, UK), mouse anti-GFAP IgG (1:1000, an astroglial marker, Millipore Corporation, Billerica, MA)/rabbit anti-TNFp55R IgG (1:1000, Abcam, Cambridge, UK), mouse anti-GFAP IgG/rabbit anti-TNFp75R IgG (1:1000, Abcam, Cambridge, UK), mouse anti-SMI-71 IgM (1:1000, Covance, Berkeley, CA)/rabbit anti-TNFp75R IgG, mouse anti-GFAP IgG/rabbit anti-NF-κB (p65-Ser276, p65-Ser311, p65-Ser529, and p65-Thr435) IgG (1:100, Abcam, Cambridge, UK), mouse anti-SMI-71 IgM/rabbit anti-p65-Thr435 NF-κB IgG, mouse anti-SMI-71 IgM/rabbit anti-GLUT-1 IgG (1:100, Abcam, Cambridge, UK), or mouse anti-GFAP IgG/rabbit anti-MIP-2 IgG (1:100) in PBS containing 0.3% triton X-100 overnight at room temperature. After washing three times for 10 minutes with PBS, sections were also incubated in a mixture of FITC- and Cy3-conjugated secondary antisera (Amersham, San Francisco, CA), diluted 1:200, for 2 hr at room temperature. The sections were washed three times for 10 min with PBS, and mounted on gelatin-coated slides. For nuclei counterstaining, we used Vectashield mounting medium with DAPI (Vector, Burlingame, CA). All images were captured using an AxioImage M2 microscope and AxioVision Rel. 4.8 software.

Fluoro-Jade B staining

Fluoro-Jade B (FJB) staining was used to identify degenerating neurons in tissues obtained from non-SE and 3 days post-SE animals in every group. In our previous [18,25] and preliminary data, neuronal damage was first detectable at 3 days after SE. Therefore, we determined 3 days after SE as the best time point to look FJB. Briefly, sections were rinsed in distilled water, and mounted onto gelatin-coated slides and then dried on a slide warmer. The slides were immersed in 100% ethanol for 3 min, followed by 70% ethanol for 2 min and distilled water for 2 min. The slides were then transferred to 0.06% potassium permanganate for 15 min and gently agitated. After rinsing in distilled water for 2 min, the slides were incubated for 30 min in 0.001% FJB (Histo-Chem Inc., Jefferson, AR), freshly prepared by adding 20 ml of a 0.01% stock FJB solution to 180 ml of 0.1% acetic acid, with gentle shaking in the dark. After rinsing for 1 min in each of three changes of distilled water, the slides were dried, dehydrated in xylene and coverslipped with DPX (Sigma-Aldrich Co., St. Louis, MO). For stereological study, every sixth section in the series throughout the entire PC was used (see below).

Volumetric analysis and cell counts

To measure vasogenic edema, the volume of anti-rat IgG positive region in PC was estimated according to the formula based on the modified Cavalieri method: $V = \Sigma a \times t_{nom} \times 1/ssf$, where a is area of the region of the delineated subfield measured by AxioVision Rel. 4.8 software, t_{nom} is the nominal section thickness (of 30 μm in this study), and ssf is the fraction of the sections sampled or section sampling fraction (of 1/6 in this study). The subfield areas were delineated with a 2.5 × objective lens [5,7,8,18,25]. The volumes are reported as mm³. An optical fractionator was used to estimate cell numbers. The optical fractionator (a combination of performing counting with the optical dissector, with fractionator sampling) is a stereological method based on a properly designed systematic random sampling method that by definition yields unbiased estimates of population number. The sampling procedure is accomplished by focusing through the depth of the tissue (the optical dissector height, h; 15 μm in all cases for this study). The number of each cell type (C) in each of the subregions is estimated as: $C = \Sigma Q^- \times t/h \times 1/asf \times 1/ssf$, where Q^- is the number of cells actually counted in the dissectors that fell within the sectional profiles of the subregion seen on the sampled sections, and Asf is the areal sampling fraction calculated by the area of the counting frame of the dissector, a(frame) (of 50 × 50 μm² in this study) and the area associated with each x, y movement, grid (x, y step) (of 250 × 250 μm² in this study) {asf = (a(frame)/a(x, y step))}. The immunoreactive cells were counted with a 40× objective lens. The immunoreactive cells were counted with a 40× objective lens. All immunoreactive cells were counted regardless the intensity of labeling. Cell counts were performed by two different investigators who were blind to the classification of tissues. SE-induced PC atrophy is evident [8], so changes in cell number may be caused by an alterations in the volume of the PC. Therefore, the total number of cells was corrected by multiplying with appropriate correction factors (CF) representing the degree of shrinkage (or swelling) compared with the Non-SE.

Quantification of data

The fluorescence intensities of SMI-71/p65-Thr435 phosphorylation or GFPA/p65-Thr435 phosphorylation were measured using a computer-assisted image analysis program (The University of Texas ImageTool program V. 3.0 and AxioVision Rel. 4.8 software). After regions were outlined, 30 areas/rat (300 μm²/area) were randomly selected within the PC, and double immunofluorescent merge images were captured from the PC (15 sections from each animal). Merge images were digitally separated to red or green image, and converted to grayscale images, respectively (n = 36 per region examined, in non-SE, 12 hr post-SE and 1 day post-SE). The range of intensity values was obtained from the selected images. Based on the mean range of intensity values, each image was normalized by adjusting the black and white range of the image. Manipulation of the images was restricted to threshold and brightness adjustments to the whole image. Intensity measurements are represented as the mean number of a 256 gray scale (NIH Image 1.59 software and AxioVision Rel. 4.8 software). Values for background staining were obtained from the corpus callosum. Optical density values were then corrected by subtracting the average values of background noise obtained from 15 image inputs.

Data analysis

Data obtained from volumetric analysis, cell counts, and quantitative measurements were analyzed using Student's t-test to determine statistical significance. Linear regression analysis was also performed to determine correlations with SMI-71/p65-Thr435 phosphorylation, and the number of MPO cells/vasogenic edema areas.

Results

TNF-α, and TNF receptor expression

In non-SE induced animals of the saline-infused groups, TNF-α immunoreactivity was weakly detected in PC neurons (data not shown). In 12 hr-post SE animals of the saline-infused group, most of the activated microglia showed strong TNF-α immunoreactivity (Figure 1A). This expression pattern was maintained up to 1 week after SE. In non-SE-induced animals of the saline-infused groups, TNFp55R and TNFp75R immunoreactivities were also weakly observed in astrocytes (data not shown). In 12 hr-post SE animals of the saline-infused group, TNFp55R immunoreactivity was observed in astrocytes (Figure 1B). Unlike TNFp55R, TNFp75R immunoreactivity was detected in endothelial cells as

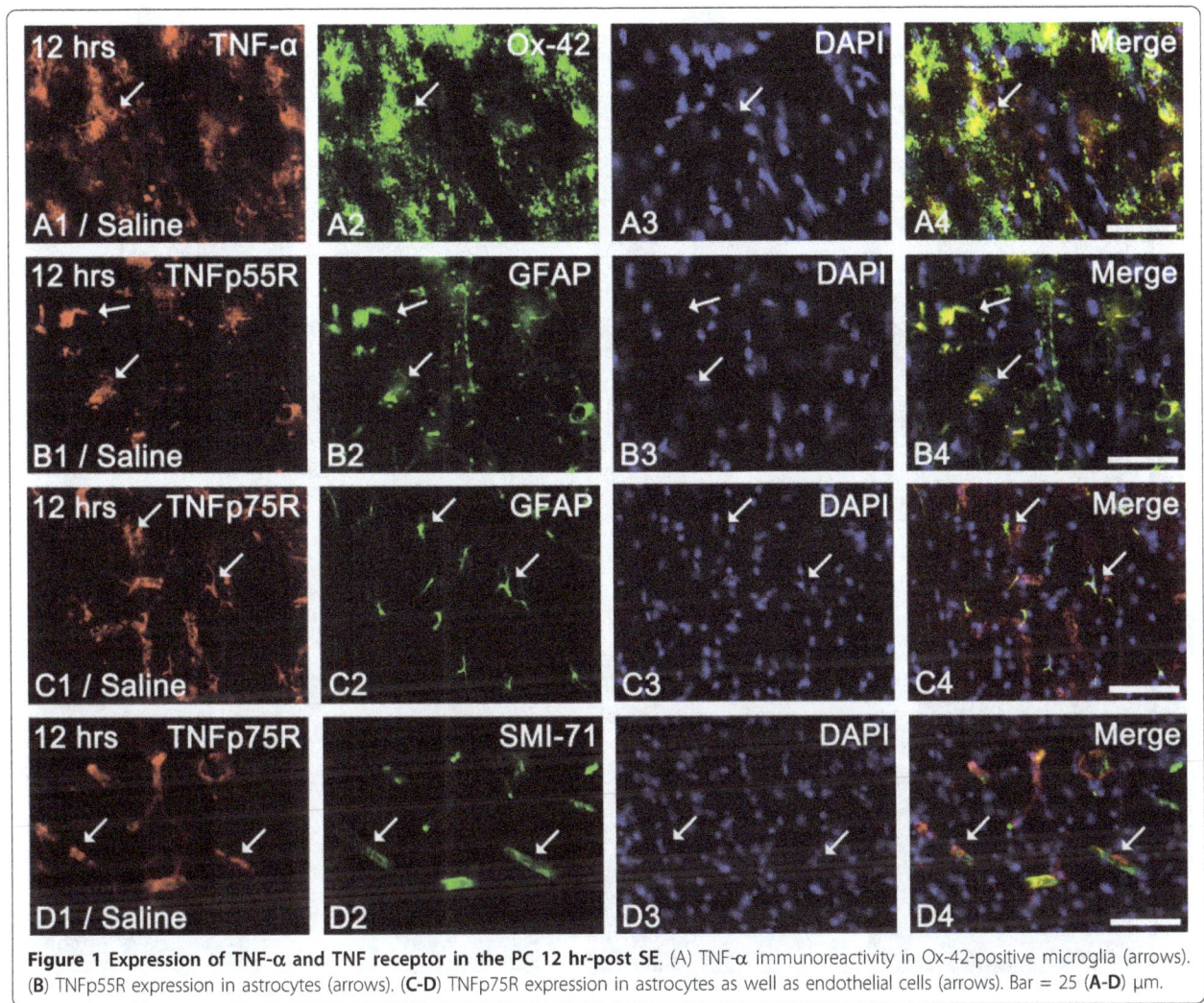

Figure 1 Expression of TNF-α and TNF receptor in the PC 12 hr-post SE. (A) TNF-α immunoreactivity in Ox-42-positive microglia (arrows). (**B**) TNFp55R expression in astrocytes (arrows). (**C-D**) TNFp75R expression in astrocytes as well as endothelial cells (arrows). Bar = 25 (**A-D**) μm.

well as astrocytes (Figures 1C-E). One day to 1 week after SE, both TNFp55R and TNFp75R immunoreactivities were significantly reduced in astrocytes, not in endothelial cells, due to massive astroglial loss (data not shown) [5,7,8,20].

Effect of sTNFp55R infusion on SE-induced serum-protein extravasation and neuronal damage

In our previous [5,7,8,20] and preliminary data, vasogenic edema and neuronal damage were noticeable at 1 day and 3 days after **SE, respectively**. Therefore, we determined that 3 days after **SE** was the best time point to evaluate the effect of sTNFp55R infusion on both vasogenic edema and neuronal damages induced by SE. In saline-treated animals, the PC was stained diffusely with anti-rat IgG (Figure 2A). The volume of vasogenic edema was 17.1 ± 1.5 mm^3 (Figure 2E). The number of FJB-positive neurons in the PC was $236,145 \pm 49,469$ (Figure 2B). In sTNFp55R-treated animals, SE-induced

vasogenic edema was attenuated to 9.8 ± 0.7 mm^3 (Figures 2C and 2E). In addition, the number of FJB-positive neurons in the PC was $89,138 \pm 5,698$ (Figures 2D-E). Thus, sTNFp55R infusion attenuated SE-induced vasogenic edema and neuronal damage compared to saline-infused animals ($p < 0.05$).

NF-κB phosphorylation

It is well established that TNF-α is one of the major stimuli toward phosphorylation of NF-κB. To confirm TNF-α-mediated signaling following SE, we performed an immunohistochemical study using five phospho-NF-κB antibodies. Compared to non-SE animals (data not shown), 12 hr-post SE animals of the saline-infused group showed p65-Ser276, p65-Ser311, p65-Ser529, and p65-Ser536 phosphorylation in astrocytes (not endothelial cells). sTNFp55R infusion effectively reduced p65-Ser276 and p65-Ser311 phosphorylation ($p < 0.05$, respectively), while it could not affect p65-Ser529 or

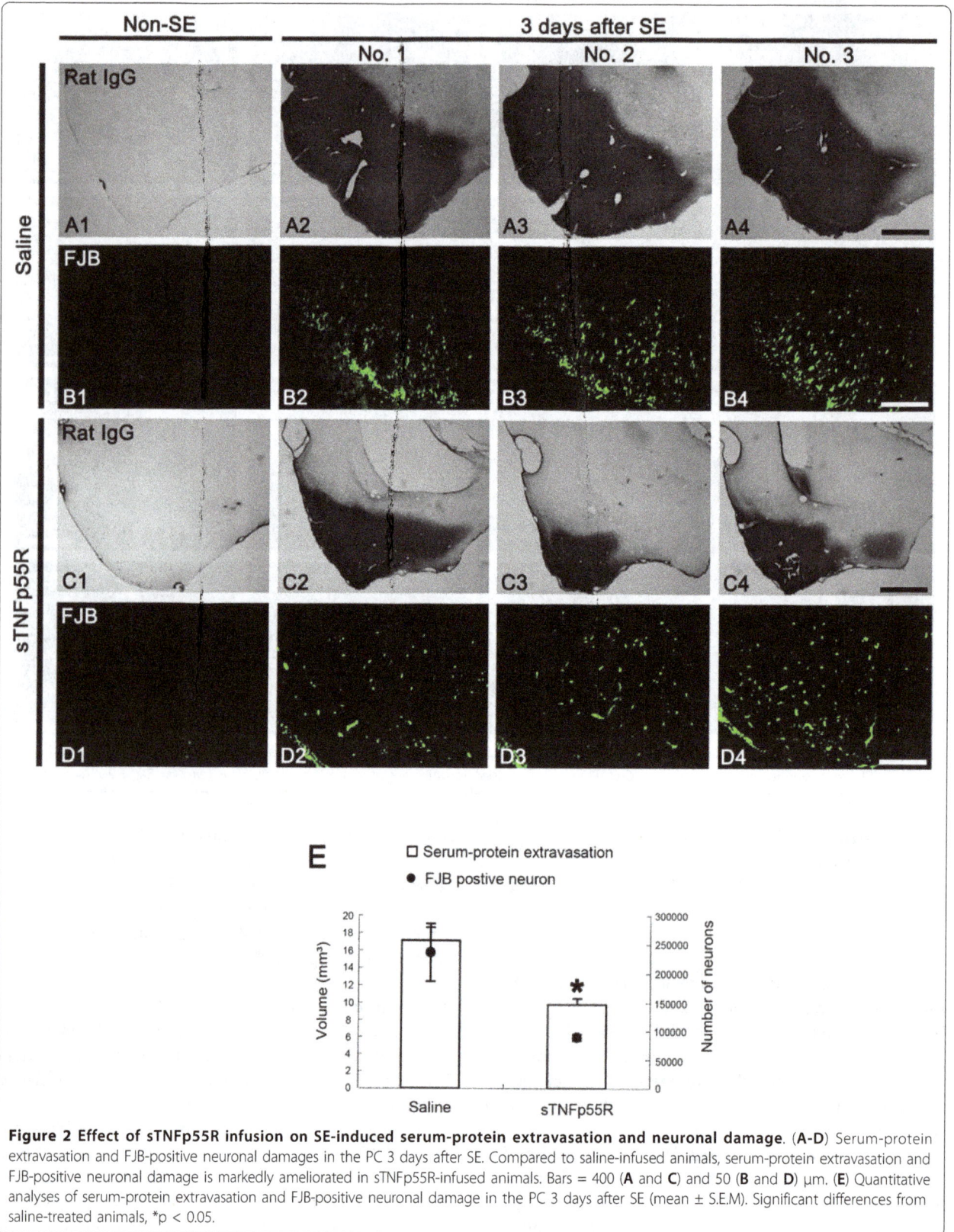

Figure 2 Effect of sTNFp55R infusion on SE-induced serum-protein extravasation and neuronal damage. (**A-D**) Serum-protein extravasation and FJB-positive neuronal damages in the PC 3 days after SE. Compared to saline-infused animals, serum-protein extravasation and FJB-positive neuronal damage is markedly ameliorated in sTNFp55R-infused animals. Bars = 400 (**A** and **C**) and 50 (**B** and **D**) μm. (**E**) Quantitative analyses of serum-protein extravasation and FJB-positive neuronal damage in the PC 3 days after SE (mean ± S.E.M). Significant differences from saline-treated animals, *p < 0.05.

p65-Ser536 phosphorylation (Figures 3 and 4A). In contrast, p65-Thr435 phosphorylation was increased in endothelial cells (not astrocytes) within the PC of saline-infused animals 12 hr after SE (Figure 5A). In addition, sTNFp55R infusion effectively alleviated SE-induced p65-Thr435 phosphorylation in endothelial cells, compared to saline infusion (p < 0.05, Figure 5B).

SMI-71 expression

Previously, we reported that SMI-71 (an endothelial barrier antigen) immunoreactivity decreased in the PC 1 day after SE [5]. Similarly, in 1 day-post SE animals of the saline-infused group, loss of SMI-71 immunoreactivity was detected in layer III/IV of the PC as compared to non-SE animals (Figures 4B and 5C-E, p < 0.05). Thus, loss of SMI-71 immunoreactivity correlated with volume of vasogenic edema following SE. This reduction in SMI-71 was accompanied by increased p65-Thr435 phosphorylation (Figures 5C-D). Therefore, the degree of SMI-71 immunoreactivity was inversely correlated to p65-Thr435 phosphorylation with a linear coefficient of correlation of -0.6324 (p < 0.05; Figure 4C). In addition, sTNFp55R infusion effectively alleviated p65-Thr435 phosphorylation and preserved SMI-71 immunoreactivity in endothelial cells following SE, as compared to saline infusion (p < 0.05; Figures 4A-B, 5D and 5F).

Neutrophil infiltration

Recent studies have reported that neutrophils infiltrate the brain under certain pathological conditions [26]. Indeed, we have reported massive neutrophil infiltration in layer III/IV of the PC 1 day after SE [20]. In the present study, 1 day-post-SE animals of the saline-infused group showed infiltration of MPO-positive neutrophils into the PC. Similarly, 1 day-post-SE animals of the sTNFp55R-infused group showed neutrophil infiltration into the PC 1 day after SE (Figure 6A). The number of neutrophils/area in the PC region (including the vasogenic edema region and the non-vasogenic edema region) of sTNFp55R-infused animals was significantly lower than that of the saline-infused group (Figure 6D, p < 0.05). However, there was no difference in neutrophil infiltration per unit area of vasogenic edema between the saline- and sTNFp55R-infused groups (Figure 6D). Furthermore, neutrophil infiltration showed a direct proportion to the area of vasogenic edema, with a linear coefficient of correlation of 0.8631 (p < 0.05, Figure 6E). Therefore, our findings indicate that SE-induced neutrophil infiltration into the PC may be correlated to TNF-α-mediated vasogenic edema formation.

MIP-2 expression

MIP-2 is a powerful chemokine that contributes to recruitment of neutrophils [27]. MIP-2 is undetectable or present at low levels under physiological conditions, and shows transient increases under pathological conditions via TNF-α and/or interleukin-1β (IL-1β)-dependent mechanisms [14]. Thus, it would be plausible that TNF-α-mediated MIP-2 expression may provoke SE-induced neutrophil infiltrations. To confirm this hypothesis, we investigated MIP-2 expression in the PC. Consistent with our previous study [20], some MIP-2-positive astrocytes were observed in the core and periphery of the vasogenic edema lesions, but not in the non-vasogenic edema region (Figure 6B and 6C). Although the number of MIP-2 positive cells per unit area in the PC region of sTNFp55R-infused animals was significantly lower than that of the saline-infused group due to reduction of the area of vasogenic edema, there was no difference in the number of MIP-2 positive cells per unit area of vasogenic edema between sTNFp55R-infused animals and saline-infused animals (Figure 6F). Furthermore, the number of MIP-2-positive cells showed a direct proportion to the unit area of vasogenic edema with a linear coefficient of correlation of 0.682 (p < 0.05, Figure 6G). Therefore, together with reduction in neutrophil infiltration in the PC region of sTNFp55R-infused animals, our findings provide evidence that TNF-α may regulate SE-induced neutrophil infiltration at least in the PC via vasogenic edema formation and not via direct TNF-α-mediated MIP-2 expression in astrocytes.

Discussion

The major findings in the present study are that TNF-α signaling showed cellular specific responses of NF-κB phosphorylation in the PC following SE, which may be related to vasogenic edema formation followed by neutrophil infiltration. BBB disruption has been reported in experimental and human epilepsy [12,13,15,16,28]. Leakage of serum-derived components into the extracellular space is associated with hyperexcitability and seizure onset [12,13,15,16,28]. Furthermore, dysfunction of the BBB leads to epileptogenesis and contributes to progression of epilepsy [12,13,15,16,28]. In the present study, TNF-α immunoreactivity was obviously observed in microglia in the PC following SE. TNF receptor expressions were also up-regulated in astrocytes (TNFp55R and TNFp75R) and endothelial cells (TNFp75R). Furthermore, blockade of TNF-α signaling by sTNFp55 infusion effectively (but not completely) reduced volumes of SE-induced vasogenic edema and neuronal damage in the PC. These findings indicate that TNF-α may participate in astroglial and endothelial responses to SE, which are relevant to SE-induced vasogenic edema formation [5-8]. Indeed, TNF-α signaling increases BBB permeability in various experimental disease models [29]. In the present study, sTNFp55

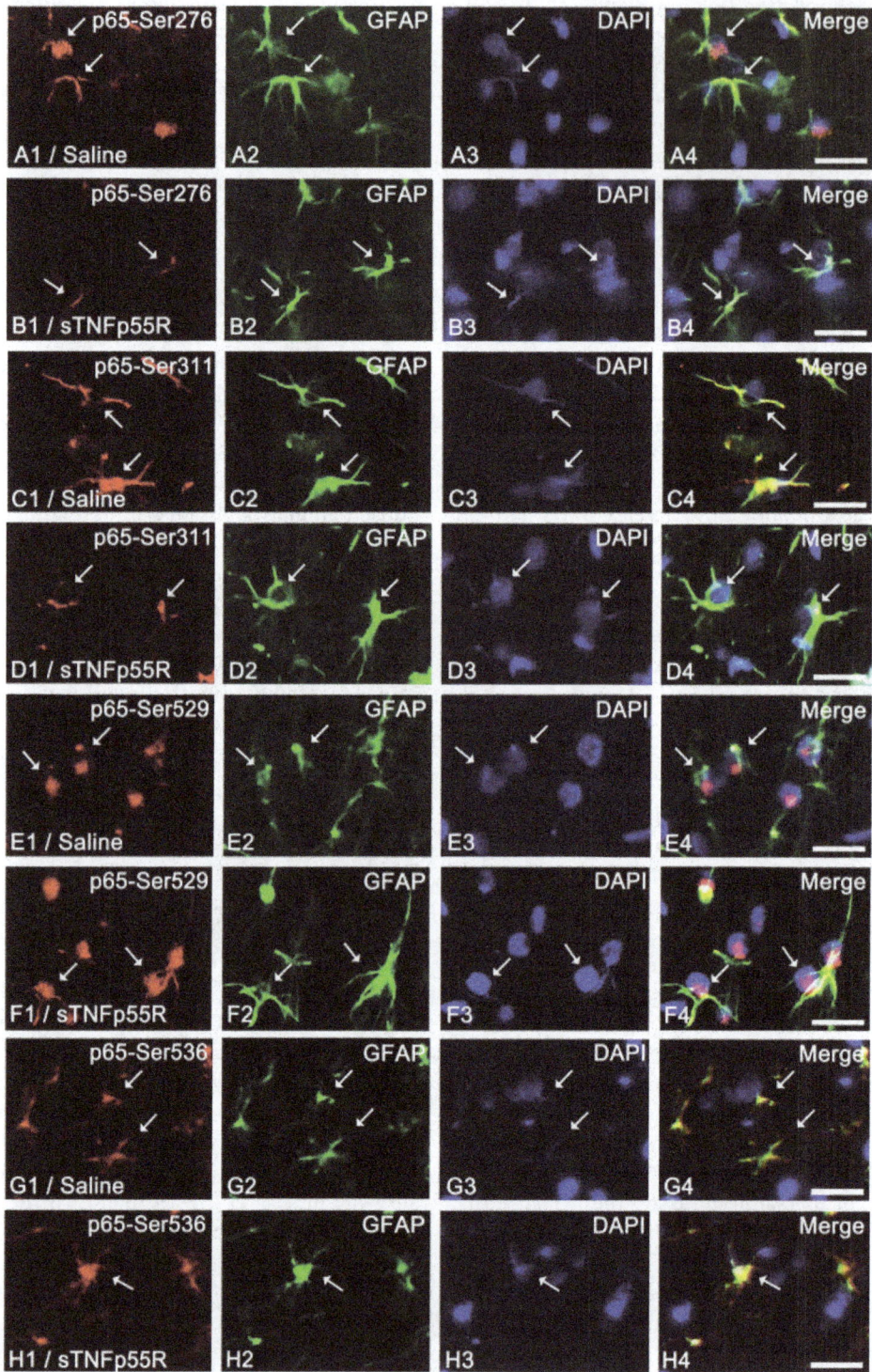

Figure 3 Effect of sTNFp55R infusion on NF-κB phosphorylation in astrocytes 12 hr after SE. In 12 hr-post SE animals of the saline-infused group (**A**, **C**, **E** and **G**), astrocytes show p65-Ser276 (**A**), p65-Ser311 (**C**), p65-Ser529 (**E**), and p65-Ser536 (**G**) phosphorylation (arrows). sTNFp55R infusion (**B**, **D**, **F** and **H**) effectively reduces p65-Ser276 (**B**) and p65-Ser311 (**D**) phosphorylation, while it does not affect p65-Ser529 (**F**) and p65-Ser536 (**H**) phosphorylation (arrows). Bar = 12.5 μm.

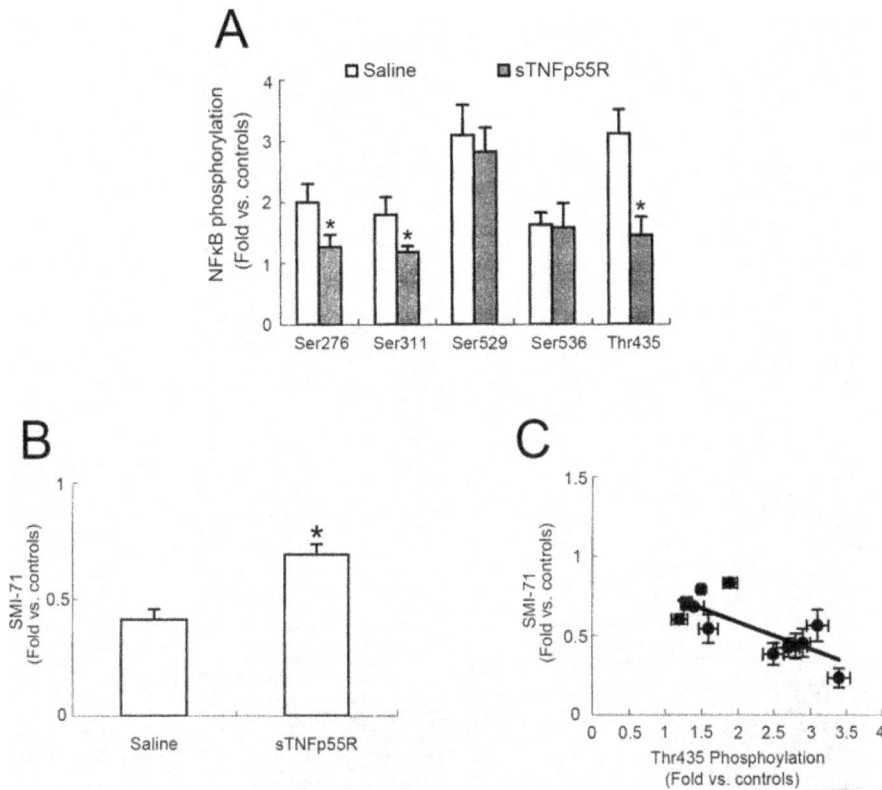

Figure 4 Quantitative analyses of the effect of sTNFp55R infusion on NF-κB phosphorylation and SMI-71 expression. (**A**) Quantitative analysis of NF-κB phosphorylation 12 hr after SE (mean ± S.E.M). Significant differences from saline-infused animals, *$p < 0.05$. (**B**) Quantitative analysis of SMI-71 expression 1 day after SE (mean ± S.E.M). Significant differences from saline-infused animals, *$p < 0.05$. (**C**) Linear regression analysis between p65-Thr435 phosphorylation and SMI-71 in the PC following SE.

infusion could not completely prevent SE-induced vasogenic edema and neuronal damage in the PC. Therefore, our findings suggest that TNF-α signaling may not be a unique upstream event in vasogenic edema development.

p65 phosphorylation of NF-κB enhances its transactivation potential, and p65 phosphorylation occurs in either the cytoplasm or the nucleus [30]. In the present study, p65-Thr435 immunoreactivity was detected in endothelial cells, and its immunoreactivity showed an inverse correlation to the degree of SMI-71 expression. SMI-71, an endothelial barrier antigen, is a protein expressed by endothelial cells of rat BBB [31]. Under pathological conditions, SMI-71 expression is lost in endothelial cells [5,7,8,30,32]. Acute phases of the above pathological conditions are accompanied by opening of the BBB and development of vasogenic edema [33]. Indeed, neutralization of SMI-71 in vivo leads to widening of intercellular junctions between endothelial cells and swelling of perivascular astrocytic processes [34], although SMI-71 is not localized at endothelial cell junctions [35-38]. In the present study, SMI-71 immunoreactivity was significantly reduced in blood vessels 1

day after SE when vasogenic edema and neuronal damage were observed. Furthermore, sTNFp55R infusion effectively prevented SE-induced SMI-71 down-regulation. With respect to the phosphorylation of p65-Thr435 by TNF-α [39], our findings indicate that TNF-α-mediated p65-Thr435 phosphorylation in endothelial cells may play an important role in vasogenic edema induction via SMI-71 degradation or its posttranslational dysfunction influencing BBB permeability.

In our previous studies [5,8], dystrophin (an actin-binding protein [40]) immunoreactivity was detected in blood vessels and in astrocytic perivascular end-feet, and was down-regulated 12 hrs after SE prior to the appearance of vasogenic edema and down-regulation of SMI-71 immunoreactivity. With respect to this previous report, changes in SMI immunoreactivity would be causes/results of interaction between endothelial cells and perivascular astrocytes. In the present study, p65-Ser276, p65-Ser311, p65-Ser529, and p65-Ser536 phosphorylation was observed in astrocytes following SE. Furthermore, sTNFp55R infusion effectively inhibited p65-Ser276 and p65-Ser311phosphorylation in astrocytes following SE. Therefore, it is likely that enhanced

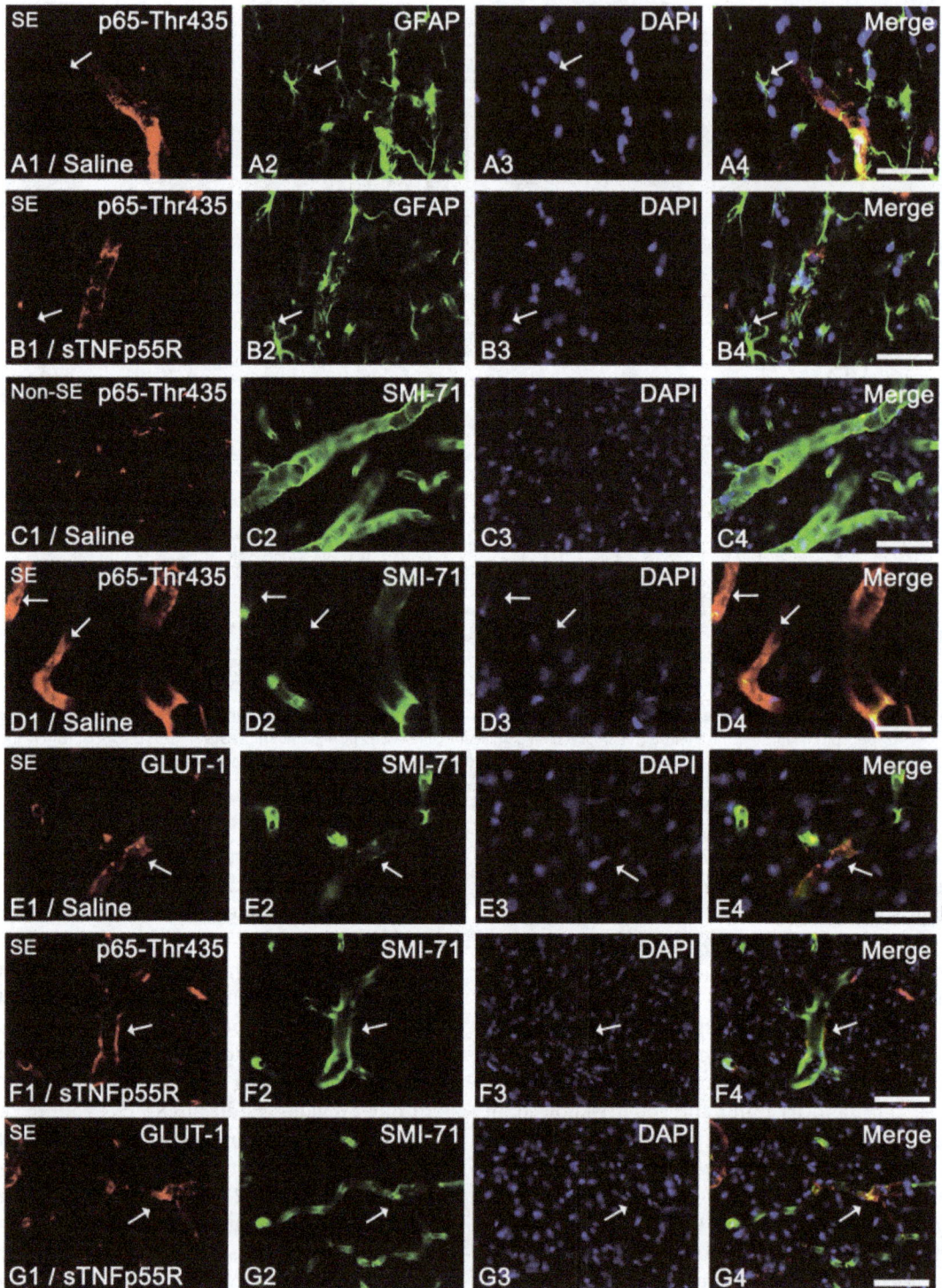

Figure 5 Effect of sTNFp55R infusion on p65-Thr435 phosphorylation in endothelial cells following SE. (**A-B**) Inhibition of p65-Thr435 phosphorylation by sTNFp55R infusion 12 hr after SE. p65-Thr435 phosphorylation is rarely observed in astrocytes (arrows). (**C**) Endothelial p65-Thr435 phosphorylation in non-SE animals. (**D-E**) Endothelial p65-Thr435 phosphorylation in saline-infused animals 1 day after SE. p65-Thr435 phosphorylation is enhanced, while SMI-71 expression is reduced in GLUT-1-positive endothelial cells (arrows). (**F-G**) Endothelial p65-Thr435 phosphorylation in sTNFp55R-infused animal 1 day after SE. sTNFp55R infusion effectively reduces p65-Thr435 and preserves SMI-71 expression in GLUT-1-positive endothelial cells (arrows). Bars = 12.5 (**A-D**) and 25 (**E-G**) μm.

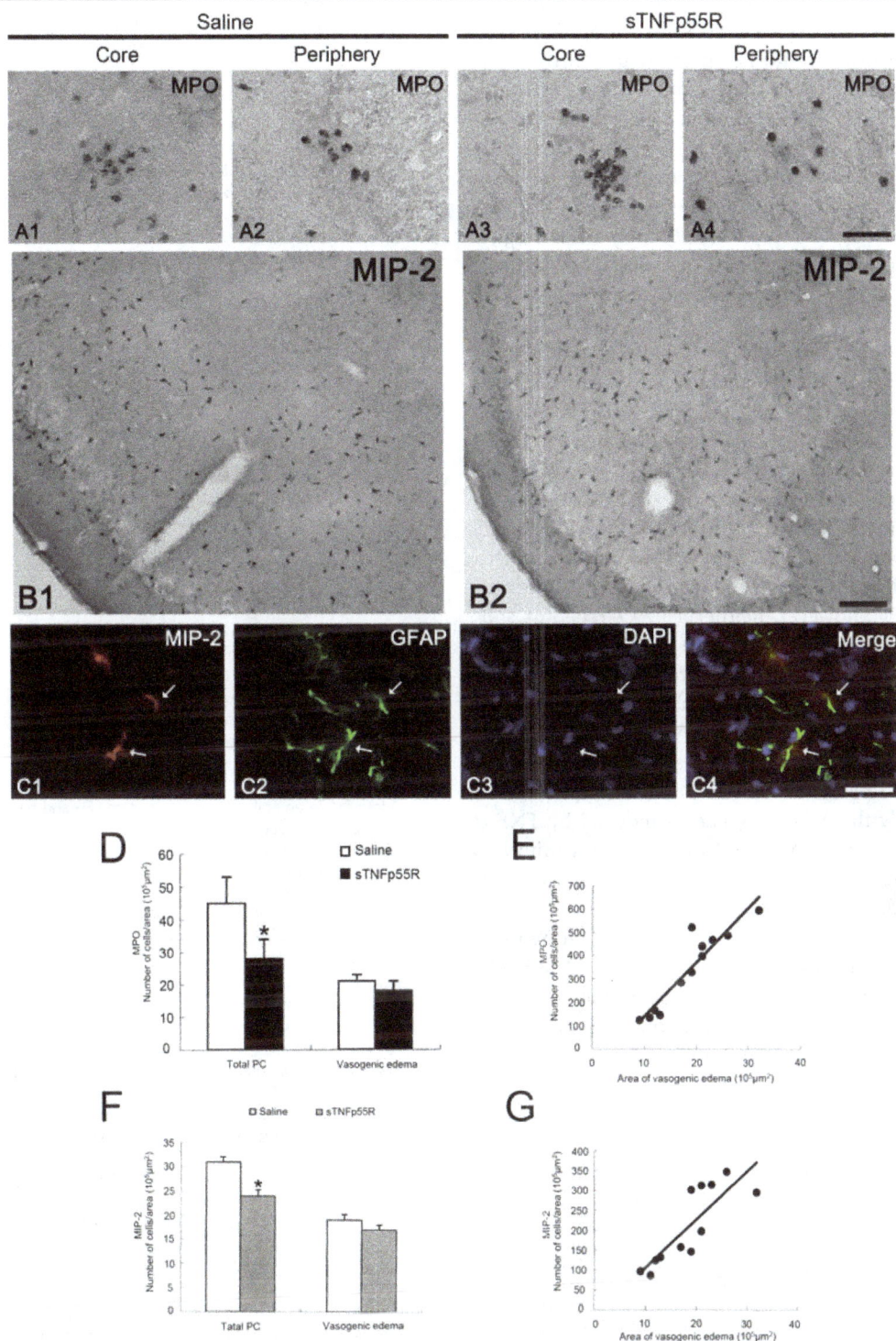

Figure 6 Effect of sTNFp55R infusion on neutrophil infiltration and MIP-2 expression following SE. (A) Neutrophil infiltration in vasogenic edema lesion 1 day after SE. (B) MIP-2 expression in the PC 1 day after SE. (C) Astroglial expression of MIP-2 (arrows). Bars = 12.5 (A and C) and 150 (B) μm. (D) Quantitative analysis of neutrophil infiltration 1 day after SE (mean ± S.E.M). Significant differences from saline-infused animals, *p < 0.05. (E) Linear regression analysis between the number of infiltrated neutrophils/area in the vasogenic edema region and the area of vasogenic edema in the PC. (F) Quantitative analysis of the number of MIP-2 positive cells per the unit area of vasogenic edema 1 day after SE (mean ± S.E.M). There is no difference in the number of MIP-2-positive cells per unit area of vasogenic edema between sTNFp55R-infused animals and saline-infused animals. (G) Linear regression analysis between the number of MIP-2 positive cells per unit area in vasogenic edema region and the area of vasogenic edema in the PC.

p65-Ser276 and p65-Ser311 phosphorylation may be involved in TNF-α-mediated BBB disruption. However, sTNFp55R infusion could not prevent p65-Ser529 and p65-Ser536 phosphorylations from SE insults. Since p65-Ser529 and p65-Ser536 are phosphorylated by TNF-α and IL-1β [41], it is likely that IL-1β-mediated p65-Ser529/Ser536 phosphorylation may also play a role in SE-induced vasogenic edema. Therefore, our findings indicate that both TNF-α and IL-1β may be synergists to play either a direct (by endothelial cells) or indirect (by astrocytes) role in the maintenance of BBB permeability.

Neutrophil infiltration into brain parenchyma is transiently observed during the acute phase of SE (4 - 36 hr after SE) and disappears thereafter [20]. SE rapidly increases synthesis and release of chemokines in various areas of the rodent brain [42]. Among them, MIP-2 is required for efficient neutrophil or lymphocyte recruitment to brain parenchyma [43]. In our previous study [20], neutrophil infiltration in the frontoparietal cortex was regulated by P2X7 receptor-mediated MIP-2 expression. In the PC, however, neither a P2X7 receptor agonist/antagonist nor IL-1Ra (an IL-1β antagonist) infusion could not affect leukocyte infiltration. In the present study, sTNFp55R infusion effectively inhibited neutrophil infiltration in the PC by reducing vasogenic edema formation in a MIP-2-independent manner. With respect to the present and our previous reports, it is therefore likely that vasogenic edema induced by TNF-α can induce neutrophil infiltration and press injury to evoke neuronal-astroglial loss in the PC, unlike other brain regions.

In conclusion, our findings reveal that impairments of endothelial cell function via TNF-α mediated p65-Thr 435 NF-κB phosphorylation may be involved in SE-induced vasogenic edema, which is relevant to neutrophil infiltration and neuronal-astroglial loss.

Acknowledgements
This study was supported by a grant of National Research Foundation of Korea (grant number: 2009-0064347, 2009-0093812 and 2010K000808)

Author details
[1]Department of Anatomy and Neurobiology, College of Medicine, Hallym University, Chunchon, Kangwon-Do 200-702, South Korea. [2]Institute of Epilepsy Research, College of Medicine, Hallym University, Chunchon, Kangwon-Do 200-702, South Korea. [3]Department of Biomedical Sciences, College of Life Science, Hallym University, Chunchon, Kangwon-Do 200-702, South Korea. [4]Department of Neurology, UCSF, and Veterans Affairs Medical Center, San Francisco, California 94121, USA.

Authors' contributions
JEK and HJR were involved in designing and performing all experiments. SYC and TCK helped in drafting the manuscript. JEK and HJR did the immunohistochemistry, the intracerebroventricular drug infusion, the seizure studies and the acquisition of data and analyses. SYC and TCK provided continuous intellectual input, and evaluation and interpretation of data. All authors read and approved the final manuscript.

Competing interests
The authors declare that they have no competing interests.

References

1. DeLorenzo RJ, Pellock JM, Towne AR, Boggs JG: Epidemiology of status epilepticus. J Clin Neurophysiol 1995, 12:316-325.
2. Rice AC, DeLorenzo RJ: NMDA receptor activation during status epilepticus is required for the development of epilepsy. Brain Res 1998, 782:240-247.
3. Stewart LS, Persinger MA: Ketamine Prevents Learning Impairment When Administered Immediately after Status Epilepticus Onset. Epilepsy Behav 2001, 2:585-591.
4. Gale K: Subcortical structures and pathways involved in convulsive seizure generation. J Clin Neurophysiol 1992, 9:264-277.
5. Sheen SH, Kim JE, Ryu HJ, Yang Y, Choi KC, Kang TC: Decrease in dystrophin expression prior to disruption of brain-blood barrier within the rat piriform cortex following status epilepticus. Brain Res 2010, 1369:173-183.
6. Turski L, Ikonomidou C, Turski WA, Bortolotto ZA, Cavalheiro EA: Review: cholinergic mechanisms and epileptogenesis. The seizures induced by pilocarpine: a novel experimental model of intractable epilepsy. Synapse 1989, 3:154-171.
7. Jo SM, Ryu HJ, Kim JE, Yeo SI, Kim MJ, Choi HC, Song HK, Kang TC: Up-regulation of endothelial endothelin-1 expression prior to vasogenic edema formation in the rat piriform cortex following status epilepticus. Neurosci Lett 2011, 501:25-30.
8. Kim JE, Yeo SI, Ryu HJ, Kim MJ, Kim DS, Jo SM, Kang TC: Astroglial loss and edema formation in the rat piriform cortex and hippocampus following pilocarpine-induced status epilepticus. J Comp Neurol 2010, 518:4612-4628.
9. Sperk G: Kainic acid seizures in the rat. Prog Neurobiol 1994, 42:1-32.
10. Nitsch C, Hubauer H: Distant blood-brain barrier opening in subfields of the rat hippocampus after intrastriatal injections of kainic acid but not ibotenic acid. Neurosci Lett 1986, 64:53-58.
11. Ates N, van Luijtelaar EL, Drinkenburg WH, Vossen JM, Coenen AM: Effects of loreclezole on epileptic activity and on EEG and behaviour in rats with absence seizures. Epilepsy Res 1992, 13:43-48.
12. Nitsch C, Suzuki R, Fujiwara K, Klatzo I: Incongruence of regional cerebral blood flow increase and blood-brain barrier opening in rabbits at the onset of seizures induced by bicuculline, methoxypyridoxine, and kainic acid. J Neurol Sci 1985, 67:67-79.
13. Cornford EM, Oldendorf WH: Epilepsy and the blood-brain barrier. Adv Neurol 1986, 44:787-812.
14. Rodgers KM, Hutchinson MR, Northcutt A, Maier SF, Watkins LR, Barth DS: The cortical innate immune response increases local neuronal excitability leading to seizures. Brain 2009, 132:2478-2486.
15. Deli MA, Abrahám CS, Kataoka Y, Niwa M: Permeability studies on in vitro blood-brain barrier models: physiology, pathology, and pharmacology. Cell Mol Neurobiol 2005, 25:59-127.
16. Sztriha L, Joó F, Szerdahelyi P, Eck E, Koltai M: Effects of dexamethasone on brain edema induced by kainic acid seizures. Neuroscience 1986, 17:107-114.
17. Sriram K, O'Callaghan JP: Divergent roles for tumor necrosis factor-alpha in the brain. J Neuroimmune Pharmaco 2007, 2:140-153.
18. Kim JE, Ryu HJ, Kang TC: P2X7 receptor activation ameliorates CA3 neuronal damage via a tumor necrosis factor-α-mediated pathway in the rat hippocampus following status epilepticus. J Neuroinflammation 2011, 8:62.
19. Fotin-Mleczek M, Henkler F, Samel D, Reichwein M, Hausser A, Parmryd I, Scheurich P, Schmid JA, Wajant H: Apoptotic crosstalk of TNF receptors: TNF-R2-induces depletion of TRAF2 and IAP proteins and accelerates TNF-R1-dependent activation of caspase-8. J Cell Sci 2002, 115:2757-2770.
20. Kim JE, Ryu HJ, Yeo SI, Kang TC: P2X7 receptor regulates leukocyte infiltrations in rat frontoparietal cortex following status epilepticus. J Neuroinflammation 2010, 7:65.
21. Hayashi M, Luo Y, Laning J, Strieter RM, Dorf ME: Production and function of monocyte chemoattractant protein-1 and other beta-chemokines in murine glial cells. J Neuroimmunol 1995, 60:143-150.
22. Otto VI, Heinzel-Pleines UE, Gloor SM, Trentz O, Kossmann T, Morganti-Kossmann MC: sICAM-1 and TNF-alpha induce MIP-2 with distinct

kinetics in astrocytes and brain microvascular endothelial cells. *J Neurosci Res* 2000, **60**:733-742.

23. Rhodes JK, Sharkey J, Andrews PJ: **The temporal expression, cellular localization, and inhibition of the chemokines MIP-2 and MCP-1 after traumatic brain injury in the rat.** *J Neurotrauma* 2009, **26**:507-525.

24. Paxinos G, Watson C: **The Rat Brain in Stereotaxic Coordinates.** San Diego, Academic Press;, 3 1997.

25. Kang TC, Kim DS, Kwak SE, Kim JE, Won MH, Kim DW, Choi SY, Kwon OS: **Epileptogenic roles of astroglial death and regeneration in the dentate gyrus of experimental temporal lobe epilepsy.** *Glia* 2006, **54**:258-271.

26. Biagas KV, Uhl MW, Schiding JK, Nemoto EM, Kochanek PM: **Assessment of posttraumatic polymorphonuclear leukocyte accumulation in rat brain using tissue myeloperoxidase assay and vinblastine treatment.** *J Neurotrauma* 1992, **9**:363-371.

27. Babcock AA, Kuziel WA, Rivest S, Owens T: **Chemokine expression by glial cells directs leukocytes to sites of axonal injury in the CNS.** *J Neurosci* 2003, **23**:7922-7930.

28. Seiffert E, Dreier JP, Ivens S, Bechmann I, Tomkins O, Heinemann U, Friedman A: **Lasting blood-brain barrier disruption induces epileptic focus in the rat somatosensory cortex.** *J Neurosci* 2004, **24**:7829-7836.

29. Farkas G, Márton J, Nagy Z, Mándi Y, Takács T, Deli MA, Abrahám CS: **Experimental acute pancreatitis results in increased blood-brain barrier permeability in the rat: a potential role for tumor necrosis factor and interleukin 6.** *Neurosci Lett* 1998, **242**:147-150.

30. Viatour P, Merville MP, Bours V, Chariot A: **Phosphorylation of NF-kappaB and IkappaB proteins: implications in cancer and inflammation.** *Trends Biochem Sci* 2005, **30**:43-52.

31. Sternberger NH, Sternberger LA: **Blood-brain barrier protein recognized by monoclonal antibody.** *Proc Natl Acad Sci USA* 1987, **84**:8169-8173.

32. Sternberger NH, Sternberger LA, Kies MW, Shear CR: **Cell surface endothelial proteins altered in experimental allergic encephalomyelitis.** *J Neuroimmunol* 1989, **21**:241-248.

33. Perdiki M, Farooque M, Holtz A, Li GL, Olsson Y: **Expression of endothelial barrier antigen immunoreactivity in blood vessels following compression trauma to rat spinal cord. Temporal evolution and relation to the degree of the impact.** *Acta Neuropathol* 1998, **96**:8-12.

34. Krum JM, Kenyon KL, Rosenstein JM: **Expression of blood-brain barrier characteristics following neuronal loss and astroglial damage after administration of anti-Thy-1 immunotoxin.** *Exp Neurol* 1997, **146**:33-45.

35. Ghabriel MN, Zhu C, Leigh C: **Electron microscope study of blood-brain barrier opening induced by immunological targeting of the endothelial barrier antigen.** *Brain Res* 2002, **934**:140-151.

36. Lawrenson JG, Ghabriel MN, Reid AR, Gajree TN, Allt G: **Differential expression of an endothelial barrier antigen between the CNS and the PNS.** *J Anat* 1995, **186**:217-221.

37. Rosenstein JM, Krum JM, Sternberger LA, Pulley MT, Sternberger NH: **Immunocytochemical expression of the endothelial barrier antigen (EBA) during brain angiogenesis.** *Dev Brain Res* 1992, **66**:47-54.

38. Sternberger NH, Sternberger LA, Kies MW, Shear CR: **Cell surface endothelial proteins altered in experimental allergic encephalomyelitis.** *J Neuroimmunol* 1989, **21**:241-248.

39. O'Shea JM, Perkins ND: **Thr435 phosphorylation regulates RelA (p65) NF-kappaB subunit transactivation.** *Biochem J* 2010, **426**:345-354.

40. Tinsley JM, Blake DJ, Zuellig RA, Davies KE: **Increasing complexity of the dystrophin-associated protein complex.** *Proc Natl Acad Sci USA* 1994, **91**:8307-8313.

41. Bird TA, Schooley K, Dower SK, Hagen H, Virca GD: **Activation of nuclear transcription factor NF-kappaB by interleukin-1 is accompanied by casein kinase II-mediated phosphorylation of the p65 subunit.** *J Biol Chem* 1997, **272**:32606-32612.

42. De Simoni MG, Perego C, Ravizza T, Moneta D, Conti M, Marchesi F, De Luigi A, Garattini S, Vezzani A: **Inflammatory cytokines and related genes are induced in the rat hippocampus by limbic status epilepticus.** *Eur J Neurosci* 2000, **12**:2623-2633.

43. Fuentes ME, Durham SK, Swerdel MR, Lewin AC, Barton DS, Megill JR, Bravo R, Lira SA: **Controlled recruitment of monocytes and macrophages to specific organs through transgenic expression of monocyte chemoattractant protein-1.** *J Immunol* 1995, **155**:5769-5776.

LncRNA H19 contributes to hippocampal glial cell activation via JAK/STAT signaling in a rat model of temporal lobe epilepsy

Chun-Lei Han[1,2], Ming Ge[3], Yun-Peng Liu[1,2], Xue-Min Zhao[1,2], Kai-Liang Wang[1,2], Ning Chen[2,4], Wen-Jia Meng[5], Wei Hu[6], Jian-Guo Zhang[2,4], Liang Li[7*] and Fan-Gang Meng[1,2*]

Abstract

Background: Astrocyte and microglia activation are well-known features of temporal lobe epilepsy that may contribute to epileptogenesis. However, the mechanisms underlying glia activation are not well understood. Long non-coding RNA (lncRNA) H19 has diverse functions depending on physiological or pathological state, and its role in epilepsy is unknown. We previously demonstrated that H19 was significantly upregulated in the latent period of epilepsy and may be associated with cell proliferation and immune and inflammatory responses. We therefore speculated that H19 is involved in the hippocampal glial cell activation during epileptogenesis.

Methods: H19 was overexpressed or knocked down using an adeno-associated viral vector delivery system. A rat status epilepticus model was induced by intra-amygdala kainic acid injection. Astrocyte and microglia activation were assessed by immunofluorescence and western blot analyses. Expression of proinflammatory cytokines and components of the Janus kinase (JAK)/signal transducer and activator of transcription (STAT) signaling pathways were evaluated with western blotting.

Results: H19 overexpression induced the activation of astrocytes and microglia and the release of proinflammatory cytokines (interleukin-1β and interleukin-6 and tumor necrosis factor-α) in the hippocampus, whereas H19 knockdown inhibited status epilepticus-induced glial cell activation. Moreover, H19 activated JAK/STAT signaling by promoting the expression of Stat3 and c-Myc, which is thought to be involved in astrocyte activation.

Conclusions: LncRNA H19 contributes to hippocampal glial cell activation via modulation of the JAK/STAT pathway and could be a therapeutic tool to prevent the development of epilepsy.

Keywords: Temporal lobe epilepsy, lncRNA H19, Astrocytes, Microglia, Inflammatory response

Background

Temporal lobe epilepsy (TLE) is one of the most common types of intractable epilepsy and is characterized by the periodic and unpredictable occurrence of seizures. Glial cell activation and proliferation, a well-described pathological feature of TLE, can alter blood-brain barrier integrity and ion and neurotransmitter homeostasis and cause an inflammatory response, resulting in neuronal hyperexcitability and the generation and spread of seizure activity [1–3]. Although impairment of these functions is thought to be associated with the pathophysiology of epilepsy, the mechanisms underlying glial cell activation are complex and are not fully understood [1].

Long non-coding RNA (lncRNA) H19, an imprinted gene, is located on human chromosome 11 and is transcribed from the maternally inherited allele [4]. Despite being identified over 20 years ago, the function of H19 remains unclear and its pathological role as a noncoding RNA has only recently been elucidated [5]. H19 has diverse functions depending on physiological and pathological state. In the central nervous system (CNS), H19 is overexpressed in glioblastoma tissue and promotes

* Correspondence: liliang@ccmu.edu.cn; mengfg@ccmu.edu.cn
[7]Department of Pathology, School of Basic Medical Sciences, Capital Medical University, No. 10 Xi TouTiao, You An Men Street, Beijing 100069, China
[1]Department of Functional Neurosurgery, Beijing Neurosurgical Institute, Capital Medical University, Beijing 100050, China

the proliferation, differentiation, migration, and invasion of glioma cells [6, 7]. However, the biological function of H19 in non-neoplastic CNS diseases including epilepsy remains unknown.

We previously showed by high-throughput microarray and bioinformatics analyses that H19 is upregulated in the latent period of TLE in rat and is involved in various aspects of epileptogenesis, including cell proliferation and immune and inflammatory responses [8]. We therefore speculated that H19 may be involved in hippocampal glial cell activation during epileptogenesis. This was investigated in the present study by gain- and loss-of-function studies in a rat model of TLE. We also examined the possible downstream targets of H19.

Methods
Animal and human samples
Male Sprague–Dawley rats weighing 200–220 g were obtained from Vital River Experimental Animal Technology Co. (Beijing, China) and were housed in a temperature-controlled room with free access to standard food and water under a 12:12-h light/dark cycle. Surgically resected hippocampus specimens were obtained from patients with intractable TLE who underwent surgical treatment at Beijing Tiantan Hospital. Control hippocampal tissue was obtained from autopsies of four patients without a history of epilepsy or other neurological diseases within 8 h after death.

H19 overexpression and knockdown
H19 was overexpressed or silencing using an adeno-associated viral (AAV) vector delivery system as previously described [8]. Briefly, a vector harboring H19 (AAV-H19) or a short hairpin RNA targeting H19 (AAV-shRNA) was constructed by Gene Chem Co. (Shanghai, China). The negative control was an empty AAV vector (AAV-NC) or one harboring a scrambled sequence (AAV-Scr: 5′-TTCTCCGAACGTGTCACGT-3′). The titers used were 1.0×10^{12} for AAV9-H19 and 4.0×10^{12} for AAV9-shRNA. A total of 6 µl AAV was infused into the right dorsal hippocampus (3.12 mm posterior to the bregma, 3.0 mm lateral to the midline, and 3.4 mm ventral to the bregma) and ventral hippocampus (5.04 mm posterior to the bregma, 5.0 mm lateral to the midline, and 6.4 mm ventral to the bregma; 3 µl at each location) [9] through a microsyringe at a speed of 0.2 µl/min.

Epilepsy model
A kainic acid (KA)-induced status epilepticus (SE) model was established by intra-amygdala microinjection of KA 14 days after AAV injection according to our previously described technique [8]. Briefly, the rats were placed in a stereotaxic apparatus (David Kopf Instruments, Tujunga,

CA, USA), and 0.7 µl KA (1 µg/µl; Sigma–Aldrich, St. Louis, MO, USA) was injected into the right amygdala (2.76 mm posterior to the bregma, 4.5 mm lateral to the midline, and 8.6 mm ventral to the bregma) [9] at a speed of 0.2 µl/min. Sham-operated controls were injected with an equal volume of saline.

Immunofluorescence analysis
Coronal sections (25 µm) were prepared at the level of the dorsal hippocampus (2.50–3.50 mm posterior to the bregma). Frozen sections were dried, washed, permeabilized, blocked in 5% goat serum, and incubated overnight with antibodies against neuronal nuclei (NeuN) (ab177487, 1:500 and ab104224, 1:200), glial fibrillary acidic protein (GFAP) (ab7260, 1:500), and OX42 (ab1211, 1:100) (all from Abcam, Cambridge, MA, USA). Immuno-labeled sections were washed and incubated with goat secondary antibodies conjugated with Alexa Fluor 594 or Alexa Fluor 488 (Merck Biosciences, Nottingham, UK). Sections were mounted with medium containing 4′,6-dia-midino-2-phenylin-dole (DAPI) (Vector Laboratories, Burlingame, CA, USA), and images were captured using an inverted fluorescence microscope (Olympus, Tokyo, Japan). GFAP+ or OX42+ cells were manually counted using ImageJ software (US National Institutes of Health, Bethesda, MD, USA).

Western blotting
Western blot analysis was performed as previously described [10] using the following primary antibodies: rabbit polyclonal anti-GFAP (ab7260, 1:1000), mouse monoclonal anti-OX42 (ab1211, 1:500), rabbit polyclonal anti-interleukin (IL)-1β (ab9722; 1:500), mouse monoclonal anti-IL-6 (ab9324; 1:500), rabbit polyclonal anti-tumor necrosis factor (TNF)-α (ab6671; 1:500), rabbit monoclonal anti-p-Stat3 (ab76315; 1:500), and rabbit polyclonal anti-c-Myc (ab39688; 1:500) (all from Abcam, Cambridge, MA, USA). Rabbit monoclonal anti-glyceraldehyde 3-phosphate dehydrogenase (GAPDH) antibody (Abcam, ab181602, 1:3000) was used as a control. Protein band density was quantified using an Epson V330 Photo scanner (Seiko Epson Co., Nagano, Japan) and Quantity One software (Bio-Rad, Hercules, CA, USA).

Statistical analysis
Data are presented as mean ± standard error of the mean. Two-group comparisons were made with the unpaired Student's t test, and multi-group comparisons were made by one-way analysis of variance followed by Sidak's multiple comparison tests using Prism 5 software (GraphPad Inc., San Diego, CA, USA). Significance was accepted at $P < 0.05$.

Results

Astrocytes and microglia are activated in the hippocampus of epileptic rats

We first examined GFAP and OX42 expression in the hippocampus of epileptic rats by immunofluorescence analysis to evaluate astrocyte and microglia activation, respectively. GFAP and OX42 immunoreactivity was detected in the ipsilateral hippocampus 7 days (latent period) (Figs. 2 and 3) or 30 days (chronic period) (Fig. 1) after KA-induced SE. The number of GFAP+ cells was increased, and activated astrocytes showed hypertrophy with a large cytoplasm and thick processes. The number of OX42+ cells was also increased, and the morphology of the activated microglia changed from spindle shape to oval with thickened processes. Fewer activated glial cells were observed in the contralateral as compared in the ipsilateral hippocampus (Fig. 1).

H19 is involved in the activation of astrocytes and microglia in the hippocampus of epileptic rats

Our previous study showed that H19 has diverse functions related to epileptogenesis [8] and is highly expressed in the seizure-free latent period of TLE. In the present study, we investigated the role of H19 in astrocyte and microglia activation by H19 overexpression and knockdown using an AAV delivery system [8]. Astrocyte and microglial activation were evaluated by GFAP and OX42 immunofluorescence and western blot analyses.

Compared to the sham group (NC + Veh or Scr + Veh), KA-induced SE (KA + Veh) or H19 overexpression (H19 + Veh) alone induced the activation of astrocytes or microglia in the stratum radiatum of the hippocampal CA3 region (Figs. 2 and 3). Moreover, more activated cells were observed in the hippocampus of rats overexpressing H19 at 7 days after SE (H19 + KA). The observed SE-induced activation of astrocytes and microglia was partly inhibited by H19 knockdown (ShRNA + KA vs Scr + KA). A quantitative analysis of GFAP and OX42 protein levels in the hippocampal CA3 region at 7 days (Figs. 2 and 3) and 60 days (Additional file 1: Figure S1) after SE confirmed these results.

We also examined proinflammatory cytokines released from the activated glia. H19 overexpression and KA-induced SE both stimulated the release of IL-1β and IL-6 and TNF-α in the CA3 subfield of the hippocampus (Fig. 4a). Cytokine release was further increased by H19 at 7 days after SE (Fig. 4a). H19 knockdown prevented the SE-induced increase in IL-1β and IL-6 and TNF-α levels (Fig. 4b). These results indicate that H19 plays an important role in astrocyte and microglia activation during epileptogenesis.

H19 induces astrocyte and microglia activation via JAK/STAT signaling

Stat3 plays a key role in astrocyte proliferation after central nervous system injury [11, 12] or SE [13]. We found

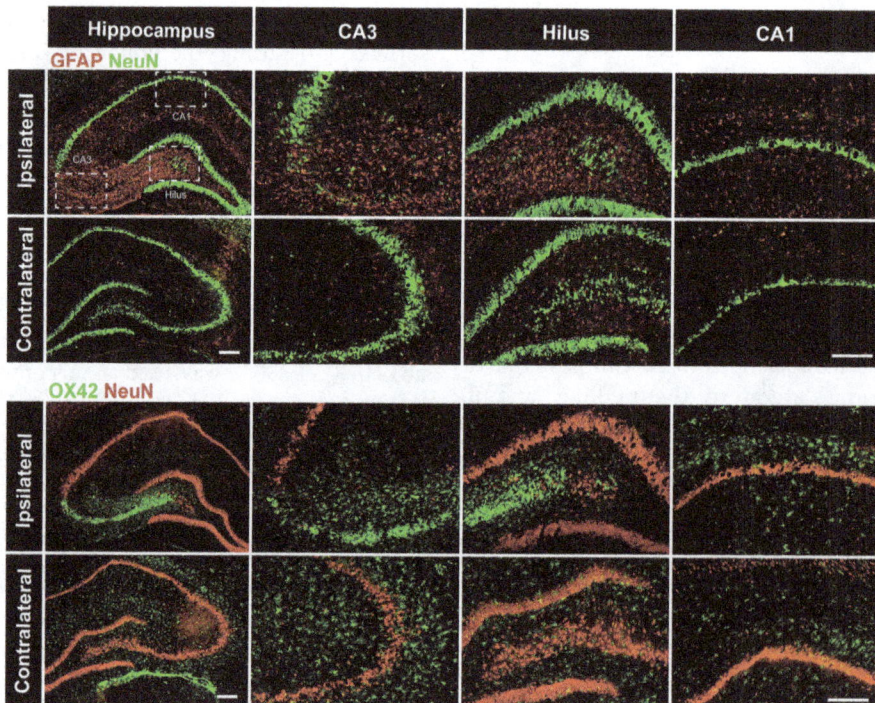

Fig. 1 Astrocytes and microglia are activated in the hippocampus of epileptic rats. Representative fluorescence micrographs of GFAP and OX42 expression in the hippocampus of rats 30 days after SE. High-magnification images correspond to the labeled boxes in the left panels. Scale bar = 200 μm

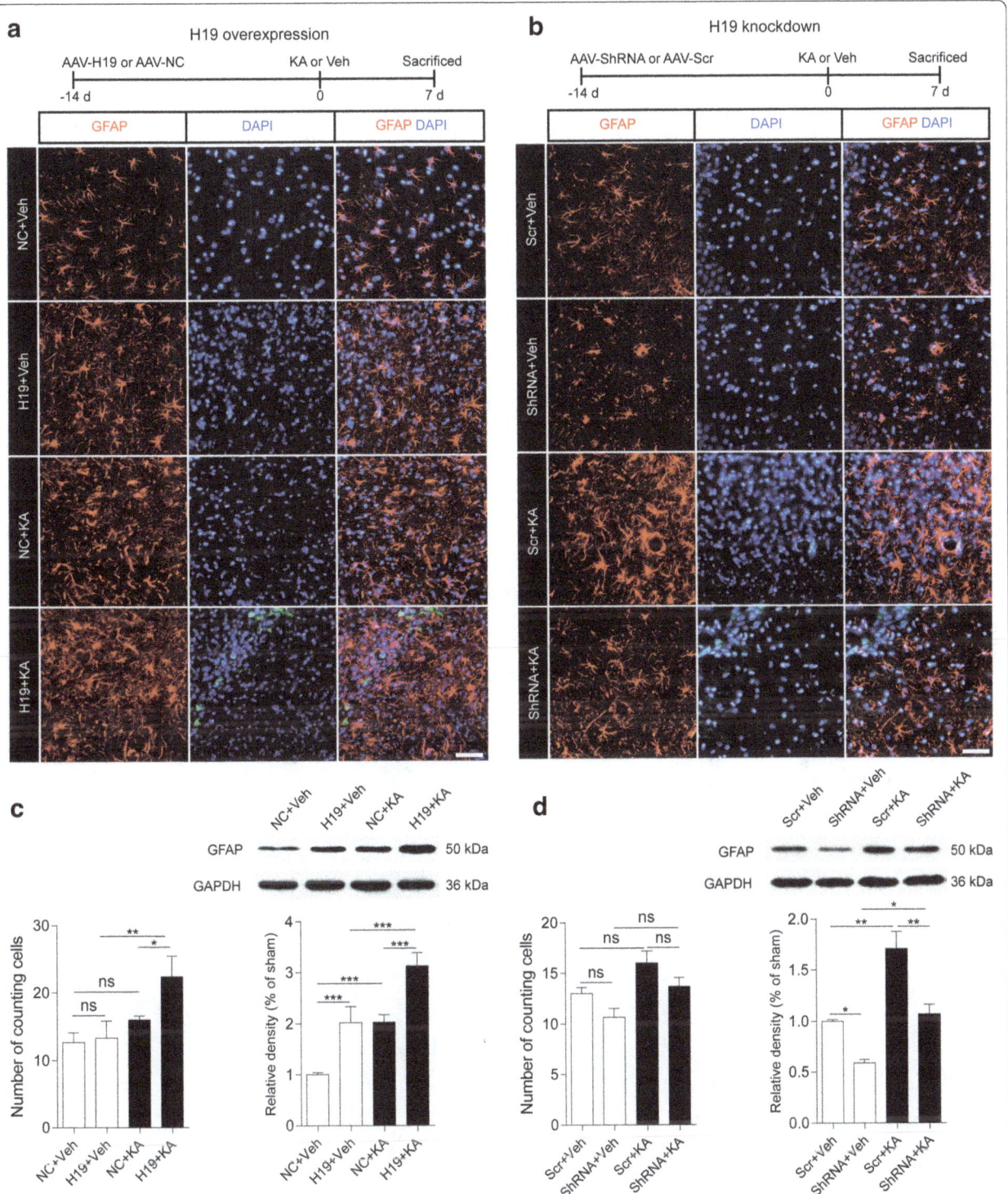

Fig. 2 H19 is involved in astrocyte activation in the hippocampus of epileptic rats. **a, b** Top: experimental timeline. Middle: representative fluorescence micrographs of GFAP expression in the hippocampus of H19 overexpression (**a**) and H19 knockdown (**b**) rats with or without KA treatment for 7 days. Scale bar = 50 μm. Bottom panels show counts of cells in the CA3 regions of the hippocampus ipsilateral to the KA injection side (*n* = 3). **c, d** Western blot analysis of GFAP protein levels in the CA3 subfield of the hippocampus of H19 overexpression (**c**) and H19 knockdown (**d**) rats with or without KA treatment for 7 days (*n* = 3–4). Protein bands were quantified by densitometry and normalized to the level of GAPDH. Data represent mean ± SEM. **P* < 0.05, ***P* < 0.01, ****P* < 0.001. NC rats injected with empty AAV vectors, Scr rats injected with scrambled AAV vectors, ShRNA rats injected with AAV vectors containing short hairpin RNA targeting H19

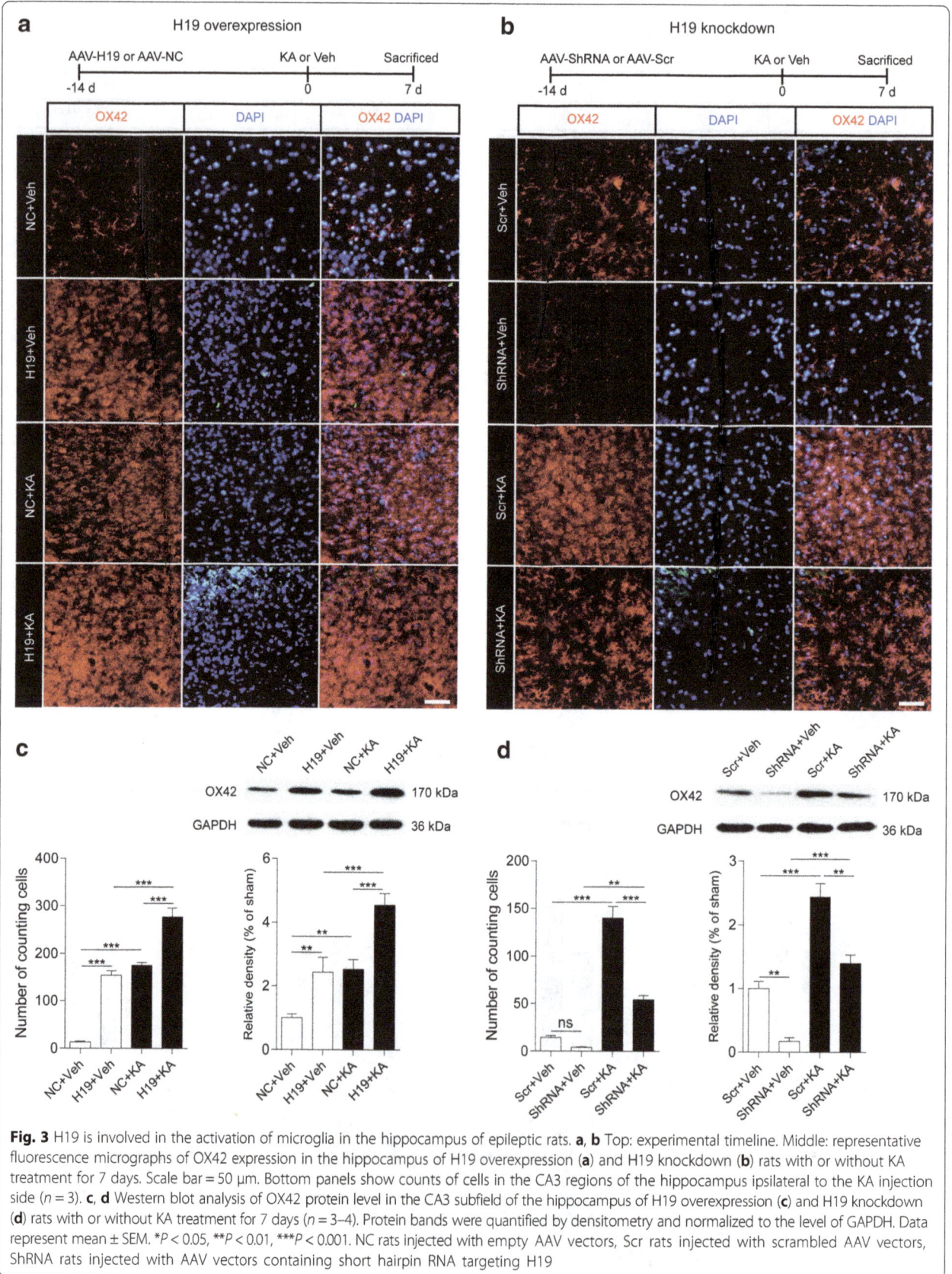

Fig. 3 H19 is involved in the activation of microglia in the hippocampus of epileptic rats. **a, b** Top: experimental timeline. Middle: representative fluorescence micrographs of OX42 expression in the hippocampus of H19 overexpression (**a**) and H19 knockdown (**b**) rats with or without KA treatment for 7 days. Scale bar = 50 μm. Bottom panels show counts of cells in the CA3 regions of the hippocampus ipsilateral to the KA injection side ($n = 3$). **c, d** Western blot analysis of OX42 protein level in the CA3 subfield of the hippocampus of H19 overexpression (**c**) and H19 knockdown (**d**) rats with or without KA treatment for 7 days ($n = 3$–4). Protein bands were quantified by densitometry and normalized to the level of GAPDH. Data represent mean ± SEM. *$P < 0.05$, **$P < 0.01$, ***$P < 0.001$. NC rats injected with empty AAV vectors, Scr rats injected with scrambled AAV vectors, ShRNA rats injected with AAV vectors containing short hairpin RNA targeting H19

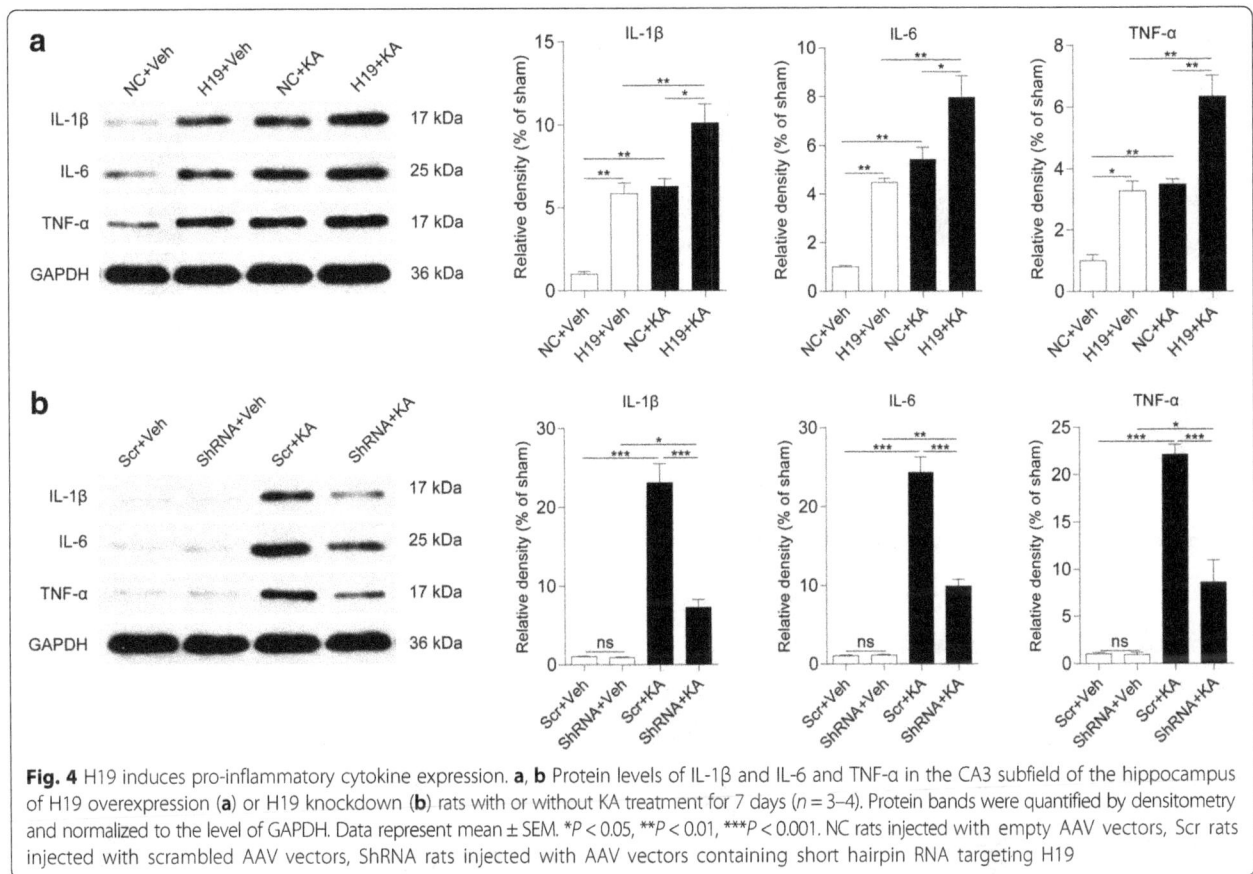

Fig. 4 H19 induces pro-inflammatory cytokine expression. **a, b** Protein levels of IL-1β and IL-6 and TNF-α in the CA3 subfield of the hippocampus of H19 overexpression (**a**) or H19 knockdown (**b**) rats with or without KA treatment for 7 days ($n = 3–4$). Protein bands were quantified by densitometry and normalized to the level of GAPDH. Data represent mean ± SEM. *$P < 0.05$, **$P < 0.01$, ***$P < 0.001$. NC rats injected with empty AAV vectors, Scr rats injected with scrambled AAV vectors, ShRNA rats injected with AAV vectors containing short hairpin RNA targeting H19

here that the levels of phosphorylated Stat3 (p-Stat3) and its downstream effector c-Myc were upregulated in hippocampal tissue samples from patients with TLE (Fig. 5a) and from rats 7 days after SE (Fig. 5b) relative to the respective control samples, as determined with western blotting, suggesting that Janus kinase (JAK)/signal transducer and activator of transcription (STAT) signaling is involved in the activation of glial cells after SE. H19 overexpression alone increased p-Stat3 and c-Myc protein levels in the CA3 subfield of the hippocampus (Fig. 5c). H19 exacerbated these protein expressions in the rats at 7 days (Fig. 5c) and 60 days (Additional file 2: Figure S2A) after SE. On the contrary, H19 knockdown abolished the SE-induced increase in p-Stat3 and c-Myc in rats at 7 days (Fig. 5d) and 60 days (Additional file 2: Figure S2B) after SE. These results indicate that H19 promotes astrocyte and microglial activation via the JAK/STAT signaling pathway.

Discussion

Most previous studies on H19 function focused on tumorigenesis. H19 was initially proposed as a tumor suppressor due to its capacity to suppress clonogenicity and tumorigenicity in tumor cells [14, 15]. However,

recent studies showed that H19 acts as an oncogene by promoting cell proliferation, migration, invasion, and metastasis in various malignancies including glioblastoma [16–18]. Apart from these functions, H19 is also implicated in several other physiological conditions or diseases, such as cartilage degeneration in osteoarthritis [19], skeletal muscle differentiation and regeneration [20], and glucose metabolism in muscle cells [21]. However, the role of H19 in non-neoplastic CNS diseases including epilepsy remains unclear. In the present study, we provide the first evidence that H19 promotes glial cell activation and stimulates inflammation in the hippocampus of rats with TLE.

Astrocyte activation is a continuum that includes changes in molecular expression, progressive cellular hypertrophy, and, in severe cases, proliferation and scar formation [22]. In mild or moderate astrocyte activation, GFAP expression is slightly upregulated and the cell body and processes undergo hypertrophy, with little or no astrocyte proliferation. However, in severe diffuse reactive astrogliosis, GFAP expression is markedly increased, which is accompanied by extensive hypertrophy of the cell body and processes and astrocyte proliferation [23]. In the present study, astrocytes in the hippocampus of epileptic rats were activated in the latent and chronic

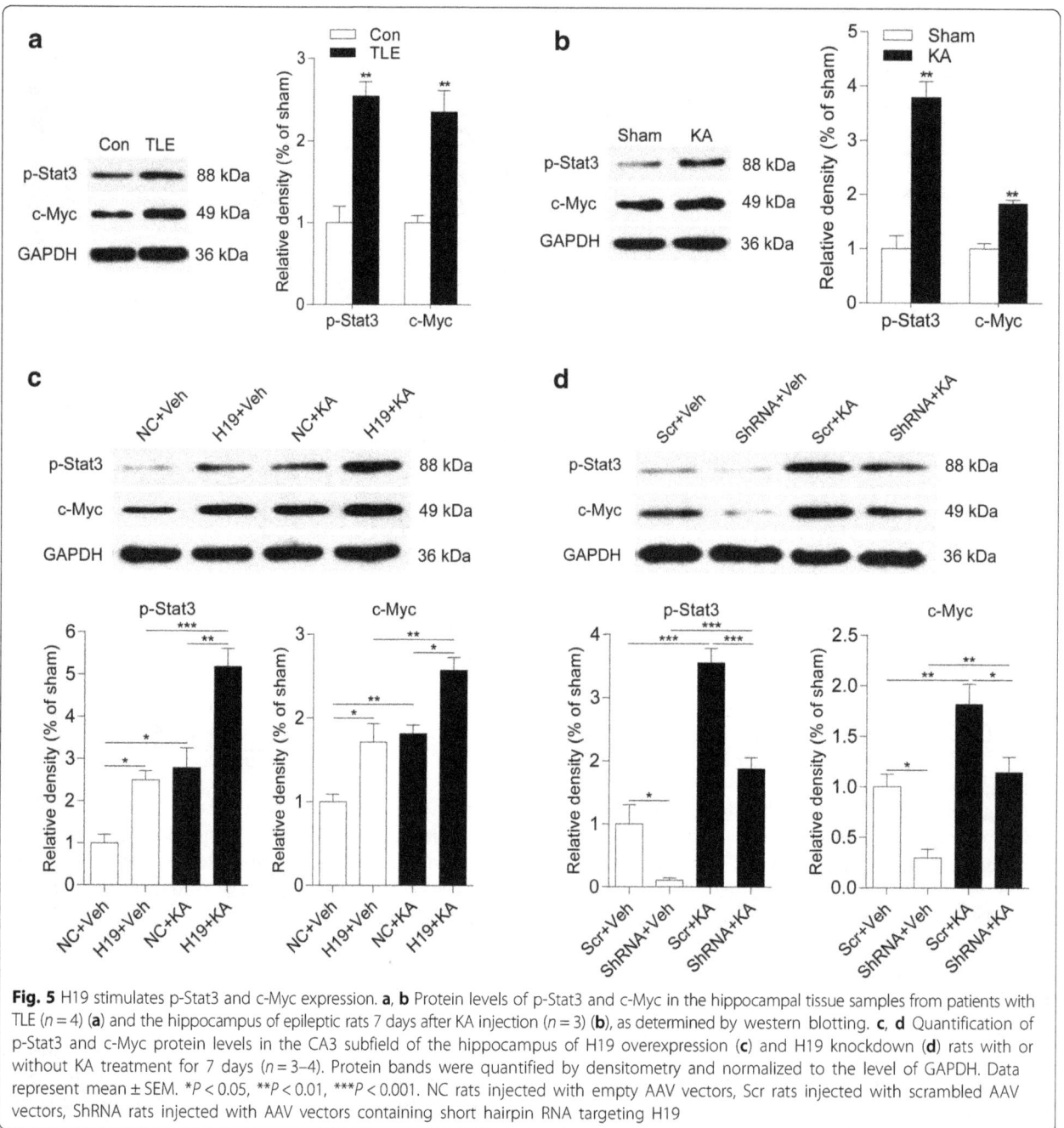

Fig. 5 H19 stimulates p-Stat3 and c-Myc expression. **a, b** Protein levels of p-Stat3 and c-Myc in the hippocampal tissue samples from patients with TLE ($n = 4$) (**a**) and the hippocampus of epileptic rats 7 days after KA injection ($n = 3$) (**b**), as determined by western blotting. **c, d** Quantification of p-Stat3 and c-Myc protein levels in the CA3 subfield of the hippocampus of H19 overexpression (**c**) and H19 knockdown (**d**) rats with or without KA treatment for 7 days ($n = 3$–4). Protein bands were quantified by densitometry and normalized to the level of GAPDH. Data represent mean ± SEM. *$P < 0.05$, **$P < 0.01$, ***$P < 0.001$. NC rats injected with empty AAV vectors, Scr rats injected with scrambled AAV vectors, ShRNA rats injected with AAV vectors containing short hairpin RNA targeting H19

phases of TLE, which is consistent with previous reports [13, 24]. Mild to moderate gliosis, which typically does not cause astrocyte proliferation, is usually observed in the early stages after SE [25]. We also found that astrocyte activation was mild or moderate, as evidenced by the upregulation of GFAP expression and cellular hypertrophy without an obvious increase in cell number in the latent period of TLE (7 days after SE). Furthermore, H19 induced an increase in GFAP expression and hypertrophy of astrocytes rather than cell proliferation in the latent period of SE. In the chronic period (30 days after

SE), astrocyte activation was extreme with severe hypertrophy of the cell body and processes; moreover, astrocyte proliferation in areas of pyramidal neuron loss was comparable to the hippocampal sclerosis observed in TLE patients [26]. Unlike astrocytes, high expression of OX42 protein and cellular hypertrophy as well as proliferation of microglia was observed in both the latent and chronic periods of TLE, as previously reported [27]. Furthermore, H19 induced the upregulation of OX42 and cellular hypertrophy and increased the number of microglia in the latent period of SE. Recent studies have shown that inflammatory cytokines are produced both by microglia and astrocytes [28]; the increased levels of proinflammatory cytokines in epileptic rats observed here is in agreement with these findings. Moreover, H19 stimulated the release of proinflammatory cytokines. However, compared to sham rats, H19 knockdown did not inhibit proinflammatory cytokine expression, possibly because under normal conditions, proinflammatory cytokine levels in the hippocampus are too low to result in an observable difference upon H19 knockdown.

Molecular triggers that lead to glial cell activation and proliferation have not been fully characterized. There is increasing evidence to suggest that H19 has a growth-promoting function, since it enhances cell proliferation in tumors [29, 30] and other diseases [20, 31]. In the present study, we showed that H19 promotes astrocyte and microglia activation and proliferation under both epileptic and normal conditions. This is consistent with earlier reports as well as with our previous research [8]. Various intracellular signaling pathways associated with Stat3, nuclear factor κB, and nuclear respiratory factor (Nrf) mediate cell hypertrophy, proliferation, and pro- or anti-inflammatory effects in astrocytes [23]. The transcription factor Stat3, a key component of the JAK/STAT pathway, is important for astrocyte proliferation in CNS diseases [11, 32, 33]. P-Stat3 is highly expressed in the rat hippocampus during different phases of epilepsy and in the temporal lobe of TLE patients [13]. Astrocyte activation can be suppressed by inhibiting JAK/STAT signaling, indicating that Stat3 activation induces GFAP expression [13]. In our study, Stat3 as well as its downstream effector c-Myc in the JAK/STAT pathway were upregulated after SE in the rat hippocampus and in TLE patients. Furthermore, H19 overexpression induced whereas its knockdown inhibited Stat3 and c-Myc protein expression in both normal and epileptic rats. Thus, H19 can itself promote gliosis via JAK/STAT signaling in addition to its role in astrocyte activation.

Conclusions

In summary, lncRNA H19 contributes to the activation of hippocampal astrocytes and microglia, as well as to the inflammatory response in epileptic rats. Furthermore, H19 may promote glial cell activation through the JAK/STAT pathway. Our findings reveal a novel lncRNA H19-mediated mechanism in seizure-induced glial cell activation and provide a basis for developing lncRNA-based strategies to prevent the development of epilepsy.

Additional files

Additional file 1: H19 promotes GFAP and OX42 expression. (a, b) Western blot analysis of GFAP and OX42 protein levels in the CA3 subfield of the hippocampus of H19 overexpression (a) or H19 knockdown (b) rats with or without KA treatment for 60 days ($n = 3$–4). Protein bands were quantified by densitometry and normalized to GAPDH level. Data represent mean ± SEM. *$P < 0.05$, **$P < 0.01$, ***$P < 0.001$. NC, rats injected with empty AAV vectors; Scr, rats injected with scrambled AAV vectors; ShRNA, rats injected with AAV vectors containing short hairpin RNA targeting H19.

Additional file 2: H19 promotes p-Stat3 and c-Myc expression. (a, b) Western blot analysis of p-Stat3 and c-Myc protein levels in the CA3 subfield of hippocampus of H19 overexpression (a) or H19 knockdown (b) rats with or without KA treatment for 60 days ($n = 3$–4). Protein bands were quantified by densitometry and normalized to GAPDH level. Data represent mean ± SEM. *$P < 0.05$, **$P < 0.01$, ***$P < 0.001$. NC, rats injected with empty AAV vectors; Scr, rats injected with scrambled AAV vectors; ShRNA, rats injected with AAV vectors containing short hairpin RNA targeting H19.

Abbreviations

AAV: Adeno-associated viral; CNS: Central nervous system; DAPI: 4′,6-diamidino-2-phenylin-dole; GAPDH: Glyceraldehyde 3-phosphate dehydrogenase; GFAP: Glial fibrillary acidic protein; IL: Interleukin; JAK: Janus kinase; KA: Kainic acid; lncRNA: Long non-coding RNA; NC: Negative control; NeuN: Neuronal nuclei; Nrf: Nuclear respiratory factor; p-Stat3: Phosphorylated Stat3; SE: Status epilepticus; shRNA: Short hairpin RNA; STAT: Signal transducer and activator of transcription; TLE: Temporal lobe epilepsy; TNF: Tumor necrosis factor

Acknowledgements
Not applicable

Funding
This study was supported by the National Natural Science Foundation of China (81471315).

Authors' contributions

CLH performed the experiments and drafted the manuscript. MG analyzed the data. YPL and XMZ established the epilepsy model. KLW performed the intro-hippocampus AAV vector injection. NC performed the immunofluorescence image analysis. WH contributed to the experimental design. WJM performed the animal experiment of AG 490. JGZ assisted with the experiment design and collected the hippocampal samples from patients with TLE. LL designed the study and revised the manuscript. FGM designed and guided the experiment. All authors have read and approved the final version of the manuscript.

Consent for publication
Not applicable

Competing interests
The authors declare that they have no competing interests.

Author details
[1]Department of Functional Neurosurgery, Beijing Neurosurgical Institute, Capital Medical University, Beijing 100050, China. [2]Beijing Key Laboratory of Neuromodulation, Beijing Municipal Science and Technology Commission, Beijing 100050, China. [3]Department of Neurosurgery, Beijing Children's Hospital, Capital Medical University, Beijing 100045, China. [4]Department of Neurosurgery, Beijing Tiantan Hospital, Capital Medical University, Beijing 100050, China. [5]The Third Division of Clinical Medicine, China Medical University, Shenyang 110122, Liaoning Province, China. [6]Department of Neurology, University of Florida, Gainesville, Florida 32607, USA. [7]Department of Pathology, School of Basic Medical Sciences, Capital Medical University, No. 10 Xi TouTiao, You An Men Street, Beijing 100069, China.

References

1. Seifert G, Carmignoto G, Steinhauser C. Astrocyte dysfunction in epilepsy. Brain Res Rev. 2010;63:212–21.

2. Perea G, Navarrete M, Araque A. Tripartite synapses: astrocytes process and control synaptic information. Trends Neurosci. 2009;32:421–31.

3. Halassa MM, Haydon PG. Integrated brain circuits: astrocytic networks modulate neuronal activity and behavior. Annu Rev Physiol. 2010;72:335.

4. Pachnis V, Belayew A, Tilghman SM. Locus unlinked to alpha-fetoprotein under the control of the murine raf and Rif genes. Proc Natl Acad Sci U S A. 1984;81:5523–7.

5. Liang WC, Fu WM, Wong CW, Wang Y, Wang WM, Hu GX, Zhang L, Xiao LJ, Wan DC, Zhang JF, Waye MM. The lncRNA H19 promotes epithelial to mesenchymal transition by functioning as miRNA sponges in colorectal cancer. Oncotarget. 2015;6:22513–25.

6. Jiang X, Yan Y, Hu M, Chen X, Wang Y, Dai Y, Wu D, Wang Y, Zhuang Z, Xia H. Increased level of H19 long noncoding RNA promotes invasion, angiogenesis, and stemness of glioblastoma cells. J Neurosurg. 2016;124:129–36.

7. Jia P, Cai H, Liu X, Chen J, Ma J, Wang P, Liu Y, Zheng J, Xue Y. Long non-coding RNA H19 regulates glioma angiogenesis and the biological behavior of glioma-associated endothelial cells by inhibiting microRNA-29a. Cancer Lett. 2016;381:359–69.

8. Han CL, Liu YP, Zhao XM, Wang KL, Chen N, Hu W, Zhang JG, Ge M, Meng FG. Whole-transcriptome screening reveals the regulatory targets and functions of long non-coding RNA H19 in epileptic rats. Biochem Biophys Res Commun. 2017;489:262–9.

9. Paxinos G, Watson C. The rat brain in stereotaxic coordinates. 5th ed. San Diego: Elsevier Academic Press; 2005.

10. Wu X, Sun J, Zhang X, Li X, Liu Z, Yang Q, Li L. Epigenetic signature of chronic cerebral hypoperfusion and beneficial effects of S-adenosylmethionine in rats. Mol Neurobiol. 2014;50:839–51.

11. Herrmann JE, Imura T, Song B, Qi J, Ao Y, Nguyen TK, Korsak RA, Takeda K, Akira S, Sofroniew MV. STAT3 is a critical regulator of astrogliosis and scar formation after spinal cord injury. J Neurosci. 2008;28:7231–43.

12. Tsuda M, Kohro Y, Yano T, Tsujikawa T, Kitano J, Tozaki-Saitoh H, Koyanagi S, Ohdo S, Ji RR, Salter MW, Inoue K. JAK-STAT3 pathway regulates spinal astrocyte proliferation and neuropathic pain maintenance in rats. Brain. 2011;134:1127–39.

13. Xu Z, Xue T, Zhang Z, Wang X, Xu P, Zhang J, Lei X, Li Y, Xie Y, Wang L, et al. Role of signal transducer and activator of transcription-3 in up-regulation of GFAP after epilepsy. Neurochem Res. 2011;36:2208–15.

14. Hao Y, Crenshaw T, Moulton T, Newcomb E, Tycko B. Tumour-suppressor activity of H19 RNA. Nature. 1993;365:764–7.

15. Yoshimizu T, Miroglio A, Ripoche MA, Gabory A, Vernucci M, Riccio A, Colnot S, Godard C, Terris B, Jammes H, Dandolo L. The H19 locus acts in vivo as a tumor suppressor. Proc Natl Acad Sci U S A. 2008;105:12417–22.

16. Yan L, Zhou J, Gao Y, Ghazal S, Lu L, Bellone S, Yang Y, Liu N, Zhao X, Santin AD, et al. Regulation of tumor cell migration and invasion by the H19/let-7 axis is antagonized by metformin-induced DNA methylation. Oncogene. 2015;34:3076–84.

17. Shi Y, Wang Y, Luan W, Wang P, Tao T, Zhang J, Qian J, Liu N, You Y. Long non-coding RNA H19 promotes glioma cell invasion by deriving miR-675. PLoS One. 2014;9:e86295.

18. Matouk IJ, DeGroot N, Mezan S, Ayesh S, Abu-lail R, Hochberg A, Galun E. The H19 non-coding RNA is essential for human tumor growth. PLoS One. 2007;2:e845.

19. Steck E, Boeuf S, Gabler J, Werth N, Schnatzer P, Diederichs S, Richter W. Regulation of H19 and its encoded microRNA-675 in osteoarthritis and under anabolic and catabolic in vitro conditions. J Mol Med (Berl). 2012;90:1185–95.

20. Dey BK, Pfeifer K, Dutta A. The H19 long noncoding RNA gives rise to microRNAs miR-675-3p and miR-675-5p to promote skeletal muscle differentiation and regeneration. Genes Dev. 2014;28:491–501.

21. Gao Y, Wu F, Zhou J, Yan L, Jurczak MJ, Lee HY, Yang L, Mueller M, Zhou XB, Dandolo L, et al. The H19/let-7 double-negative feedback loop contributes to glucose metabolism in muscle cells. Nucleic Acids Res. 2014;42:13799–811.

22. Sofroniew MV, Vinters HV. Astrocytes: biology and pathology. Acta Neuropathol. 2010;119:7–35.

23. Sofroniew MV. Molecular dissection of reactive astrogliosis and glial scar formation. Trends Neurosci. 2009;32:638–47.

24. Shapiro LA, Wang L, Ribak CE. Rapid astrocyte and microglial activation following pilocarpine-induced seizures in rats. Epilepsia. 2008;49(Suppl 2):33–41.

25. Gibbons MB, Smeal RM, Takahashi DK, Vargas JR, Wilcox KS. Contributions of astrocytes to epileptogenesis following status epilepticus: opportunities for preventive therapy? Neurochem Int. 2013;63:660–9.

26. Thom M. Review: hippocampal sclerosis in epilepsy: a neuropathology review. Neuropathol Appl Neurobiol. 2014;40:520–43.

27. Avignone E, Ulmann L, Levavasseur F, Rassendren F, Audinat E. Status epilepticus induces a particular microglial activation state characterized by enhanced purinergic signaling. J Neurosci. 2008;28:9133–44.

28. Rizzi M, Perego C, Aliprandi M, Richichi C, Ravizza T, Colella D, Veliskova J, Moshe SL, De Simoni MG, Vezzani A. Glia activation and cytokine increase in rat hippocampus by kainic acid-induced status epilepticus during postnatal development. Neurobiol Dis. 2003;14:494–503.

29. Tan D, Wu Y, Hu L, He P, Xiong G, Bai Y, Yang K. Long noncoding RNA H19 is up-regulated in esophageal squamous cell carcinoma and promotes cell proliferation and metastasis. Dis Esophagus. 2017;30:1–9.

30. lempridee T. Long non-coding RNA H19 enhances cell proliferation and anchorage-independent growth of cervical cancer cell lines. Exp Biol Med (Maywood). 2017;242:184–93.

31. Xu X, Ji S, Li W, Yi B, Li H, Zhang H, Ma W. LncRNA H19 promotes the differentiation of bovine skeletal muscle satellite cells by suppressing Sirt1/FoxO1. Cell Mol Biol Lett. 2017;22:10.

32. Satriotomo I, Bowen KK, Vemuganti R. JAK2 and STAT3 activation contributes to neuronal damage following transient focal cerebral ischemia. J Neurochem. 2006;98:1353–68.

33. Ben Haim L, Ceyzeriat K, Carrillo-de Sauvage MA, Aubry F, Auregan G, Guillermier M, Ruiz M, Petit F, Houitte D, Faivre E, et al. The JAK/STAT3 pathway is a common inducer of astrocyte reactivity in Alzheimer's and Huntington's diseases. J Neurosci. 2015;35:2817–29.

Monocyte chemoattractant protein-1 affects migration of hippocampal neural progenitors following status epilepticus in rats

Yu-Wen Hung[1,5], Ming-Tsong Lai[2,5], Yi-Jhan Tseng[1,5], Chien-Chen Chou[2,5] and Yung-Yang Lin[1,2,3,4,5,6*]

Abstract

Background: Epilepsy is a common brain disorder characterized by a chronic predisposition to generate spontaneous seizures. The mechanisms for epilepsy formation remain unknown. A growing body of evidence suggests the involvement of inflammatory processes in epileptogenesis. In the present study, we investigated the involvement of monocyte chemoattractant protein-1 (MCP-1) in aberrant migration of hippocampal progenitors in rats after the insult of status epilepticus (SE).

Methods: SE was induced with pilocarpine in Sprague–Dawley rats. Transcriptional expression of MCP-1 in the dentate gyrus (DG) was measured using quantitative real-time PCR. From 1 to 28 days after SE, the temporal profiles of MCP-1 protein expression in DG were evaluated using enzyme-linked immunosorbent assay. Chemokine (C-C motif) receptor 2 (CCR2) expression in doublecortin-positive neuronal progenitors was examined using double-labeling immunohistochemistry. The involvement of MCP-1/CCR2 signaling in aberrant neuronal progenitor migration in the epileptic hippocampus was assessed in the SE rats using a CCR2 antagonist, RS102895, and the ectopic migration of neuronal progenitors was determined using Prox1/doublecortin double immunostaining.

Results: After SE, MCP-1 gene was significantly upregulated and its corresponding protein expression in the DG was significantly increased on days 1 and 3. Some hilar ectopic progenitor cells of SE rats expressed the MCP-1 receptor, CCR2. Notably, the ectopic migration of neuronal progenitors into hilus was attenuated by a blockade of the MCP-1/CCR2 interaction with a selective CCR2 inhibitor, RS102895.

Conclusions: An increase in dentate MCP-1 is associated with seizure-induced aberrant migration of neuronal progenitors through the interaction with CCR2. The upregulation of MCP-1 after an insult of SE may play a role in the generation of epilepsy.

Keywords: Chemokine (C-C motif) receptor 2 (CCR2), Dentate gyrus, Epileptogenesis, Monocyte chemoattractant protein-1 (MCP-1), Neuroinflammation, Neuronal progenitor migration, Pilocarpine-induced status epilepticus, Rats

Background

Mesial temporal lobe epilepsy (MTLE) is a common type of epilepsy; more than half of patients with MTLE continue to experience seizures despite intensive medical treatment [1]. In some MTLE patients, a medical history-taking reveals an early precipitating brain insult and a following seizure-free latent period before the

occurrence of unprovoked recurrent seizures in later childhood or adolescence. Epileptogenic insults may induce molecular and pathophysiological alterations in the hippocampus, including selective neuronal loss in the CA1, CA3 and dentate hilus, dentate neurogenesis, synaptic reorganization, gliosis and inflammatory responses [2-5]. These structural and functional changes in the hippocampal formation are potentially involved in the development of MTLE [2,3,6]. According to previous pathological studies in MTLE, the neuroplastic changes in the hippocampal dentate gyrus (DG) are important for local hyperexcitability and subsequent development

* Correspondence: yylin@vghtpe.gov.tw
[1]Institute of Physiology, National Yang-Ming University, No.155, Sec. 2, Linong Street, Taipei 112, Taiwan
[2]Institute of Brain Science, National Yang-Ming University, No.155, Sec. 2, Linong Street, Taipei 112, Taiwan

of epilepsy [6]. However, the exact mechanisms underlying the epileptogenic structure alterations remain unclear.

Previous studies in experimental animals and human patients [5] have suggested a potential contribution of inflammatory process to seizure-related pathologies and the induction of epilepsy [7,8]. Seizures may trigger significant inflammatory responses, including activation of glial cells and secretion of inflammatory mediators by microglia, astrocytes and affected neurons [5]. Pathological alterations in animal models of epilepsy, such as neuronal cell death, reactive gliosis and neuroplastic changes, might be associated with these neuroinflammatory responses [9]. Therefore, neuroinflammation may participate in epileptogenesis [5,7-9].

Several chemokines and chemokine receptors expressed in normal brain participate in various physiological processes, including the regulation of neuronal development and migration, synaptic activity and cellular communication [10,11]. These molecules can be up-regulated in response to inflammatory brain insults [11-13]. The chemokine monocyte chemoattractant protein-1 (MCP-1) is increased in patients with intractable epilepsy, suggesting its possible involvement in the pathogenesis of epilepsy [14-16]. In animal studies, MCP-1 expression in the hippocampus was up-regulated after acute seizures [17,18]. MCP-1, one of the most commonly expressed chemokines in the inflamed brain [19], belongs to a member of the cysteine-cysteine (CC) chemokine gene family. Members of this gene family attract monocytes and activate T cells and B cells through their interaction with the seven-transmembrane domain, G protein-coupled receptors chemokine (C-C motif) receptor 2 (CCR2) or CCR9 [20]. Elevated MCP-1 expression in the inflamed brain is related to the activation and recruitment of macrophages/microglia and granulocytes near the site of injury [18] and is also related to the breakdown of the blood-brain barrier [19,21]. Accordingly, MCP-1 in the epileptic brain might participate in the inflammation-related epileptogenesis of MTLE.

In addition to involving inflammatory response, MCP-1 may enhance the migration of adult neural progenitors *in vitro* [22,23]. MCP-1 may induce neural progenitor migration from the subventricular zone toward the damaged brain regions after focal ischemia, since expression of MCP-1 receptor CCR2 has been identified in the migrating neuroblasts [23]. Also, MCP-1 is important in attracting neural progenitors toward sites of neuroinflammation in the hippocampus [13,24]. Thus, MCP-1 is a potential regulator of neuronal progenitor migration in response to brain insults [23]. In the epileptic hippocampus, ectopic granule cells derived from newborn neurons were observed in the dentate hilus following seizure activity [25,26]. The aberrant migration of neuronal progenitors may contribute to the formation of epileptic

neuronal circuits and hyperexcitability in the hippocampus [25-27]. In response to these findings, we hypothesized that MCP-1 participates in epileptogenesis through its attraction of neural progenitors in the subgranular zone (SGZ) to form hilar ectopic granule cells.

To study the pro-epileptogenic role of MCP-1 in the seizure-induced aberrant reorganization of the dentate hilus, we evaluated the temporal profiles of MCP-1 expression in the DG after pilocarpine-induced status epilepticus (SE) and determined whether MCP-1 enhances the migration of adult neural progenitors towards ectopic locations.

Methods
Animals
Adult male Sprague-Dawley rats weighing 200 to 350 g were housed in a controlled environment (lights on from 8:00 A.M. to 8:00 P.M.) and given free access to food and water. Animal protocols were approved by the Taipei Veterans General Hospital Institutional Animal Care and Use Committee (Permit Number: 97-100), Taipei, Taiwan, and conformed to the National Institutes of Health (NIH) Guidelines of USA for the care and use of laboratory animals.

Pilocarpine-induced status epilepticus
In order to assess MCP-1 gene expression profiles of hippocampal DG in response to a SE insult, pilocarpine hydrochloride (325 mg/kg; Sigma, St. Louis, MO, USA) was intraperitoneally (i.p.) administered in 6 rats, while normal saline of the same volume was i.p. injected in 7 control rats. In a separate experiment for the analysis of protein and histopathological alterations, rats were pretreated with scopolamine methylnitrate (1 mg/kg, i.p.; Sigma) to reduce peripheral cholinergic side effects [28]. Thirty minutes later, pilocarpine hydrochloride was given to induce SE. In age-matched control rats, pilocarpine was replaced with normal saline. Animal behavior was monitored, and only the rats exhibiting convulsive SE at stage 5 of Racine's scale were enrolled for subsequent experimental manipulations [25]. Two hours after SE onset, rats were treated with diazepam (10 mg/kg, i.p.; China Chemical & Pharmaceutical Co., Ltd., Taipei, Taiwan) to terminate seizures.

Administration of RS102895, an antagonist of CCR2b
As a potent and specific antagonist of CCR2b, RS102895 (Tocris Bioscience, Ellisville, MO, USA) can inhibit MCP-1/CCR2 signaling in rodents [29,30]. One day after SE induction, SE rats were subcutaneously treated with 10 mg/kg of RS102895 (in a solution of 10% dimethyl sulfoxide (DMSO; Sigma) and 90% normal saline) for 3 days. Then the dose of RS102895 was 5 mg/kg for subsequent days until one day prior to sacrifice.

Preparation of the DG

Animals were deeply anesthetized via isoflurane inhalation (AErrane, Baxter, Guayama, PR, USA) and decapitated. The brain was quickly removed from the skull and placed into ice-cold phosphate-buffered saline (PBS). Hippocampal DG tissue was carefully dissected out from each cerebral hemisphere by sliding 30-gauge needles superficially along the boundaries of the DG and Ammon's horn within the hippocampus [31]. The left or right DG was chosen at random for total RNA isolation and protein extraction.

RNA isolation and quantitative real-time reverse transcriptase PCR (qRT-PCR)

To obtain hippocampal dentate RNA for qRT-PCR, SE rats were sacrificed 30 min after diazepam injection. Total RNA was isolated using TRIzol reagent (Invitrogen, Carlsbad, CA, USA) according to the manufacturer's instructions. The integrity of each RNA sample was confirmed using agarose gel electrophoresis and an Agilent 2100 Bioanalyzer (Agilent Technologies, Santa Clara, CA, USA).

qRT-PCR was performed in triplicate to validate the expression of MCP-1 [32]. First, total RNA was reverse-transcribed into cDNA. A 20 μL reaction volume containing 2.5 μg of total RNA was used in the first-strand cDNA synthesis reaction. Oligo dT (0.5 μg) and dNTP mix (1 μL, 10 mM) were added to total RNA. The mixture was heated to 65°C for 5 min and quickly chilled on ice for 2 min. Then, 5× first-strand buffer (5 μL), dTT (1 μL) and SuperScript III reverse transcriptase (1 μL, 200U, Invitrogen) were added to the reverse transcription reaction mixture. Following incubation of the mixture at 42°C for 60 min and then 70°C for 15 min, first-strand cDNA was generated. Next, qRT-PCR was carried out using the SYBR Green chemistry for amplicon detection on the LightCycler 480 Real-Time PCR System (Roche Applied Science, Indianapolis, IN, USA). Each sample for qRT-PCR contained the following: 10 μL 2× FastStart Universal Probe Master (Roche Applied Science), 1 μL primers for MCP-1 (forward: TGAACTT GACCCATAAATCTGAAG, reverse: AAGGCATCACA TTCCAAATCAC) and for GAPDH (forward: CTCCCA TTCTTCCACCTTTG, reverse: CTTGCTCTCAGTATC CTTGC), and 1 μL cDNA. The final volume was adjusted to 20 μL with the addition of H_2O. Temperature cycling was performed as follows: 3 min polymerase activation at 95°C followed by 45 cycles of denaturation at 95°C for 30 sec, annealing at 55°C for 30 sec and extension at 72°C for 30 sec. The fluorescence signal was read during the extension step of each cycle. To distinguish between the specific and non-specific products and primer dimers, melting curves were obtained by ramping the temperature 1°C every second from 55°C to 95°C after PCR amplification.

The relative fold change of gene expression was calculated by the value of $2^{\wedge}\Delta C_T$ (compared to the control group) and normalized to the expression of the housekeeping gene GAPDH.

Detection of MCP-1 protein in the DG by enzyme-linked immunosorbent assay (ELISA)

DG tissue was dissected at 1, 3, 7, 14 and 28 days after SE in SE rats (n = 6 per time points) and at 1 day after saline treatment in control rats (n = 6). Total protein was extracted using T-PER tissue protein extraction reagent (Pierce Biotechnology, Inc., Rockford, IL, USA) containing EDTA-free Complete protease inhibitors (Roche Applied Science), according to the manufacturer's recommendations. Total protein concentration was determined using the Bio-Rad protein assay kit (Bio-Rad, Hercules, CA, USA). MCP-1 protein concentration from each sample was evaluated using the BD OptEIA Rat MCP-1 ELISA kit (BD Biosciences Pharmingen, San Diego, CA, USA), according to the manufacturer's instructions, and then normalized to the total protein content. The data of MCP-1 protein concentration were presented as pg/μg of total protein.

Tissue preparation and immunohistochemistry

Rats were deeply anesthetized with Zoletil 50 anesthesia (10 mg/kg, i.p.; Virbac Laboratories, Carros, France) and perfused transcardially with ice-cold normal saline, followed by 4% paraformaldehyde in PBS (10 mM, pH 7.4). Brain tissue was removed immediately after perfusion, post-fixed in 4% paraformaldehyde overnight at 4°C and cryoprotected with 30% (w/v) sucrose in PBS. Coronal sections (40 μm) through the dorsal hippocampus (AP = –1.8 to –6.12 mm) were prepared using a freezing microtome (CM1900, Leica, Heidelberg, Germany) and stored in an antifreeze solution (50 mM phosphate buffer, 15% glucose, 30% (v/v) ethylene glycol, 0.05% sodium azide; pH 7.4) at –20°C until further testing [33]. Every 12th section (480 μm apart) through the hippocampus was selected in each rat.

To detect the expression patterns of MCP-1 and prospero homeobox protein 1 (Prox1), free-floating tissue sections were incubated in 3% H_2O_2 for 30 min to block endogenous peroxidase. After a PBS rinse for 10 min, sections were placed in 3% NHS at room temperature (RT) for 30 min. The sections were then incubated overnight at 4°C with goat polyclonal MCP-1 primary antibody (1:100; sc-1785, Santa Cruz Biotechnology, Santa Cruz, CA, USA) and rabbit polyclonal Prox1 primary antibody (1:2000; ab5475, Millipore, Temecula, CA, USA). Sections were then washed and incubated for 1 hr at RT in biotinylated-secondary anti-goat antibody (1:300; Vector Laboratories, Burlingame, CA, USA) and anti-rabbit antibody (1:300; Vector Laboratories), respectively. After washing three times, the sections were incubated in the avidin-biotin complex (Vector Laboratories) for 30 min. The sections were then washed three times and reacted with diaminobenzidine tetrahydrochloride (DAB; Sigma) (in 1.5% NaCl containing 0.015% hydrogen peroxide) for 5 min. The color reaction was stopped with ice-cold PBS.

To characterize the cellular source of MCP-1, tissue sections were blocked in 3% normal horse serum (NHS) (in 0.1 M Tris, 0.1% Triton X-100) for 30 min at RT and then incubated overnight at 4°C with a goat polyclonal MCP-1 primary antibody (1:100; sc-1785, Santa Cruz Biotechnology). Following primary antibody treatment, sections were washed in PBS, incubated with DyLight 594-conjugated secondary anti-goat antibody (1:500; Jackson ImmunoResearch Laboratories, West Grove, PA, USA) for 1 hr at RT, washed in PBS and incubated in mouse monoclonal primary antibodies as follows: CD11b antibody (1:100; ab1211, Abcam, Cambridge, MA, USA), neuronal neuclei protein (NeuN) antibody (1:500; MAB377, Millipore), and glial fibrillary acidic protein (GFAP) antibody (1:1000; MAB360, Millipore) at 4°C overnight. After washing in PBS, sections were incubated in DyLight 488-conjugated secondary anti-mouse antibody (1:500; Jackson ImmunoResearch Laboratories) for 1 hr at RT and then washed in PBS.

To determine whether neuronal progenitors in DG express MCP-1 receptor CCR2, immunofluorescent double staining was performed. The tissue sections were first blocked in 3% NHS for 30 min at RT and then incubated with rabbit polyclonal CCR2 antibody (1:100; ab21667, Abcam) for 48 hr at 4°C. Following primary antibody treatment, sections were washed in PBS, incubated with DyLight 488-conjugated secondary anti-rabbit antibody (1:500; Jackson ImmunoResearch Laboratories) for 1 hr at RT, and washed in PBS. Negative controls for CCR2 immunochemistry were performed by blocking with the CCR2 peptide (ab22407, Abcam) that was used as an immunogen for the CCR2 antibody production and also by omitting the primary CCR2 antibody. The tissue sections were then incubated with a goat polyclonal doublecortin (Dcx) antibody (1:100; sc-8066, Santa Cruz Biotechnology) for 48 hr at 4°C. After washing in PBS, sections were incubated in DyLight 594-conjugated secondary anti-goat antibody (1:500; Jackson ImmunoResearch Laboratories) for 1 hr at RT and then washed in PBS.

Double-immunofluorescence labeling for Prox1 and CCR2 was performed using 1:200 mouse monoclonal Prox1 antibody (MAB5652, Millipore) and 1:500 DyLight 549-conjugated secondary anti-mouse antibody (Jackson ImmunoResearch Laboratories), followed by rabbit polyclonal CCR2 antibody (1:100; ab21667, Abcam) and DyLight 488-conjugated secondary anti-rabbit antibody (1:500; Jackson ImmunoResearch Laboratories). To ensure that the hilar ectopic Prox1-expressing cells are neuronal

progenitors, double-immunofluorescence staining for Prox1 and Dcx was performed. The sections were incubated in a rabbit polyclonal Prox1 antibody (1:1000; ab5475, Millipore) and DyLight 488 -conjugated secondary anti-rabbit antibody (1:500; Jackson ImmunoResearch Laboratories), followed by a goat polyclonal Dcx antibody (1:100; sc-8066, Santa Cruz Biotechnology) and DyLight 594-conjugated secondary anti-goat antibody (1:500; Jackson ImmunoResearch Laboratories).

All of the tissue sections were then mounted on gelatin-coated slides and air-dried. The sections for immunoperoxidase staining were coverslipped with DPX Mountant (Fluka, Buchs, Switzerland), and those for immunofluorescent staining were coverslipped with Vectashield HardSet mounting medium with DAPI (H-1500; Vector Laboratories). Immunoperoxidase-stained sections were detected using a bright-field microscope (Olympus BX61, Olympus Optical Co. Ltd.) and photomicrographs were captured using a digital camera (Olympus CC12, Olympus Optical Co. Ltd.) with a 10× objective.

To confirm the types of MCP-1 expressing cells, fluorescent images were detected using an epi-fluorescent microscope (Olympus BX61, Olympus Optical Co. Ltd.)

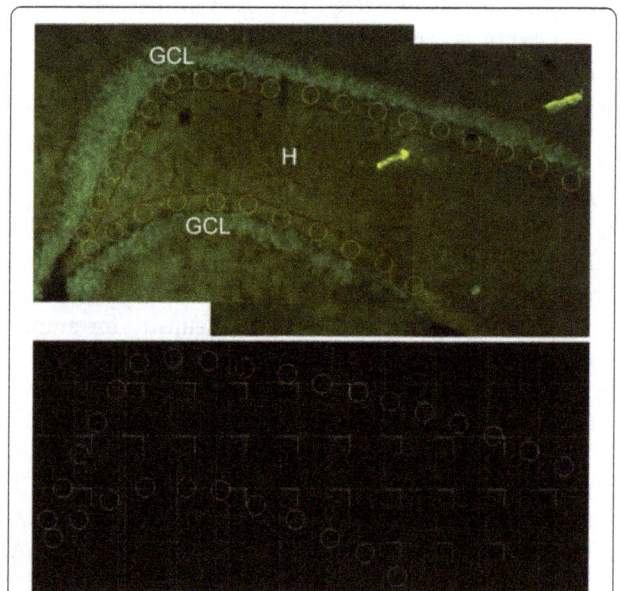

Figure 1 Schematic illustration of the stereological methods for quantification of Prox1/Dcx-positive cells in hilus. The upper panel represents the tracing procedure for the contour of the hilar region. Some 50 μm diameter circles were placed on the interior of the granule cell layer to exclude the SGZ. The boundaries of hilus was traced along the edge of the circles in hilus, from the vertex of the granule cell layer to a straight line drawn between the two lateral tips of the granule cell layer. The lower panel demonstrates a counting frame of 50×50 μm distributed in a randomly oriented 150×150 μm XY grid. Only the grids within the traced contour were included. GCL: granule cell layer; H: hilus.

and photomicrographs were captured using a digital camera (Olympus CC12, Olympus Optical Co. Ltd.) with a 10× objective. In addition, the hilar ectopic Dcx/CCR2-expressing neuroblasts, Prox1/CCR2-expressing cells and Prox1/Dcx-expressing progenitors, were verified by a laser scanning confocal microscope (Olympus FV1000, Olympus Optical Co. Ltd.) with 20× and 60× objectives.

Stereology of Prox1/Dcx double-labeled cells

The number of Prox1/Dcx-positive cells in the bilateral dentate hilus was estimated in every 12th section using the optical fractionator [34] with StereoInvestigator 9

software (Microbrightfield, Williston, VT, USA). The sections were viewed in an epi-fluorescent microscope (Olympus BX51, Olympus Optical Co. Ltd.) with a motorized stage. The contours around regions of interest were traced with a 10× objective and the Prox1/Dcx double-labeled cells were counted with a 40× objective. The hilus was demarcated by the border of the upper and lower blades of the granule cell layer, and a straight line drawn between the two lateral tips of granule cell layer. Because it was difficult to determine the border between CA3c and hilus in Prox1/Dcx immunostained sections, the immunoreactive cells in CA3c were included in this study.

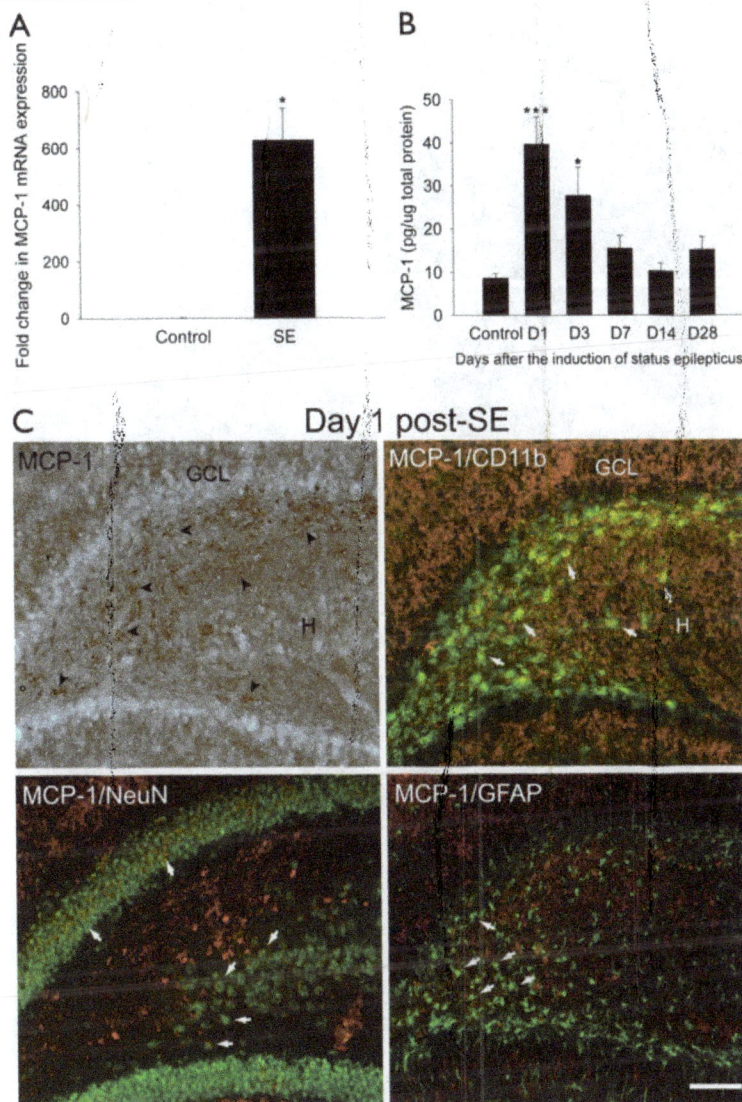

Figure 2 Upregulated MCP-1 expression in the DG after SE. (**A**) Mean fold-change (+ SEM) of MCP-1 gene expression in SE rats with respect to control rats. *P <0.05 compared with the control group. (**B**) Mean concentration (+ SEM) of MCP-1 protein at 1 to 28 days after SE. *P <0.05, ***P <0.001 compared with the control group. (**C**) Distribution patterns in the DG of MCP-1 expression (left upper panel) and its co-labeling with CD11b (right upper panel), NeuN (left lower panel) and GFAP (right lower panel) on day 1 after SE. Arrowheads denote MCP-1-positive cells in hilus. Arrows denote MCP-1-positive cells (red) co-labeled with CD11b, GFAP and NeuN (green), respectively. Scale bar: 100 μm. GCL: granule cell layer; H: hilus.

To exclude the Prox1/Dcx-positive cells at the border of the granule cell layer and hilus, 50 μm diameter circles were placed on the interior of the granule cell layer and the contour of the hilus was traced along the edge of these circles in hilus, from the vertex of the granule cell layer to a straight line drawn between the two lateral tips of granule cell layer [35]. Within the contour of the hilus, a counting frame of 50×50 μm was distributed in a randomly oriented 150×150 μm XY grid (Figure 1). The Prox1/Dcx double-labeled cells at each counting frame were counted within the optical dissector height (20 μm) centered between top and bottom guard zones (5 μm) to estimate the number of hilar ectopic neuronal progenitors. In each section, the cell count and total volume of traced hilar region were estimated according to the formula developed by West *et al.* [34,36] and Cavalieri's principle [37], as described previously [35,38]. The data were expressed as the number of Prox1/Dcx-positive cell per unit volume of the hilus (cells/mm^3 + SEM).

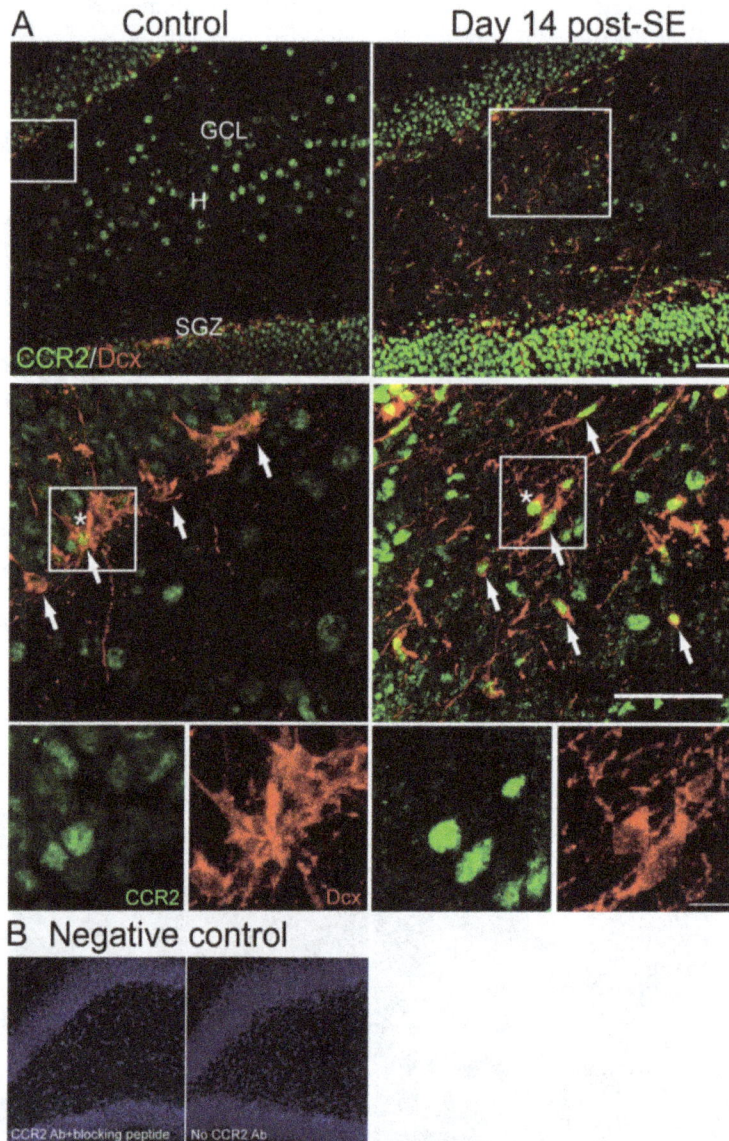

Figure 3 Confocal micrographs of MCP-1 receptor, CCR2 and Dcx in the hippocampal DG. (A) As shown in top panels, CCR2-positive cells (green) appeared in the GCL, SGZ and hilus. Within the SGZ, CCR2-positive cells were double-labeled with a neuroblast marker Dcx (red). Note that Dcx-positive cells appeared ectopically within the hilus after SE, and a subset of these cells expressed CCR2. The middle and bottom panels show projected z-stack confocal images to demonstrate colocalization of CCR2 with Dcx. White brackets mark the magnified views of the area. Arrows denote CCR2/Dcx-positive cells. The cell denoted by the asterisk is enlarged to illustrate the pattern of CCR2 and Dcx labeling. Scale bar: top and middle, 50 μm; bottom, 10 μm. GCL: granule cell layer; H: hilus; SGZ: subgranular zone. **(B)** Negative control immunostaining images for CCR2 when the CCR2 primary antibody was omitted (right) or eliminated by a blocking peptide (left). Nuclei were counterstained with DAPI (blue).

Statistical analysis

The qRT-PCR data were statistically analyzed by independent-samples t-test. MCP-1 protein concentrations in the DG at the indicated time points in the SE groups were compared with those in the control group using one-way ANOVA followed by Dunnett's *post hoc* test. The density of hilar ectopic Prox1/Dcx-positive cells in all groups was statistically analyzed using one-way ANOVA followed by the Scheffe *post hoc* test. The data were shown as the mean + SEM. The significance level was set at $P <0.05$.

Results

MCP-1 expression in the hippocampal DG after SE

There was a significant increase in MCP-1 gene expression in response to seizure insults compared with the control ($P = 0.022$; independent-samples t-test; n = 6 to 7 rats per group) (Figure 2A). Compared with the control levels, MCP-1 protein expression in the DG was significantly increased one day ($P = 0.000052$) and three days ($P = 0.013$) post-SE (one-way ANOVA, $F_{(df = 5, 30)} = 8.17$, $P = 0.000058$, Dunnett's *post hoc* test; n = 6 rats per time point) (Figure 2B). Double-labeling immunohistochemical analysis at one day after SE showed that MCP-1 expression was mainly found in CD11b-positive reactive microglia within the hilar area and that some MCP-1 expressing cells were co-labeled with GFAP and NeuN (Figure 2C).

Distribution of MCP-1 receptor CCR2 in the hippocampal DG after SE

In the DG, CCR2-positive cells were found in the hilus, the SGZ and the granule cell layer. In the SGZ, CCR2-expressing cells were double-labeled with Dcx in control and SE rats, indicating that neural progenitors express CCR2. Furthermore,

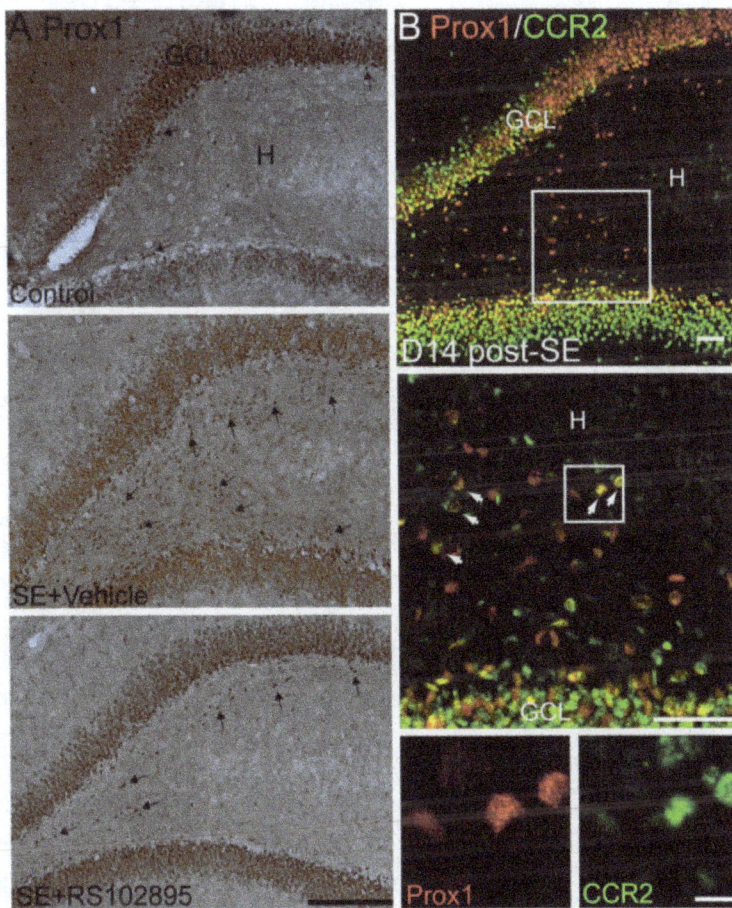

Figure 4 Effects of MCP-1/CCR2 inhibition on the formation of hilar-ectopic granule cells. (**A**) Granule cells were immunolabeled with the granule cell-specific marker Prox1 in controls, vehicle-treated SE rats, and RS102895-treated SE rats. In SE rats, Prox1 expression was observed not only in the granule cell layer but also in the hilus. Note that the number of Prox1-expressing cells in the hilus was reduced in the SE rats treated with RS102895. Arrows denote the Prox1-positive cells. Scale bar: 200 μm. (**B**) Confocal micrographs for Prox-1 (red) and CCR2 (green) showing a co-expression of CCR2 in Prox-1-expressing cells in the hilus at 14 days post-SE. The middle and bottom panels show projected z-stack confocal images to demonstrate colocalization of Prox1 with CCR2, as denoted by arrows. White brackets mark the magnified views of the area. Scale bar: top and middle, 50 μm; bottom, 10 μm. GCL: granule cell layer; H: hilus.

we also found the ectopically located Dcx-positive cells in the hilar region of SE rats, and a subset of these cells also expressed CCR2 (Figure 3A). CCR2 immunostaining was abolished either by pretreatment with a synthetic immunogenic peptide or by omitting the primary antibody (Figure 3B).

Effect of a CCR2 antagonist RS102895 on the ectopic migration of neuronal progenitors after SE

As shown in Figure 4A, Prox1 expression in the controls was found throughout the granule cell layer. In the SE rats, Prox1-expressing cells in the hilus at 14 days post-SE also expressed CCR2 (Figure 4B). According to double-immunofluorescence staining for Prox1 and Dcx,

Prox1/Dcx-expressing neuronal progenitors were found primarily within the SGZ in controls. In SE rats, the number of Prox1/Dcx-expressing neuronal progenitors in the hilus was decreased after administration of a CCR2 antagonist RS102895 (Figure 5).

Quantitative stereological analysis further confirmed that the density of Prox1/Dcx-expressing neuronal progenitors in the hilus was significantly higher in the SE rats treated with vehicle compared with control rats ($P = 0.0001$; one-way ANOVA, $F(df = 2, 9)$, $P = 0.00010$, Scheffe *post hoc* test; n = 5 sections per rat, 4 rats per group) and the SE rats treated with RS102895 ($P = 0.018$; one-way ANOVA, $F(df = 2, 9)$,

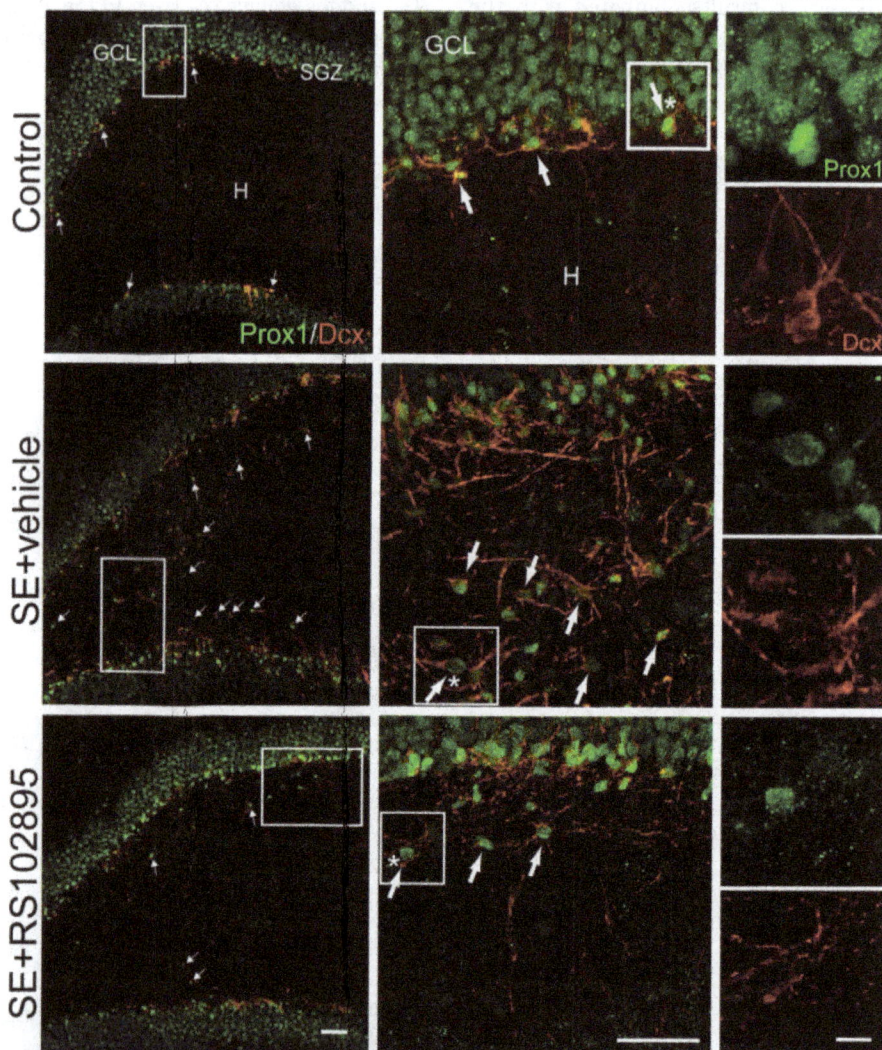

Figure 5 Confocal micrographs of Prox1-expressing progenitors (green) co-labeled with Dcx (red) in the hilus regions of control rats, vehicle-treated SE rats, and RS102895-treated SE rats on Day 14 after SE. The middle and right panels show projected z-stack confocal images to demonstrate colocalization of Prox1 with Dcx. Prox1/Dcx-expressing progenitors appeared within the SGZ in control and SE rats. Note that Prox1/Dcx-expressing progenitors appeared ectopically within the hilus after SE, and the formation of these hilar ectopic neuronal progenitors was attenuated by administration of RS102895. Arrows denote the Prox1/Dcx-positive cells. White brackets mark the magnified views of the area. The cell denoted by the asterisk is enlarged to illustrate the pattern of Prox1 and Dcx labeling. Scale bar: left and middle, 50 μm; right, 10 μm. GCL: granule cell layer; H: hilus; SGZ: subgranular zone.

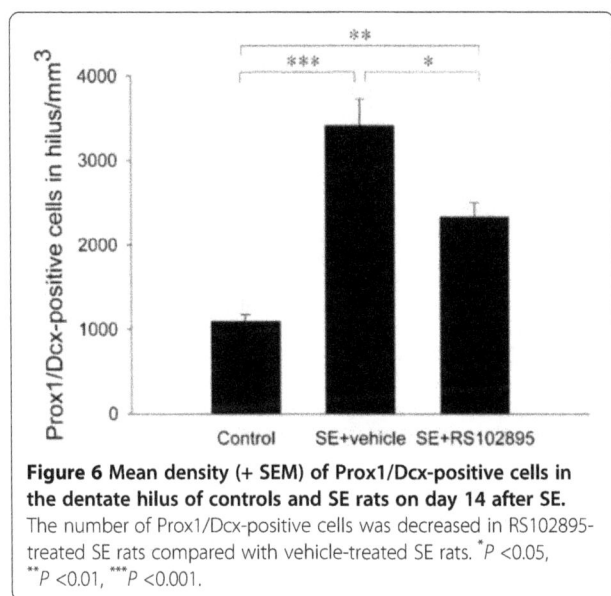

Figure 6 Mean density (+ SEM) of Prox1/Dcx-positive cells in the dentate hilus of controls and SE rats on day 14 after SE. The number of Prox1/Dcx-positive cells was decreased in RS102895-treated SE rats compared with vehicle-treated SE rats. $^*P$ <0.05, $^{**}P$ <0.01, $^{***}P$ <0.001.

$P = 0.00010$, Scheffe *post hoc* test; n = 5 sections per rat, 4 rats per group) (Figure 6). Table 1 shows a summary of the estimation of Prox1/Dcx-expressing cell density in the hilus.

Discussion

Following SE, MCP-1 expression was up-regulated in the DG and CCR2-exhibiting neuroblasts appeared ectopically in the hilus. Notably, the ectopic migration of neuronal progenitors into hilus was significantly decreased by inhibiting the MCP-1/CCR2 interaction. These findings suggest an important role of MCP-1 in the aberrant migration of neuronal progenitors after SE.

Abnormalities in DG and epileptogenesis

The pathogenic mechanisms of MTLE remain largely unknown. As a gating structure in the hippocampal circuit [6], the DG has been an important target in human and experimental studies. Mossy fiber sprouting, selective neuron loss and abnormal neurogenesis have been considered to be histopathological changes contributing to synaptic reorganization and local hyperexcitability in

Table 1 Estimates of Prox1/Dcx-positive cells in the hilus

	Control	SE-vehicle	SE-RS102895
Cells counted/rat[a]	9.25 ±0.48	28.50 ±5.11	20.25 ±1.03
Estimated cell number[a]	1726.26 ±87.51	5498.83 ±917.25	3916.08 ±294.36
Total area (mm²)[a]	3.85 ±0.21	3.99 ±0.35	4.00 ±0.18
Mean CE[b]	0.13	0.08	0.09

CE is coefficient of error.
[a]Values are mean ± SEM.
[b]Mean CE is calculated as √Mean CE² [34].

the DG [6]. Several recent studies have implicated aberrant neurogenesis in the DG in the development of epilepsy. Acute seizure activity promotes the rate of dentate neurogenesis [4,39,40], and prolonged seizures may dysregulate the migration of the DG progenitor cells and lead to hilar-ectopic granule cells [25,26,41,42]. Consistent with previous research, the present study found ectopic Dcx-positive neuroblasts and Prox1-positive granule cells in the hilus after SE induction (Figures 3, 4, 5). These ectopic and pre-existing granule neurons may integrate abnormally with each other and contribute to network hyperexcitability [25].

MCP-1 related neuroinflammation in epilepsy

The interaction of MCP-1 and its receptor CCR2 in the brain can mediate monocyte infiltration and microglial recruitment [43] and contribute to tissue injury via the modulation of blood–brain barrier permeability [18,19] under neuroinflammatory conditions. Increased MCP-1 expression has been detected in rodent brains after acute seizures [17,18,44] and in pathological brain tissue of epilepsy patients [14-16]. In the present study, MCP-1 expression in the DG was upregulated significantly by pilocarpine-induced SE, and this change persisted for at least 28 days (Figure 2A and B).

Our present study further showed that MCP-1 was expressed mainly by CD11b-positive reactive microglia within the hilus after SE. Interestingly, the MCP-1 expressing reactive microglia were localized near the ectopic locations of neuroblasts (Figure 2C). In line with our observation of the linkage between MCP-1 expression and microglia, one recent study in MCP-1-deficient mice has demonstrated a reduction in microglial migration to the site of excitatory neurotransmitter release and a reduction in excitotoxic neuron loss [43]. Taken together, reactive microglia might be involved in seizure-induced dentate MCP-1 upregulation and aberrant migration of neuronal progenitors. Moreover, MCP-1 expression was increased in neurons and astrocytes in SE rats of the present study. We have previously proposed that the upregulated MCP-1 expression in various cell types might participate in the neuroplastic and neuroinflammatory alterations following SE [17].

Mechanisms of aberrant migration of neural progenitors

In the present study, Dcx-positive neuroblasts in the SGZ expressed the MCP-1 receptor, CCR2, in both control and SE rats, and ectopic Dcx/CCR2-positive cells in the hila were found exclusively in SE rats (Figure 3). The findings suggest that MCP-1 upregulation in the DG might be associated with aberrant migration of neural progenitors. Furthermore, the attenuating effect of a CCR2 antagonist (RS102895) on the formation of hilar-ectopic Prox1/Dcx-positive cells (Figures 5 and 6) suggests an interactive involvement of both MCP-1 and CCR2 in the ectopic migration of neural progenitors toward the hilar region.

However, Prox1/Dcx-expressing neuronal progenitors were still found in the hila of SE rats when CCR2 was inhibited (Figure 5). The migration of neural progenitors in SE rats may be related to several factors. For example, the chemokine stromal cell-derived factor-1α (SDF-1α/CXCL12) has been reported to regulate the migration of dentate granule cells [45] and embryonic stem cell-derived neuronal progenitors through the CXCR4 receptor in the hippocampus [46]. One recent study has further identified a co-expression of CXCR4 and CCR2 in neurogenic cells of mouse brain [45]. Increased expression of SDF-1α/CXCL12 following seizures may influence the migration and/or differentiation of neural progenitors during embryogenesis and in the adult hippocampus [46]. Moreover, Reelin has been reported to modulate neural progenitor migration in rodent and human hippocampal DG. Loss of Reelin might contribute to ectopic chain migration and to aberrant integration of newborn neurons in the epileptic adult hippocampus [41].

Conclusions

In conclusion, the MCP-1/CCR2 chemokine-receptor interaction may lead to aberrant migration of neuronal progenitors and subsequently contribute to abnormal synaptic integration and epileptogenesis. Further studies are needed to clarify the underlying signaling pathways of aberrant neuronal progenitor migration affected by MCP-1 following SE. This study supports the involvement of neuroinflammation in epileptogenesis.

Abbreviations

CCR2: Chemokine (C-C motif) receptor 2; Dcx: Doublecortin; DG: Dentate gyrus; ELISA: Enzyme-linked immunosorbent assay; MCP-1: Monocyte chemoattractant protein-1; MTLE: Mesial temporal lobe epilepsy; Prox1: Prospero homeobox protein 1; qRT-PCR: Quantitative real-time reverse transcriptase PCR; SE: Status epilepticus; SGZ: Subgranular zone.

Competing interests

The authors declare that they have no competing interests.

Authors' contributions

YWH contributed to the design and performance of experiments, acquisition and analysis of data, preparing figures, and drafting the manuscript. MTL, YJT and CCC helped to perform experiments, collect qRT-PCR and immunohistochemistry data, and prepare the manuscript. YYL conceived the study, participated in its design and coordination, was involved in drafting the manuscript and revising it critically for important intellectual content. All authors have read and approved the final version of the manuscript.

Acknowledgements

This study was supported in part by research grants from the Taipei Veterans General Hospital (V96S4-010, V96C1-123, V97S4-011, V97C1-034, V98S4-001, V98C1-095, V99S4-004, V99C1-156, V100E6-003, V100C-146), from the National Science Council (NSC-96-2628-B-010-030-MY3, NSC 98-2321-B-010-007, NSC 99-2321-B-010 -004, NSC-99-2628-B-010-011-MY3, NSC 100-2321-B-010-004, NSC 101-2314-B-010 -068-MY3), and from the Ministry of Education, Aim for the Top University Plan, Taipei, Taiwan. The authors acknowledge the technical services provided by the National Yang-Ming University Genome Research Center (YMGC) and the Imaging Core Facility of Nanotechnology of the UST-YMU, and thank the staff of TC5 Bio-Image Tools, Technology Commons, College of Life Science, National Taiwan University, for help with the use of the stereological system.

Author details

[1]Institute of Physiology, National Yang-Ming University, No.155, Sec. 2, Linong Street, Taipei 112, Taiwan. [2]Institute of Brain Science, National Yang-Ming University, No.155, Sec. 2, Linong Street, Taipei 112, Taiwan. [3]Institute of Clinical Medicine, National Yang-Ming University, No.155, Sec. 2, Linong Street, Taipei 112, Taiwan. [4]Brain Research Center, National Yang-Ming University, No.155, Sec. 2, Linong Street, Taipei 112, Taiwan. [5]Laboratory of Neurophysiology, Taipei Veterans General Hospital, No. 201, Sec. 2, Shih-Pai Rd, Taipei 112, Taiwan. [6]Department of Neurology, Taipei Veterans General Hospital, No. 201, Sec. 2, Shih-Pai Rd, Taipei 112, Taiwan.

References

1. Spencer SS: When should temporal-lobe epilepsy be treated surgically? *Lancet Neurol* 2002, 1:375–382.
2. Buckmaster PS: Laboratory animal models of temporal lobe epilepsy. *Comp Med* 2004, 54:473–485.
3. Dalby NO, Mody I: The process of epileptogenesis: a pathophysiological approach. *Curr Opin Neurol* 2001, 14:187–192.
4. Parent JM, Yu TW, Leibowitz RT, Geschwind DH, Sloviter RS, Lowenstein DH: Dentate granule cell neurogenesis is increased by seizures and contributes to aberrant network reorganization in the adult rat hippocampus. *J Neurosci* 1997, 17:3727–3738.
5. Vezzani A, Granata T: Brain inflammation in epilepsy: experimental and clinical evidence. *Epilepsia* 2005, 46:1724–1743.
6. Chang BS, Lowenstein DH: Epilepsy. *N Engl J Med* 2003, 349:1257–1266.
7. Turrin NP, Rivest S: Innate immune reaction in response to seizures: implications for the neuropathology associated with epilepsy. *Neurobiol Dis* 2004, 16:321–334.
8. Vezzani A, French J, Bartfai T, Baram TZ: The role of inflammation in epilepsy. *Nat Rev Neurol* 2011, 7:31–40.
9. Vezzani A, Balosso S, Ravizza T: The role of cytokines in the pathophysiology of epilepsy. *Brain Behav Immun* 2008, 22:797–803.
10. Asensio VC, Campbell IL: Chemokines in the CNS: plurifunctional mediators in diverse states. *Trends Neurosci* 1999, 22:504–512.
11. Cartier L, Hartley O, Dubois-Dauphin M, Krause KH: Chemokine receptors in the central nervous system: role in brain inflammation and neurodegenerative diseases. *Brain Res Brain Res Rev* 2005, 48:16–42.
12. Huang D, Han Y, Rani MR, Glabinski A, Trebst C, Sorensen T, Tani M, Wang J, Chien P, O'Bryan S, Bielecki B, Zhou ZL, Majumder S, Ransohoff RM: Chemokines and chemokine receptors in inflammation of the nervous system: manifold roles and exquisite regulation. *Immunol Rev* 2000, 177:52–67.
13. Miller RJ, Rostene W, Apartis E, Banisadr G, Biber K, Milligan ED, White FA, Zhang J: Chemokine action in the nervous system. *J Neurosci* 2008, 28:11792–11795.
14. Choi J, Nordli DR Jr, Alden TD, DiPatri A Jr, Laux L, Kelley K, Rosenow J, Schuele SU, Rajaram V, Koh S: Cellular injury and neuroinflammation in children with chronic intractable epilepsy. *J Neuroinflammation* 2009, 6:38.
15. van Gassen KL, de Wit M, Koerkamp MJ, Rensen MG, van Rijen PC, Holstege FC, Lindhout D, de Graan PN: Possible role of the innate immunity in temporal lobe epilepsy. *Epilepsia* 2008, 49:1055–1065.
16. Wu Y, Wang X, Mo X, Xi Z, Xiao F, Li J, Zhu X, Luan G, Wang Y, Li Y, Zhang J: Expression of monocyte chemoattractant protein-1 in brain tissue of patients with intractable epilepsy. *Clin Neuropathol* 2008, 27:55–63.
17. Foresti ML, Arisi GM, Katki K, Montanez A, Sanchez RM, Shapiro LA: Chemokine CCL2 and its receptor CCR2 are increased in the hippocampus following pilocarpine-induced status epilepticus. *J Neuroinflammation* 2009, 6:40.
18. Manley NC, Bertrand AA, Kinney KS, Hing TC, Sapolsky RM: Characterization of monocyte chemoattractant protein-1 expression following a kainate model of status epilepticus. *Brain Res* 2007, 1182:138–143.
19. Stamatovic SM, Shakui P, Keep RF, Moore BB, Kunkel SL, Van Rooijen N, Andjelkovic AV: Monocyte chemoattractant protein-1 regulation of

blood–brain barrier permeability. *J Cereb Blood Flow Metab* 2005, **25**:593–606.

20. Yadav A, Saini V, Arora S: MCP-1: chemoattractant with a role beyond immunity: a review. *Clin Chim Acta* 2010, **411**:1570–1579.

21. Iyer AM, Zurolo E, Boer K, Baayen JC, Giangaspero F, Arcella A, Di Gennaro GC, Esposito V, Spliet WG, van Rijen PC, Troost D, Gorter JA, Aronica E: Tissue plasminogen activator and urokinase plasminogen activator in human epileptogenic pathologies. *Neuroscience* 2010, **167**:929–945.

22. Widera D, Holtkamp W, Entschladen F, Niggemann B, Zanker K, Kaltschmidt B, Kaltschmidt C: MCP-1 induces migration of adult neural stem cells. *Eur J Cell Biol* 2004, **83**:381–387.

23. Yan YP, Sailor KA, Lang BT, Park SW, Vemuganti R, Dempsey RJ: Monocyte chemoattractant protein-1 plays a critical role in neuroblast migration after focal cerebral ischemia. *J Cereb Blood Flow Metab* 2007, **27**:1213–1224.

24. Belmadani A, Tran PB, Ren D, Miller RJ: Chemokines regulate the migration of neural progenitors to sites of neuroinflammation. *J Neurosci* 2006, **26**:3182–3191.

25. Overstreet-Wadiche LS, Bromberg DA, Bensen AL, Westbrook GL: Seizures accelerate functional integration of adult-generated granule cells. *J Neurosci* 2006, **26**:4095–4103.

26. Walter C, Murphy BL, Pun RY, Spieles-Engemann AL, Danzer SC: Pilocarpine-induced seizures cause selective time-dependent changes to adult-generated hippocampal dentate granule cells. *J Neurosci* 2007, **27**:7541–7552.

27. Parent JM: Adult neurogenesis in the intact and epileptic dentate gyrus. *Prog Brain Res* 2007, **163**:529–540.

28. Zheng Y, Moussally J, Cash SS, Karnam HB, Cole AJ: Intravenous levetiracetam in the rat pilocarpine-induced status epilepticus model: behavioral, physiological and histological studies. *Neuropharmacology* 2010, **58**:793–798.

29. Elmarakby AA, Quigley JE, Olearczyk JJ, Sridhar A, Cook AK, Inscho EW, Pollock DM, Imig JD: Chemokine receptor 2b inhibition provides renal protection in angiotensin II - salt hypertension. *Hypertension* 2007, **50**:1069–1076.

30. Mirzadegan T, Diehl F, Ebi B, Bhakta S, Polsky I, McCarley D, Mulkins M, Weatherhead GS, Lapierre JM, Dankwardt J, Jr Morgans D, Wilhelm R, Jarnagin K: Identification of the binding site for a novel class of CCR2b chemokine receptor antagonists: binding to a common chemokine receptor motif within the helical bundle. *J Biol Chem* 2000, **275**:25562–25571.

31. Hagihara H, Toyama K, Yamasaki N, Miyakawa T: Dissection of hippocampal dentate gyrus from adult mouse. *J Vis Exp* 2009, **33**:e1543.

32. Holland PM, Abramson RD, Watson R, Gelfand DH: Detection of specific polymerase chain reaction product by utilizing the 5′–3′ exonuclease activity of Thermus aquaticus DNA polymerase. *Proc Natl Acad Sci U S A* 1991, **88**:7276–7280.

33. Kralic JE, Ledergerber DA, Fritschy JM: Disruption of the neurogenic potential of the dentate gyrus in a mouse model of temporal lobe epilepsy with focal seizures. *Eur J Neurosci* 2005, **22**:1916–1927.

34. West MJ, Slomianka L, Gundersen HJ: Unbiased stereological estimation of the total number of neurons in thesubdivisions of the rat hippocampus using the optical fractionator. *Anat Rec* 1991, **231**:482–497.

35. McCloskey DP, Hintz TM, Pierce JP, Scharfman HE: Stereological methods reveal the robust size and stability of ectopic hilar granule cells after pilocarpine-induced status epilepticus in the adult rat. *Eur J Neurosci* 2006, **24**:2203–2210.

36. West MJ: New stereological methods for counting neurons. *Neurobiol Aging* 1993, **14**:275–285.

37. Mouton PR: *Principles and practices of unbiased stereology: an introduction for bioscientists*. Baltimore: Johns Hopkins University Press; 2002.

38. Wong-Goodrich SJ, Mellott TJ, Glenn MJ, Blusztajn JK, Williams CL: Prenatal choline supplementation attenuates neuropathological response to status epilepticus in the adult rat hippocampus. *Neurobiol Dis* 2008, **30**:255–269.

39. Scharfman HE: Functional implications of seizure-induced neurogenesis. *Adv Exp Med Biol* 2004, **548**:192–212.

40. Scharfman HE, Goodman JH, Sollas AL: Granule-like neurons at the hilar/CA3 border after status epilepticus and their synchrony with area CA3 pyramidal cells: functional implications of seizure-induced neurogenesis. *J Neurosci* 2000, **20**:6144–6158.

41. Gong C, Wang TW, Huang HS, Parent JM: Reelin regulates neuronal progenitor migration in intact and epileptic hippocampus. *J Neurosci* 2007, **27**:1803–1811.

42. Parent JM, Elliott RC, Pleasure SJ, Barbaro NM, Lowenstein DH: Aberrant seizure-induced neurogenesis in experimental temporal lobe epilepsy. *Ann Neurol* 2006, **59**:81–91.

43. Sheehan JJ, Zhou C, Gravanis I, Rogove AD, Wu YP, Bogenhagen DF, Tsirka SE: Proteolytic activation of monocyte chemoattractant protein-1 by plasmin underlies excitotoxic neurodegeneration in mice. *J Neurosci* 2007, **27**:1738–1745.

44. Kalehua AN, Nagel JE, Whelchel LM, Gides JJ, Pyle RS, Smith RJ, Kusiak JW, Taub DD: Monocyte chemoattractant protein-1 and macrophage inflammatory protein-2 are involved in both excitotoxin-induced neurodegeneration and regeneration. *Exp Cell Res* 2004, **297**:197–211.

45. Tran PB, Banisadr G, Ren D, Chenn A, Miller RJ: Chemokine receptor expression by neural progenitor cells in neurogenic regions of mouse brain. *J Comp Neurol* 2007, **500**:1007–1033.

46. Hartman NW, Carpentino JE, LaMonica K, Mor DE, Naegele JR, Grabel L: CXCL12-mediated guidance of migrating embryonic stem cell-derived neural progenitors transplanted into the hippocampus. *PLoS One* 2010, **5**:e15856.

Permissions

All chapters in this book were first published in JNI, by BioMed Central; hereby published with permission under the Creative Commons Attribution License or equivalent. Every chapter published in this book has been scrutinized by our experts. Their significance has been extensively debated. The topics covered herein carry significant findings which will fuel the growth of the discipline. They may even be implemented as practical applications or may be referred to as a beginning point for another development.

The contributors of this book come from diverse backgrounds, making this book a truly international effort. This book will bring forth new frontiers with its revolutionizing research information and detailed analysis of the nascent developments around the world.

We would like to thank all the contributing authors for lending their expertise to make the book truly unique. They have played a crucial role in the development of this book. Without their invaluable contributions this book wouldn't have been possible. They have made vital efforts to compile up to date information on the varied aspects of this subject to make this book a valuable addition to the collection of many professionals and students.

This book was conceptualized with the vision of imparting up-to-date information and advanced data in this field. To ensure the same, a matchless editorial board was set up. Every individual on the board went through rigorous rounds of assessment to prove their worth. After which they invested a large part of their time researching and compiling the most relevant data for our readers.

The editorial board has been involved in producing this book since its inception. They have spent rigorous hours researching and exploring the diverse topics which have resulted in the successful publishing of this book. They have passed on their knowledge of decades through this book. To expedite this challenging task, the publisher supported the team at every step. A small team of assistant editors was also appointed to further simplify the editing procedure and attain best results for the readers.

Apart from the editorial board, the designing team has also invested a significant amount of their time in understanding the subject and creating the most relevant covers. They scrutinized every image to scout for the most suitable representation of the subject and create an appropriate cover for the book.

The publishing team has been an ardent support to the editorial, designing and production team. Their endless efforts to recruit the best for this project, has resulted in the accomplishment of this book. They are a veteran in the field of academics and their pool of knowledge is as vast as their experience in printing. Their expertise and guidance has proved useful at every step. Their uncompromising quality standards have made this book an exceptional effort. Their encouragement from time to time has been an inspiration for everyone.

The publisher and the editorial board hope that this book will prove to be a valuable piece of knowledge for researchers, students, practitioners and scholars across the globe.

List of Contributors

Juha T Järvelä, Francisco R Lopez-Picon, Anna Plysjuk, Saku Ruohonen and Irma E Holopainen
Department of Pharmacology, Drug Development, and Therapeutics, Institute of Biomedicine, University of Turku, Itäinen Pitkäkatu 4B, FIN-20014 Turku, Finland

Francisco R Lopez-Picon
Turku PET Center, Preclinical imaging, Tykistökatu 6A, 4th Floor, FIN-20520 Turku, Finland

Irma E Holopainen
Medicity Research Laboratory, Tykistökatu 6A, 4th Floor, Institute of Biomedicine, University of Turku, FIN-20014 Turku, Finland

Wan-Yu Huang and Kuei-Sen Hsu
Institute of Basic Medical Sciences, College of Medicine, National Cheng Kung University, Tainan, Taiwan

Wan-Yu Huang
Pediatrics of Kung-Ten General Hospital, Taichung City, Taiwan

Shankung Lin, Hsuan-Ying Chen, Ya-Ping Chen, Ting-Yu Chen and Hung-Ming Wu
Inflammation Research & Drug Development Center, Changhua Christian Hospital, Changhua, Taiwan

Hung-Ming Wu
Department of Neurology, Changhua Christian Hospital, Changhua City, Taiwan
Institute of Acupuncture, School of Chinese Medicine, China Medical University, Taichung City, Taiwan

Ya-Jun Li, Bei Zhang, Xiao Zhe, Ming-Jue Wang, Shao-Ting Shi, Jing Bai, Tao Lin, Chang-Jiang Guo, Shi-Jun Zhang, Xiang-Li Kong, Xing Zuo and Hang Zhao
Department of Neurology, The Affiliated Hospital of Xián Medical University, No. 48, West Fenghao Road, Xián 710077, Shaanxi Province, China

Zheng-Hai Wang
Department of Neurology, The General Hospital of Ningxia Medical University, Ningxia, China

Kenneth I. Strauss
College of Human Medicine, Michigan State University, 333 Bostwick Ave NE, Grand Rapids, MI, USA

Kost V. Elisevich
Department of Clinical Neurosciences, Spectrum Health System, Grand Rapids, MI, USA
Division of Neurosurgery, Michigan State University, East Lansing, USA

Ying Liu, Teng Wang, Xi Liu, Tao Xu, Xinyuan Yu, Xin Wei, Xueying Ding, Lijuan Mo, Maojia Yin, Xinjie Tan and Lifen Chen
Department of Neurology, The Second Affiliated Hospital of Chongqing Medical University, 74 Linjiang Road, Yuzhong District, Chonqing 400010, China

Yuetao Wen
Department of Neurosurgery, The University-Town Hospital of Chongqing Medical University, Chongqing 401331, China

Jieun Choi
Department of Pediatrics, Seoul National University Boramae Hospital, Seoul National University, College of Medicine, Seoul, Korea

Hyun Jin Min and Jeon-Soo Shin
Department of Microbiology, Yonsei University College of Medicine, Seoul, Korea

Jeon-Soo Shin
Severance Biomedical Science Institute and Institute for Immunology and Immunological Diseases, Yonsei University College of Medicine, Seoul, Korea

Amna Rana and Alberto E. Musto
Department of Pathology and Anatomy, Department of Neurology, Eastern Virginia Medical School, 700 W. Olney Road, Lewis Hall, Office 2174, Norfolk, VA 23507, USA

Nina Dupuis, Béatrice Desnous, Vibol Chhor, Bobbi Fleiss, Tifenn Le Charpentier, Sophie Lebon, Zsolt Csaba, Pierre Gressens, Pascal Dournaud and Stéphane Auvin
INSERM, U1141, 75019 Paris, France

Nina Dupuis, Béatrice Desnous, Vibol Chhor, Bobbi Fleiss, Tifenn Le Charpentier, Sophie Lebon, Zsolt Csaba, Pierre Gressens, Pascal Dournaud and Stéphane Auvin
Université Paris Diderot, Sorbonne Paris Cité, INSERM UMR1141, 75019 Paris, France

Andrey Mazarati
Department of Pediatrics, Neurology division and Children's Discovery and Innovation Institute, David Geffen School of Medicine at UCLA, Los Angeles, CA 90095, USA

Béatrice Desnous, Pierre Gressens and Stéphane Auvin
AP-HP, Hôpital Robert Debré, Service de Neurologie Pédiatrique, 75019 Paris, France

Nina Dupuis, Béatrice Desnous, Vibol Chhor, Bobbi Fleiss, Tifenn Le Charpentier, Sophie Lebon, Zsolt Csaba, Pierre Gressens, Pascal Dournaud and Stéphane Auvin
INSERM, U1141, 75019 Paris, France

Nina Dupuis, Béatrice Desnous, Vibol Chhor, Bobbi Fleiss, Tifenn Le Charpentier, Sophie Lebon, Zsolt Csaba, Pierre Gressens, Pascal Dournaud and Stéphane Auvin
Université Paris Diderot, Sorbonne Paris Cité, INSERM UMR1141, 75019 Paris, France

Andrey Mazarati
Department of Pediatrics, Neurology division and Children's Discovery and Innovation Institute, David Geffen School of Medicine at UCLA, Los Angeles, CA 90095, USA

Béatrice Desnous, Pierre Gressens and Stéphane Auvin
AP-HP, Hôpital Robert Debré, Service de Neurologie Pédiatrique, 75019 Paris, France

Daniela M. Magalhães, Noémia Pereira, Diogo M. Rombo, Cláudia Beltrão-Cavacas, Ana M. Sebastião and Cláudia A. Valente
Instituto de Farmacologia e Neurociências, Faculdade de Medicina, Universidade de Lisboa, Lisboa, Portugal
Instituto de Medicina Molecular, Faculdade de Medicina, Universidade de Lisboa, Lisboa, Portugal

Xiang-Fei Meng, Lan Tan, Chen-Chen Tan, Meng-Meng Li and Jin-Tai Yu
Department of Neurology, Qingdao Municipal Hospital, School of Medicine,Qingdao University, Qingdao, PR China

Lan Tan, Hui-Fu Wang and Jin-Tai Yu
Department of Neurology, Qingdao Municipal Hospital, Nanjing Medical University, Nanjing, PR China

Meng-Shan Tan
Department of Neurology, Qingdao Municipal Hospital, College of Medicine and Pharmaceutics, Ocean University of China, Qingdao, PR China

Teng Jiang
Department of Neurology, Nanjing First Hospital, Nanjing Medical University, Nanjing, PR China

Jin-Tai Yu
Department of Neurology, Memory and Aging Center, University of California, San Francisco, CA, USA

Erik A Johnson, Thuy L Dao, Michelle A Guignet, Claire E Geddes, Andrew I Koemeter-Cox and Robert K Kan
Research Division, Pharmacology Branch, US Army Medical Research Institute of Chemical Defense (USAMRICD), Aberdeen Proving Ground, MD 21010, USA

Xinjian Zhu, Mengyi Zhu, Kangni Xu, Li Yang, Bing Han, Rongrong Huang and Honghong Yao
Department of Pharmacology, Medical School of Southeast University, Dingjiaqiao 87th, Nanjing 210009, China

Xiaolin Li
Department of Geriatrics, The First Affiliated Hospital of Nanjing Medical University, Nanjing, China

Aifeng Zhang
Department of Pathology, Medical School of Southeast University, Nanjing, China

Chen-Chen Tan, Xiang-Fei Meng, Zhen Sun, Meng-Meng Li, Jin-Tai Yu and Lan Tan
Department of Neurology, Qingdao Municipal Hospital, School of Medicine, Qingdao University, No.5 Donghai Middle Road, Qingdao 266071, China

Jian-Guo Zhang and Da-Wei Meng
Department of Functional Neurosurgery, Beijing Neurosurgical Institute, Capital Medical University, No.6, Tiantan Xili, Beijing 100050, China

Jian-Guo Zhang and Da-Wei Meng
Department of Neurosurgery, Beijing Tiantan Hospital, Capital Medical University, No.6, Tiantan Xili, Beijing 100050, China

Jin-Tai Yu, Lan Tan, Meng-Shan Tan, Jin-Tai Yu and Lan Tan
College of Medicine and Pharmaceutics, Ocean University of China, No.5 Yushan Road, Qingdao 266003, China

Hua Chen and Ying Li
Department of Pathology, Qingdao Municipal Hospital, School of Medicine, Qingdao University, No.5 Donghai Middle Road, Qingdao 266071, China

Teng Jiang, Jin-Tai Yu and Lan Tan
Department of Neurology, Qingdao Municipal Hospital, Nanjing Medical University, No.5 Donghai Middle Road, Qingdao 266071, China

Jin-Tai Yu
Memory and Aging Center, Department of Neurology, University of California, San Francisco, CA 94158, USA

Ji-Eun Kim, Hea Jin Ryu and Tae-Cheon Kang
Department of Anatomy and Neurobiology, College of Medicine, Hallym University, Chunchon, Kangwon-Do 200-702, South Korea

Ji-Eun Kim, Hea Jin Ryu, Tae-Cheon Kang and Soo Young Choi
Institute of Epilepsy Research, College of Medicine, Hallym University, Chunchon, Kangwon-Do 200-702, South Korea

Soo Young Choi
Department of Biomedical Sciences, College of Life Science, Hallym University, Chunchon, Kangwon-Do 200-702, South Korea

Ji-Eun Kim
Department of Neurology, UCSF, and Veterans Affairs Medical Center, San Francisco, California 94121, USA

Chun-Lei Han, Yun-Peng Liu, Xue-Min Zhao, Kai-Liang Wang and Fan-Gang Meng
Department of Functional Neurosurgery, Beijing Neurosurgical Institute, Capital Medical University, Beijing 100050, China

Chun-Lei Han, Yun-Peng Liu, Xue-Min Zhao, Kai-Liang Wang, Ning Chen, Jian-Guo Zhang and Fan-Gang Meng
Beijing Key Laboratory of Neuromodulation, Beijing Municipal Science and Technology Commission, Beijing 100050, China

Ming Ge
Department of Neurosurgery, Beijing Children's Hospital, Capital Medical University, Beijing 100045, China

Ning Chen and Jian-Guo Zhang
Department of Neurosurgery, Beijing Tiantan Hospital, Capital Medical University, Beijing 100050, China

Wen-Jia Meng
The Third Division of Clinical Medicine, China Medical University, Shenyang 110122, Liaoning Province, China

Wei Hu
Department of Neurology, University of Florida, Gainesville, Florida 32607, USA

Liang Li
Department of Pathology, School of Basic Medical Sciences, Capital Medical University, No. 10 Xi TouTiao, You An Men Street, Beijing 100069, China

Yu-Wen Hung, Yi-Jhan Tseng and Yung-Yang Lin
Institute of Physiology, National Yang-Ming University, No.155, Sec. 2, Linong Street, Taipei 112, Taiwan

Ming-Tsong Lai, Chien-Chen Chou and Yung-Yang Lin
Institute of Brain Science, National Yang- Ming University, No.155, Sec. 2, Linong Street, Taipei 112, Taiwan

Yung-Yang Lin
Institute of Clinical Medicine, National Yang-Ming University, No.155, Sec. 2, Linong Street, Taipei 112, Taiwan
Brain Research Center, National Yang-Ming University, No.155, Sec. 2, Linong Street, Taipei 112, Taiwan
Laboratory of Neurophysiology, Taipei Veterans General Hospital, No. 201, Sec. 2, Shih-Pai Rd, Taipei 112, Taiwan
Department of Neurology, Taipei Veterans General Hospital, No. 201, Sec. 2, Shih-Pai Rd, Taipei 112, Taiwan

Index

www.ingramcontent.com/pod-product-compliance
Lightning Source LLC
Chambersburg PA
CBHW082016190326
41458CB00010B/3204